Yearbook of
Vascular and Endovascular Surgery 2016

Yearbook of Vascular and Endovascular Surgery 2016

R Sekhar
MS FRCS (Edin) FRCS (Glasg) FVSI
Consultant Vascular and Endovascular Surgeon
Kokilaben Dhirubhai Ambani Hospital and
Medical Research Institute, Mumbai
Maharashtra, India

Foreword

Pradip K Datta

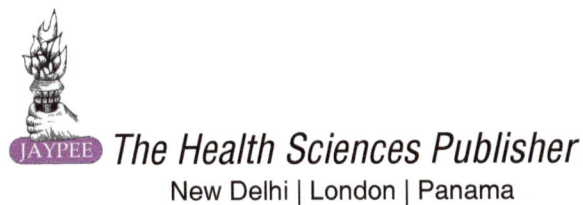

The Health Sciences Publisher
New Delhi | London | Panama

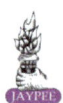
Jaypee Brothers Medical Publishers (P) Ltd

Headquarters

Jaypee Brothers Medical Publishers (P) Ltd
4838/24, Ansari Road, Daryaganj
New Delhi 110 002, India
Phone: +91-11-43574357
Fax: +91-11-43574314
Email: jaypee@jaypeebrothers.com

Overseas Offices

J.P. Medical Ltd
83 Victoria Street, London
SW1H 0HW (UK)
Phone: +44 20 3170 8910
Fax: +44 (0)20 3008 6180
Email: info@jpmedpub.com

Jaypee-Highlights Medical Publishers Inc
City of Knowledge, Bld. 235, 2nd Floor, Clayton
Panama City, Panama
Phone: +1 507-301-0496
Fax: +1 507-301-0499
Email: cservice@jphmedical.com

Jaypee Brothers Medical Publishers (P) Ltd
17/1-B Babar Road, Block-B, Shaymali
Mohammadpur, Dhaka-1207
Bangladesh
Mobile: +08801912003485
Email: jaypeedhaka@gmail.com

Jaypee Brothers Medical Publishers (P) Ltd
Bhotahity, Kathmandu
Nepal
Phone: +977-9741283608
Email: kathmandu@jaypeebrothers.com

Website: www.jaypeebrothers.com
Website: www.jaypeedigital.com

© 2017, Jaypee Brothers Medical Publishers

The views and opinions expressed in this book are solely those of the original contributor(s)/author(s) and do not necessarily represent those of editor(s) of the book.

All rights reserved. No part of this publication may be reproduced, stored or transmitted in any form or by any means, electronic, mechanical, photocopying, recording or otherwise, without the prior permission in writing of the publishers.

All brand names and product names used in this book are trade names, service marks, trademarks or registered trademarks of their respective owners. The publisher is not associated with any product or vendor mentioned in this book.

Medical knowledge and practice change constantly. This book is designed to provide accurate, authoritative information about the subject matter in question. However, readers are advised to check the most current information available on procedures included and check information from the manufacturer of each product to be administered, to verify the recommended dose, formula, method and duration of administration, adverse effects and contraindications. It is the responsibility of the practitioner to take all appropriate safety precautions. Neither the publisher nor the author(s)/editor(s) assume any liability for any injury and/or damage to persons or property arising from or related to use of material in this book.

This book is sold on the understanding that the publisher is not engaged in providing professional medical services. If such advice or services are required, the services of a competent medical professional should be sought.

Every effort has been made where necessary to contact holders of copyright to obtain permission to reproduce copyright material. If any have been inadvertently overlooked, the publisher will be pleased to make the necessary arrangements at the first opportunity.

Inquiries for bulk sales may be solicited at: jaypee@jaypeebrothers.com

Yearbook of Vascular and Endovascular Surgery 2016

First Edition: **2017**

ISBN: 978-93-86261-25-0

Dedicated to

My mother, wife Meena, daughter Rohini and my extended family, India and abroad.
Blessed to be a member of this illustrious group of wonderful human beings.

CONTRIBUTORS

Amman Bolia MBChB DMRD FRCR
Consultant Interventional
Radiologist
Department of Radiology,
Heartlands Hospital
Heart of England NHS Foundation
Trust, Birmingham, UK

Aniket Pradhan DNB (Gen Surg) DNB
(Vascular Surgery)
Senior Fellow in Vascular Surgery
Vascular and Endovascular Surgery
Unit,
The Royal Adelaide Hospital
(Discipline of Surgery, The
University of Adelaide)
North Terrace
Adelaide, SA

Ashwini Naveen Gangadharan DNB
Senior Registrar
Vascular and Endovascular Services
Kokilaben Dhirubhai Ambani
Hospital and Medical Research
Institute
Mumbai, Maharashtra, India

Cho Ee Ng MRCS
Senior Clinical Fellow in Vascular
Surgery
Queen Elizabeth Hospital NHS
Foundation Trust
Gateshead, United Kingdom

Dayananda Shamurailatpam
Chief Physicist and Radiation
Safety Officer
Kokilaben Dhirubhai Ambani
Hospital and
Medical Research Institute
Mumbai, Maharashtra, India

Dovile Gudzinskaite- Brar MD
Senior Vascular Fellow
King's College Hospital
London

G Atturu FRCS
Leeds Vascular Institute
Leeds General Infirmary
United Kingdom

Harshal Vora MD DNB (Nephro)
Senior Registrar
Centre for Kidney Disease
Kokilaben Dhirubhai Ambani
Hospital and
Medical Research Institute
Mumbai, Maharashtra, India

J De Siqueira MRCS
Leeds Vascular Institute
Leeds General Infirmary
United Kingdom

Jessica Shah DNB
Registrar
Vascular and Endovascular Services
Kokilaben Dhirubhai Ambani
Hospital and Medical Research
Institute
Mumbai, Maharashtra, India

Kapil Mathur MS MCh (Vascular Surgery)
Associate Professor
Department of Vascular Surgery
Sri Ramachandra University
Chennai, Tamil Nadu, India

Krishna Gummalla DMRD EDIR FRCR
Consultant
Department of Radiology
Tan Tock Seng Hospital
11 Jalan TanTock Seng
Singapore

Lauren D Giamberardino MHA
Palmetto Health – University of
South Carolina Medical Group
Department of Neurology
Columbia, South Carolina
USA

Marzanna T Zaleska
Medical Research Centre
Polish Academy of Sciences
Warsaw, Poland

Neghal Kandiyil MBChB MRCS FRCR PhD
Consultant Interventional Radiologist
Department of Radiology, University Hospitals of Leicester NHS Trust,
Leicestershire, UK

Neil Patel MD
Palmetto Health – University of
South Carolina Medical Group
Department of Neurology
Columbia, South Carolina
USA

Niranjan Kulkarni MD DM
Consultant Nephrologist
Centre for Kidney Disease,
Kokilaben Dhirubhai Ambani
Hospital and Medical Research
Institute, Mumbai
Maharashtra, India

Paul Scott MD FRCR
Consultant Vascular Radiologist
Hull and East Yorkshire Hospitals
NHS Trust, Hull, UK

Pranav Thusay DNB
Senior Registrar
Vascular and Endovascular Services
Kokilaben Dhirubhai Ambani
Hospital and Medical Research
Institute, Mumbai
Maharashtra, India

R Sekhar MS FRCS (Glasg)FRCS (Edin) FVSI
Consultant Vascular and
Endovascular Surgeon
Kokilaben Dhirubhai Ambani
Hospital and Medical Research
Institute
Mumbai, Maharashtra, India

Raghvinder Pal Singh Gambhir MS DNB FRCS (Ed & Eng) FACS
Consultant Vascular Surgeon
King's College Hospital
London

Raghuram Lakshminarayan DMRD DNB FRCR FRANZCR EBIR
Consultant Vascular Radiologist
Hull and East Yorkshire Hospitals
NHS Trust, Hull, UK

Rajesh Hydrabadi MS MCh
Vein Clinic
Ahmedabad, Gujarat, India

Ravish Kothari MD
Palmetto Health–University of South
Carolina Medical Group
Department of Neurology
Columbia, South Carolina, USA

Ritu K Kashikar MD
Consultant Radiologist
Department of Imaging and
Interventional Radiology
Jaslok Hospital and Research Center.
Mumbai, Maharashtra, India

Riza Ibrahim FRCS (Gen Surg) FRCS (Vascular Surgery)
Consultant Vascular and
Endovascular Surgeon
Clinical Director for Vascular and
Endovascular Services
The Pennine Acute Hospitals NHS
Trust, UK

Robert Fitridge MS FRACS
Professor of Vascular Surgery
Vascular and Endovascular Surgery Unit,
The Royal Adelaide Hospital
(Discipline of Surgery
The University of Adelaide)
North Terrace, Adelaide, SA

Sameer Tulpule MD MRCP (UK) FRCPath (UK)
Consultant
Clinical Hematology
Kokilaben Dhirubhai Ambani Hospital and Medical Research Institute, Mumbai
Maharashtra, India

Satheesh Ramamurthy MD
Department of Interventional Radiology
Sri Ramachandra University
Chennai, Tamil Nadu, India

S Homer-Vanniasinkam
BSc MD FRCSEd FRCS
Consultant Vascular Surgeon
The General Infirmary at Leeds
Clinical Sub-Dean
University of Leeds Medical School
Professor of Surgery (Founding)
University of Warwick Medical School and University Hospitals Coventry and Warwickshire NHS Trust
Professor of Engineering and Surgery, University College London
United Kingdom

Shrinivas B Desai MD
Director and Head
Department of Imaging and Interventional Radiology
Jaslok Hospital and Research Center
Mumbai, Maharashtra, India

Siddharth Rajput DNB MSc (Neuro)
Intensive Care Unit
Westmead Hospital NSW
Australia

Simit Vora DNB FVES
Vascular Associate
Kokilaben Dhirubhai Ambani Hospital and Medical Research Institute
Mumbai, Maharashtra, India

Souvik Sen MD MS MPH FAHA
Professor and Chair
Department of Neurology
University of South Carolina School of Medicine
Columbia, South Carolina, USA

Sundeep Punamiya MD FSIR FAMS
Senior Consultant and Head
Vascular and Interventional Radiology
Department of Radiology
Tan Tock Seng Hospital
11 Jalan TanTock Seng
Singapore

T Vidyasagaran MS MCh (Vascular Surgery)
Head
Department of Vascular Surgery
Sri Ramachandra University,
Chennai, Tamil Nadu, India

Vish Bhattacharya FRCS (Glas and Edin) FRCS (Gen Surg)
Consultant in Vascular Surgery
Clinical Lead in Surgery
Queen Elizabeth Hospital NHS Foundation Trust
Gateshead
United Kingdom
Associate Clinical Lecturer
Newcastle University

Waldemar Olszewski
Medical Research Centre
Polish Academy of Sciences
Warsaw, Poland

WNDP Chinthaka Appuhamy MBBS
MD MMed FRCR
Clinical Associate
Department of Neuroradiology
National Neuroscience Institute
11 Jalan Tan Tock Seng
Singapore

FOREWORD

Dr R Sekhar should be congratulated for editing this *Yearbook of Vascular and Endovascular Surgery 2016*. The vascular and endovascular surgical world in the subcontinent would be most grateful to him for his immense efforts. He should justly be compared with the conductor of a finely tuned orchestra in which the players are truly international. The contributors that he has gathered come from Australia, Poland, Singapore, UK and USA; some of them would rightly get a mention in *'Who's Who in Vascular Surgery.'*

This book reminds me of another monumental work in vascular surgery of yesteryear (1999) called *The Evidence for Vascular Surgery* by J J Earnshaw and J A Murie. Although the purpose of both these books are slightly different, their value as a font of knowledge in the speciality cannot be overestimated. This particular yearbook touches upon most aspects of recent advances and controversies, besides every chapter is extensively referenced. I dare say that the knowledge imparted will continue to be useful in future years.

Vascular surgery is now regarded as a speciality in its own right in the National Health Service in the UK. Gone are the days when there were 'general surgeons with an interest in vascular surgery'. It is high time that vascular surgery is recognised as a superspeciality, and this yearbook testifies to that concept. Like other specialities, vascular surgery in particular works very closely as a team with the interventional radiologist, cardiologist and haematologist. This book reflects that ethos as Dr Sekhar has recruited into his team of collaborators, such specialists with great success.

As one who has edited and authored several books to do with MRCS and FRCS, I can appreciate the huge amount of work the editor has to put in, particularly to liaise with all the contributors in getting their chapters on time to meet the deadline. Dr Sekhar, previously a consultant vascular surgeon at a busy government hospital in Mumbai, has brought to bear his vast experience from that teaching hospital in publishing this book. The readers of this book and vascular surgeons in the Indian subcontinent should be indebted to him for this publication which hopefully will be the first of others to follow.

Pradip K Datta
MBE MS FRCS(Ed) FRCS(Eng) FRCS(Irel) FRCS(Glasg) FIMSA(Hon FCSSL(Hon)
Honorary Consultant Surgeon
Caithness General Hospital
Wick, Scotland, UK
Honorary Secretary (2003-2007)
Member of Council (2000-2012)
Royal College of Surgeons of Edinburgh

PREFACE

Yearbook of Vascular and Endovascular Surgery 2016 is an effort to give vascular practitioners access to recent concepts in vascular and endovascular therapy based on current evidences and consensus statements accepted internationally. Vascular surgery when I took it up several years ago has evolved a great deal, and despite what detractors might say or wish, endovascular work is slowly and steadily becoming the backbone of the practicing vascular surgeon worldwide. Thus, keeping abreast with changing concepts and backing procedures with evidence has become mandatory. The contributors to this book include vascular surgeons, most of whom are doing their own endovascular work, radiologists who function as part of a well-knit team of vascular specialists, clinical haematologists and nephrologists.

Bringing out a book of this nature was always a dream for me since taking up this subspeciality. The fulfilment of this dream can be attributed to several things. The good wishes of my teacher Professor Dipak Ghosh at the beginning of my career as a surgeon, the inspirational teaching methods of Mr Pradip Dutta when I was in the UK, the encouragement to teach and share knowledge that I got from Professor Gautam Sen and the resilience to struggle and succeed despite adversity from my late father Professor RC Sekhar come foremost to mind.

I am extremely indebted to the doyens in vascular surgery in India whose vision has kept the speciality evolving in India and helped grow to a stature it is today. Some like Professor Vidyasagaran have contributed to this book and I am humbled. Surgeons like Surg. Comm (Retd) Dr VS Bedi, Professor Ramesh Tripathi, Dr KR Suresh, and Dr Rajiv Parakh have taken endovascular work to a different level in India and their zeal to spread and share knowledge with trainees and mentor them has been an inspiration for me.

I am indebted to the management of Kokilaben Dhirubhai Ambani Hospital, my "karmabhoomi", in particular Dr Ram Narain and Dr Santosh Shetty, who believed in my abilities when I joined them and continue to support me in all my academic and professional endeavours, vascular and endovascular included.

My trainee registrars, both past and present, have been brilliant. They make me proud and emotional. They have risen to the occasion time and again and their contribution to this book has been immense, to say the least.

Thank you to all the contributors, the quality and class of your chapters speaks for itself. I sincerely apologise for the pressures to meet the deadlines. A big thanks to Mr Kumaresh Menon and Mr Sabarish Menon (Mumbai branch) of M/s Jaypee Brothers Medical Publishers (P) Ltd., New Delhi India, whose support has been amazing.

R Sekhar

CONTENTS

Chapter 1	**Advances in Translational Vascular Research**	1
	J De Siqueira, G Atturu, S Homer-Vanniasinkam	

- Regression of Atherosclerosis 1
- Angiogenesis 3
- Chronic Foot Ulcers 5
- Aneurysmal Disease 7

Chapter 2	**Newer Oral Anticoagulants**	15
	Sameer Tulpule	

- Newer Oral Anticoagulants 15
- Pharmacology 16
- Prevention of Venous Thromboembolism in Surgical Patients 18
- Dabigatran 19
- Atrial Fibrillation 23
- Rivaroxaban 24
- Apixaban 25
- Practical Management 26
- Elective Surgery 27
- Complex Clinical Scenarios 28
- Management of Bleeding Complications/Overdose 29
- Reversal Agents 30

Chapter 3	**Statins in Peripheral Vascular Disease**	37
	Siddharth Rajput	

- Statins: 3-Hydroxy-3-Methylglutaryl-Coenzyme A Reductase Inhibitors 38

Chapter 4	**Endovascular Management of Abdominal Aortic Aneurysms: Devices Available and Evidence for Use**	49
	Riza Ibrahim	

- Basic Design and Principles of Endovascular Stent Grafts for Abdominal Aortic Aneurysm (AAA) Repair 50

Chapter 5	**Current Concepts in the Management of Type B Aortic Dissections**	62
	Raghuram Lakshminarayan, Paul M Scott	

- Imaging of Type B Aortic Dissection (Type B AD) 63
- Established Indications for Treatment of Type B Dissections 65

Chapter 6	**Managing Superficial Femoral Artery Lesions: Metal, Drugs or More**	75
	Aniket Pradhan, Robert Fitridge	

- Selecting Patients for Open Surgical or Endovascular Treatment of the Superficial Femoral Artery 76
- Anatomical Classification of Arterial Lesions 76
- Bypass vs Endovascular Options 78
- Endovascular Treatment 78
- Treatment Outcomes 80
- Other Therapies 89

| Chapter 7 | Subintimal Angioplasty | 96 |

Neghal Kandiyil, Amman Bolia

- Clinical Relevance 96
- Indications 97
- Contraindications 101
- Equipment 102
- Technique 103
- Post-procedural and Follow-Up Care 107
- Complications 110
- Outcomes 111

| Chapter 8 | Current Concepts in Managing Tibial Vessel Disease | 117 |

Kapil Mathur, Satheesh Ramamurthy, T Vidyasagaran

- Surgery vs Endovascular Debate 117
- Endovascular Adjuncts—Drug-coated Balloons 119
- Balloon Angioplasty Techniques 122
- Ongoing BTK Trials Worldwide 125

| Chapter 9 | Failing Vascular Grafts | 129 |

Cho Ee Ng, Vish Bhattacharya

- Pathophysiology 129
- Predictors of Graft Failure 130
- Duplex US Scanning after Vein Grafting 130
- Methods of Preventing Graft Failure 131
- Management of Failing Grafts 132
- Management of Completely Occluded Grafts 133

| Chapter 10 | Recent Advances in Management of Ischaemic Stroke | 137 |

Souvik Sen, Ravish Kothari, Neil Patel, Lauren D Giamberardino

- Stroke Prevention 138
- Stroke Treatment 140
- Recent Advancement in Stroke Treatment 141
- Analysis and Conclusion 145
- Future of Endovascular Stroke Treatment 146
- Recommendations from Guidelines 153

| Chapter 11 | Protection Devices in Endovascular Practice | 156 |

WNDP Chinthaka Appuhamy, Sundeep Punamiya

- Distal Embolisation 156
- Embolic Protection Devices 157
- Clinical Applications 166

| Chapter 12 | Status of CEA in an Endovascular Era | 172 |

Dovile Gudzinskaite-Brar, Raghvinder Pal Singh Gambhir

- Guidelines 172
- Timing of Intervention 172
- Technique 174
- Best Medical Therapy 174
- Carotid artery Stenting 174
- Asymptomatic Carotid Disease 175

Chapter 13	**Role of Interventions in Acute Lower Limb Deep Venous Thrombosis: Current Options**	180

Krishna Gummalla, Sundeep Punamiya

- Triaging Patients with DVT 181
- Interventions for Acute DVT 181
- Commonly Used Thrombectomy Devices 188
- Post-procedure Management 194

Chapter 14	**Current Concepts in Management of Pulmonary Embolism**	198

R Sekhar, Simit Vora, Pranav Thusay

- Triaging of Pulmonary Embolism in the Accident and Emergency Department 199
- Catheter-based Management of High-risk PE 203
- Role of Open Surgery in Acute Pulmonary Embolism 211
- Management of Acute Pulmonary Embolism without Hypotension 211
- Strategy for Non-high Risk Pulmonary Embolism 214
- Prognostic Scoring In Pulmonary Embolism 215
- Geneva Prognostic Scoring 216
- Oral Anticoagulation Schedule 217
- Key Points for Clinical Practice 218

Chapter 15	**Contrast-induced Nephropathy**	225

Niranjan Kulkarni, Harshal Vora

- Summary of Recommendations for Prevention of CIN 230
- Key Points for Clinical Practice 231

Chapter 16	**Carbon Dioxide Angiograpy and the Vascular Surgeon**	237

Ashwini Naveen Gangadharan, Jessica Shah, R Sekhar

- Principles of CO_2 Angiography 237
- Technical Aspects 238
- Practical Experiences With CO_2 244
- Key Points for Clinical Practice 248

Chapter 17	**Radiation Safety in Clinical Practice**	250

Dayananda Shamurailatpam, R Sekhar

- Understanding The Hazards 251
- Radiation Protection Equipment 254
- Practical Advice to Reduce or Minimise Occupational Radiation Dose 258
- Occupational Dosimetry in the Interventional Laboratory 260
- Evaluation of Personal Dosimetry Data 262
- What is the Role of the Institution 263
- Key Points for Safe Practice 263

Chapter 18	**Current Management of Lymphoedema of Limbs**	268

Rajesh Hydrabadi, Waldemar L Olszewski, Marzanna T Zaleska

- History and Clinical Examination 271
- Clinical Classification 271
- Investigation 272
- Dermato-lymphangio-adenitis 274

**Chapter 19 A Novel Noninvasive Tool for Interventions: Magnetic
Resonance-guided Focussed Ultrasound Surgery   285**
Shrinivas B Desai, Ritu K Kashikar
- Physics Principles of MRgFUS 285
- Equipment Configuration 287
- Uterine Fibroids 288
- MR-guided Focussed Ultrasound Procedure 289
- Complications 293
- Results 293
- Adenomyosis 296

Index   **301**

CHAPTER

1

Advances in Translational Vascular Research

J De Siqueira, G Atturu, S Homer-Vanniasinkam

INTRODUCTION

Cardiovascular science is a broad and complex field ranging from the interaction of microRNA molecules in the cell nucleus to the clinical evaluation of large vessel grafts and stents. Given the breadth of practice of a modern vascular surgeon (arterial, venous and lymphatic pathology; aneurysmal and occlusive disease; ulcer management; medical, endovascular and open surgical treatment), it is indeed a challenge to cover the entire topic in a single chapter.

We have chosen to focus on some of the more recent advances in research in arterial pathology which should be of interest to the general vascular surgeon: regression of atherosclerosis, angiogenesis, chronic foot ulcers and the modulation of aneurysmal dilatation. The advances in translational research described in this chapter have the potential to impact future management strategies for the prevention and treatment of vascular disease.

REGRESSION OF ATHEROSCLEROSIS

Atherosclerotic cardiovascular disease remains the leading cause of morbidity and mortality in most countries. Atherogenesis, the process of plaque formation, is complex and involves systemic and local factors. It generally runs a benign indolent course until the plaque ruptures, when the patient presents with acute symptoms.[1] Currently, research efforts in this area focus on (i) identifying the vulnerable plaque[2,3] in an attempt to prevent plaque rupture and thrombosis, and (ii) atherosclerosis regression. Achieving atherosclerosis regression, although it seems implausible, has been at the centre of research efforts for approximately 60 years.[4] In translational clinical studies, both the lipid theory[5] and the inflammation theory[6] of atherosclerosis have been put to the test.

Dyslipidaemia is a well-known modifiable risk factor for atherosclerosis. Lowering the total plasma cholesterol level using statin therapy has been shown to reduce the incidence of fatal and non-fatal cardiovascular events by

25%.[7] Currently, there are approximately 24 different antilipidaemic drugs on the market with five different modes of action.[8] The commonly used class of drugs are the statins, which act on the enzyme 3-hydroxy-3-methylglutaryl-coenzyme A reductase (HMG-Co-Reductase inhibitors). Other drugs act on different pathways of lipid metabolism such as: inhibiting intestinal cholesterol absorption (ezetimibe), increasing hepatic bile acid synthesis (bile acid sequestrants – cholestyramine) and activation of peroxisome proliferator activator receptor α (PPAR α – the fibrates). Vitamin B3 (nicotinic acid or niacin) is a potent lipid-modifying drug that acts on multiple targets. In spite of the availability of a large number of antilipidaemic drugs, this therapeutic modality achieves only about 30% cardiovascular risk reduction in clinical practice. Efforts in this area continue, with over 50 novel drug candidates in the development pipeline, aimed at different molecular targets. Current antilipidaemic drugs are orally active small organic molecules, in contrast to several of the newer agents which are biological products ranging from monoclonal antibodies to gene therapy, requiring invasive routes of administration.

One of the commonest target molecules for these newer generation drugs is proprotein convertase subtilisin/kexin type 9 (PCSK9). PCSK9 is a serine protease synthesised by the liver and intestine, which binds to the LDL receptor and promotes its degradation. Heterozygous loss-of-function mutation of PCSK9 is seen in around 3% of Afro-Americans and is associated with hypocholesterolaemia and an 88% reduction in cardiovascular risk.[9] Alirocumab and evolocumab are two monoclonal anti-PCSK9 antibodies that have successfully completed Phase 3 trials and are awaiting approval. In the ODYSSEY trial, addition of 150 mg of alirocumab, administered subcutaneously every fortnight with a statin, was shown to reduce the low-density lipoprotein (LDL)-C by 61% from baseline, compared to a placebo which caused a reduction of 0.8%, with a 54% risk reduction in the absolute rate of cardiovascular events.[10] In the DESCARTES study, which is a multicentre, randomised double-blind, placebo-controlled Phase 3 trial, addition of 420 mg of evolocumab (subcutaneously every 4 weeks) to other lipid-modifiying therapies, such as diet control, low-dose and high-dose atorvastatin and ezetimibe, achieved an additional reduction of 48.5–61.2% in low-density lipoprotein (LDL) cholesterol.[11]

A further area of lipid research interest focuses on increasing high-density lipoprotein (HDL-C) levels by the development of inhibitors of cholesterol ester transfer protein (CETP).[12] CETP catalyses the transfer of cholesterol ester from HDL particles to LDL and VLDL (very low-density lipoprotein) particles. Anacetrapib, a potent HDL-C increasing drug, when used at a dose of 100 mg per day in addition to a statin, has been shown to increase the HDL-C by 138% and decrease LDL-C by 40% without significant toxicity, in a multicentre double-blind placebo-controlled Phase 3 trial (DEFINE trial).[13] Evacetrapib is another potent inhibitor of CETP that is proven to increase HDL-C levels in a randomised control trial.[14] However, both these drugs, in addition to increasing the HDL-C levels also reduce the plasma LDL-C levels, making it difficult to differentiate the specific effect of increased HDL-C levels in reducing cardiovascular risk.

Gene modulation using antisense oligonucleotide or ribonucleic acid (RNA)-silencing technologies is a powerful way of inhibiting specific target proteins.[15] Mipomersen (KYNAMRO®) is the first FDA-approved anti-apolipoprotein B (ApoB) antisense oligonucleotide for treating patients with familial hypercholesterolaemia. Volanesorsen is another apolipoprotein CIII (ApoCIII) antisense oligonucleotide that has reached Phase 3 clinical trials. The results of the two large placebo-controlled randomised trials, APPROACH and BROADEN, are awaited with interest.

In contrast to the lipid-modifying drug trials, those exploring the effect of anti-inflammatory properties in reducing cardiovascular events have met with little success.[16] Highly-sensitive C-reactive protein (hs-CRP), a biomarker of inflammation, is shown to independently predict the risk of cardiovascular disease. Clinical studies such as CARE and JUPITER[17] have shown that statins reduce both the LDL-C and CRP levels; however, it was difficult to attribute the individual contribution of these two effects to the overall reduction in cardiovascular events.

Peroxisome proliferator-activated receptor-γ (PPARγ) factor is shown to affect glucose metabolism and vascular inflammation. Two PPARγ agonists (also known as insulin sensitisers), rosiglitazone and pioglitazone, were studied in large randomised controlled trials. In the RECORD trial, rosiglitazone did not show any significant reduction in cardiovascular events.[18] In the PROactive study, pioglitazone was shown to significantly reduce the occurrence of fatal and non-fatal myocardial infarction.[19]

Interleukins (IL), mainly IL-1β and IL-6, are other targets of anti-inflammatory clinical trials in atherosclerosis. Canakinumab is a monoclonal antibody against IL-1β. The efficacy of canakinumab in reducing cardiovascular events is the subject of a large study, the Canakinumab Anti-inflammatory Thrombosis Outcome Study (CANTOS), involving 17,200 patients.[20] Similarly, the efficacy in reducing cardiovascular events of low-dose methotrexate, by its effect on the IL-6 pathway, is being studied in the Cardiovascular Inflammation Reduction Trial (CIRT) involving 7,000 patients.[21] The results from both these studies are awaited.

ANGIOGENESIS

Therapeutic angiogenesis is an exciting field of translational research for clinicians who manage patients with occlusive arterial disease. As evidenced by serial imaging, patients on best medical therapy are able to bypass occlusive or stenotic disease by vessel proliferation. The attempt to reproduce or accelerate this process is called therapeutic angiogenesis, which can be brought about by the delivery of angiogenic factors (growth factors, cytokines) locally or by inducing cells in ischaemic tissues to secrete the proteins of interest (gene therapy). Gene therapy carries an inherent advantage over protein delivery – if cells can be programmed to secrete a protein of interest continuously, its delivery can be sustained more easily than with multiple administrations.[22] From evidence gathered in pre-clinical studies, five angiogenic factors have been investigated in clinical trials of peripheral arterial disease.

Vascular endothelial growth factor (VEGF) promotes endothelial cell migration, proliferation and angiogenesis. Although initial small studies showed promising results with angiographic evidence of increased vascularity, the Phase 2 randomised controlled trial using VEGF121 (RAVE trial) in patients with disabling intermittent claudication did not show significant changes in peak walking time or ankle brachial pressure index (ABPI).[23] In a more recent randomised clinical trial, intramuscular injection of VEGF165 gene in patients with diabetes mellitus and critical limb ischaemia (CLI) showed improvements in healing of skin ulceration, ABPI and toe brachial pressure index (TBPI) without significant changes in amputation rates or rest pain.[24]

Fibroblast growth factor (FGF) is another angiogenic factor that enhances blood vessel formation. The initial Phase 2 TALISMAN trial was encouraging with decreased amputation rates.[25] However, these results were not reproduced in the follow-up Phase 3 TAMARIS trial.[26]

Hepatocyte growth factor (HGF), in addition to promoting angiogenesis, has an established role in myogenesis and wound-healing. It is also more potent than VEGF and has fewer side-effects, particularly the risk of oedema. In Phase 1 and 2 trials, intramuscular administration of HGF in patients with CLI improved ulcer healing, rest pain and ABPI.[27] These beneficial effects were maintained even after a two-year follow-up, encouraging further clinical trials. Hypoxia-inducible factor 1- alpha (HIF 1α)[28] and developmental endothelial locus-1 (DEL-1)[29] are the other two angiogenic factors which showed promising results in pre-clinical studies but failed to show clinical benefit in Phase 1 and 2 clinical trials.

The other well-explored option in therapeutic angiogenesis is stem cell therapy. The key concept is that stem cells can proliferate and generate new blood vessels in ischaemic tissues. Stem cells can be subclassified by their lineage: embryonic stem cells (ESC) and adult stem cells (ASC). Of particular interest in the context of angiogenesis is the endothelial progenitor cell;[30] however, this term has fallen out of favour and instead it is now more common to refer to mononuclear cells (MNC), either harvested from bone marrow (BMMNC) or peripheral blood (PBMNC).

Two landmark trials reported the use of stem cells: TACT and PROVASA. TACT[31] showed that injection of BMMNC into the gastrocnemius muscle led to an improvement in CLI. In its second stage, TACT also investigated whether effects brought about by BMMNC were superior to those from PBMNC. At 4 and 24 weeks, there were significant improvements in ABPI, rest pain and walking time. PROVASA,[32] on the other hand, demonstrated that intra-arterial administration of BMMNC did not lead to significant increases in ABPI. Nonetheless, there were notable improvements in ulcer healing and rest pain at 6 months. More recently, Inei and colleagues have reported 4-year data on amputation-free survival in patients with CLI or Buerger's disease after intramuscular injection of BMMNC. Of note, amputation rates were halved in the CLI group (100% vs 52%). Most recently, a meta-analysis of 12 randomised trials[33] has shown improvements in amputation (8 treatments to prevent a single event), ABPI, ulcer healing and walking distance, following stem cell therapy. For these reasons, stem cell therapy is the most promising new technology in the management of peripheral arterial disease.

One of the limitations of BMMNC therapy is the need for invasive and painful bone marrow aspiration to procure the cells. PBMNC therapy aims to overcome this limitation by mobilising BMMNC to the peripheral blood using granulocyte-colony stimulating factor (G-CSF) and harvesting them from the peripheral blood circulation. The therapeutic potential of these peripherally-harvested MNC were evaluated in few clinical trials. Huang et al [34] and Ozturk et al [35] performed autologous transplantation of PBMNC in diabetic patients with CLI and found that the pain scores and ABPIs were significantly improved. In another small clinical trial, Mohammadzadeh et al reported improved ABPIs and amputation rates by transplanting autologous PBMNC in diabetic patients with CLI.[36] A direct comparison of the therapeutic potential of BMMNC and PBMNC was performed in a few clinical trials with variable results.[37-39]

CHRONIC FOOT ULCERS

In the studies described in the preceding section, it is clear that stem cells have shown great translational potential in the management of peripheral arterial disease. There is some evidence that they may also have a future in ulcer healing, beyond improving limb vascularity. However, this area of research is not as advanced as that of therapeutic angiogenesis and much of the evidence for the use of stem cells to treat lower limb ulcers comes from preclinical models and small clinical case series.

The role of stem cells in foot ulcers is not only to propagate and differentiate into skin tissues but also to promote an environment where the native cells may proliferate and eventually cover the ulcer area. Analysis of animal models of stem cell transplantation has shown that this is achieved by the release of a cascade of growth factors including vascular endothelial growth factor and epithelial growth factor.[40] The choice of stem cell is just as important in ulcer management as it is in angiogenesis. Embryonic stem cells are a default option given their pluripotent ability to differentiate into any cell type. However, this treatment raises a number of ethical controversies, given the need to sacrifice human embryos to procure the cells. Hence, an obvious alternative is autologous bone marrow as a source of stem cells.

Kataoka[41] conducted an elegant experiment where bone marrow mesenchymal stem cells were harvested from green fluorescent protein (GFP) transgenic mice (a breed of mice that have been genetically engineered so that their cells express proteins which fluoresce under the appropriate light wavelengths) and transplanted onto wounds on genetically bald mice. After three weeks, the wounds had healed and hair was growing in the transplantation area. Furthermore, histological analysis of the treated skin revealed GFP visible in the dermis, epidermis and hair follicles, demonstrating that the stem cells had successfully differentiated into multiple cell lines. The effectiveness of bone-marrow derived mesenchymal stem cells has been shown in other murine models[42] and in a small series of 8 patients,[43] which demonstrated that bone-marrow derived mesenchymal stem cells helped to reduce ulcer size. The use of bone-marrow derived haematopoietic stem cells also led to positive effects on ulcer healing, when applied topically,[44] in a murine model.

There has also been some interest in the use of adipose-derived stem cells (ADSC). These are harvested by performing liposuction and using selection enzymes to separate them from 'contaminating' adipocytes.[45] Studies with ADSC have not reached clinical trials, though early animal data have shown improvements in wound healing in different preclinical models.[46]

The above studies have investigated the topical application of stem cells to wounds. However, the simple application of stem cells to a wound bed is insufficient to promote healing; the ulcer environment is, by default, hostile to the cell through a combination of inflammation, ischaemia and oxidative stress. Biological scaffolds are being increasingly tested to encourage both cell seeding and their uptake on the ulcer bed. Fibrin scaffolds are marketed as haemostatic sealants,[47] and as such are perhaps the most widely available. However, there is evidence to suggest that these inhibit the proliferation of stem cells, and their use has not led to uniformly positive results.[48] Another approach is to use collagen scaffolds. Collagen is one of the most abundant components of the extracellular matrix in mammals. There are 16 types of collagen; skin and vascular tissues are predominantly composed of types I and III. Collagen is laid down in staggered, end-to-end arrangements, as well as by cross-linking, giving collagen-containing tissues a high tensile strength. Hence, applying the stem cell within a collagen-based gel is analogous to transplanting a cell within its native biological scaffold. Indeed, collagen biogels have been shown to bring about enhanced engraftment of stem cells in animal models.[49] However, this has not yet been translated into human studies.

An alternative approach is to manage wounds primarily with extracellular matrices without the contemporaneous use of stem cells. Such matrices can be biological scaffolds as described earlier, or decellularised matrices (DCMs). The mechanism of action of DCMs is not fully understood but it has been suggested that they work by binding matrix metalloproteinases (enzymes which work to breakdown the wound bed) and nullifying their biological effects. It is also thought that DCMs promote the recruitment of epithelial cells and vascular endothelial cells. Sources for DCMs include porcine intestinal submucosa and human dermal matrices, many of which are available commercially. Whilst no randomised controlled trials have been carried out to assess the effectiveness of these products, the manufacturer-sponsored literature demonstrates encouraging results. However, it is difficult to judge these studies without proper controls; in a study of 23 patients who were treated with surgical wound debridement and topical application of equine pericardium, there was a 94% wound improvement rate.[50] However, it is not clear to what extent this was brought about by debridement alone.

The true clinical effect of DCMs remains elusive. One of the most recent advances in ECM engineering has been the development of hybrid biological/synthetic matrices such as the Integra Dermal Regeneration Template.™ This template combines a glycogen and glycosaminoglycan (dermal) layer with a silicone (epidermal) layer. These templates have been predominantly developed for the management of burns,[51] but recent evidence suggests that they may also have an application in the management of the diabetic foot ulcer.[52]

The gold standard in the management of foot ulcers will continue to be infection control, offloading and revascularisation of ischaemic tissues. However, there are clearly emerging technologies and treatments on the horizon which may help to manage more effectively this frequent and disabling complication of peripheral vascular disease.

ANEURYSMAL DISEASE

The surgical management of aortic aneurysmal disease has fundamentally changed over the last two decades. Lessons learnt from the UK small aneurysm study,[53] MASS trial[54] and EVAR 1 and 2 trials[55] have served to reduce the mortality associated with abdominal aortic aneurysm rupture and interventions carried out to prevent it. Nonetheless, the fundamental biology of aneurysm development (as opposed to its risk factors), still eludes most clinicians.

The aorta contains a high proportion of collagen and elastin, which serve to give it tensile strength and elasticity, both of which are vital for the carriage of pulsatile blood. Histological studies have demonstrated that aortic elastin is altered in Marfan's syndrome[56] and in the elderly population.[57] Additionally, there is a lower concentration of elastin in aneurysmal aortas compared to healthy vessels.[58] It is, therefore, natural to presume that there is an association, if not causation, between collagen, elastin and aneurysm development.

The variability in collagen types (as described in the ulcer management section) has led to studies of the differential composition of collagen in aneurysmal and healthy aortas. In particular, there has been an interest in the two most common types: I and III. Bode[59] has described the distribution of collagen types in aneurysmal aortas: his group found that the media from abdominal aortic aneurysms had a higher concentration of type III collagen than those from healthy aortas. Similarly, there is some evidence of a higher rate of collagen III breakdown in patients with aneurysmal disease, as evidenced by higher circulating concentrations of its fragments.[60,61]

The changes in collagen and elastin composition in aneurysmal aortas have driven researchers to investigate the mechanism behind their catabolism in the hope of inhibiting this process. Matrix metalloproteinases (MMPs) are a group of zinc-dependent enzymes responsible for the degradation of extracellular proteins. Interstitial collagen degradation is associated with increased expression of the collagenases MMP 1 and 13, whilst the elastases MMP 2, 9 and 12 have been noted in the wall of aneurysmal aortas. As MMPs have also been linked with tumour invasion, the study of MMP inhibition is well established in the field of cancer research. MMP inhibitors work by targeting the catalytic zinc ion within the enzyme with a number of zinc-binding molecules demonstrating in vitro and in vivo MMP inhibition.[62] However, to date, Phase 3 trials have mostly met with disappointing results,[63] often due to the side-effect profiles of these compounds.[64]

In recent years, aneurysm researchers have become interested in the MMP inhibitory effects of tetracyclines, a discovery that was made and developed in the field of periodontal disease.[65] Petrinec[66] was among the first to study the effects of doxycycline on mice. He demonstrated a significant reduction in the rate of aneurysm development and growth in an experimental model. Further work in this field successfully explored the use of low-dose regimes[67] before translating into human studies.[68] However, trials exploring this therapeutic strategy have not shown unanimously positive results.[69] Initial results were encouraging, with significant reductions in aneurysm expansion, but the Pharmaceutical Aneurysm Stabilization Trial revealed no difference in aneurysm expansion or rate of repair over 18 months in patients taking doxycycline.[70] Nonetheless, the effectiveness of doxycycline in modulating aneurysm development is still of interest to the clinical community with a Phase 2 North American randomised trial currently recruiting patients.

Another strategy for the attenuation of aneurysms is the inhibition of elastases. As has been established, elastin content is altered in aneurysmal aortas. Indeed, pancreatic elastase infusion is an established method of developing aneurysms in animal models.[71] Elastase inhibition has historically been of interest for the prevention of emphysema[72] and in wound healing.[73] However, it is only recently that the effects of elastin inhibitors have been studied for aneurysmal disease. Delbosc and colleagues have published an interesting animal study using a rat model of aneurysm development, wherein the administration of a synthetic elastase inhibitor led to an attenuation in infective (*Porphyromonas gingivalis*) aneurysm progression.[74] They propose that it may have a role in the future management of aneurysms, though it is worth noting that such inhibition was not observed in the absence of infection, and the management of mycotic aneurysms presents an entirely different set of clinical challenges.

In summary, the pathophysiological processes responsible for the development of aneurysms are not as well understood as those of atherosclerotic disease. However, there appears to be a clear role for the catabolism of collagen and elastin. The enzymes that degrade these proteins have been implicated in the development of aneurysmal disease, but the inhibition of these enzymes has not yet led to clinically significant improvements in outcomes. As the evidence to date is equivocal, the results of large clinical trials are awaited. Future research could elucidate the missing links in the development and medical management of aortic aneurysms.

CONCLUSION

This chapter has described some of the important advances in research in the management of diseases commonly encountered by vascular surgeons. The overview of the four research topics covered is by no means comprehensive; rather, it is designed to provide readers with an introduction to the areas of ongoing vascular research. Most of the therapies discussed are some years away from entering routine clinical practice. Clinical efficacy and cost will be important factors in bringing these therapies to market. However, 'a journey of a thousand miles begins with a single step': many modern clinical therapies would not have been possible without translational research.

Clinical and pre-clinical research depends crucially on external funding and the provision of such financial support remains a challenge, with a multitude of scientists and clinicians competing for funds from what seems to be an ever-decreasing pool of resources. Even the concepts which show great initial promise may not progress to the bedside, i.e. move 'from concept to clinic', without adequate and timely funding. On a positive note, we are witnessing greater collaboration between surgeons and scientists with each contributing to, and enhancing, the other's work. Such collaboration is at the heart of translational vascular research.

REFERENCES

1. Falk E. Pathogenesis of atherosclerosis. J Am Coll Cardiol. 2006;47(8 Suppl):C7-12.
2. Dweck MR, Aikawa E, Newby DE, Tarkin JM, Rudd JH, Narula J, et al. Noninvasive Molecular Imaging of Disease Activity in Atherosclerosis. Circ Res. 2016;119(2):330-40.
3. Tarkin JM, Dweck MR, Evans NR, Takx RA, Brown AJ, Tawakol A, et al. Imaging Atherosclerosis. Circ Res. 2016;118(4):750-69
4. Friedman M, Byers SO, Rosenman RH. Resolution of aortic atherosclerotic infiltration in the rabbit by phosphatide infusion. Proc Soc Exp Biol Med. 1957;95(3):586-8.
5. Steinberg D. In celebration of the 100th anniversary of the lipid hypothesis of atherosclerosis. J Lipid Res. 2013;54(11):2946-9.
6. Tuttolomondo A, Di Raimondo D, Pecoraro R, Arnao V, Pinto A, Licata G. Atherosclerosis as an inflammatory disease. Curr Pharm Des. 2012;18(28):4266-88.
7. Taylor FC, Huffman M, Ebrahim S. Statin therapy for primary prevention of cardiovascular disease. JAMA. 2013;310(22):2451-2.
8. Kramer W. Antilipidemic drug therapy today and in the future. Handb Exp Pharmacol. 2016;233:373-435.
9. Seidah NG, Awan Z, Chretien M, Mbikay M. PCSK9: a key modulator of cardiovascular health. Circ Res. 2014;114(6):1022-36.
10. Robinson JG, Farnier M, Krempf M, Bergeron J, Luc G, Averna M, et al. Efficacy and safety of alirocumab in reducing lipids and cardiovascular events. N Engl J Med. 2015;372(16):1489-99.
11. Blom DJ, Hala T, Bolognese M, Lillestol MJ, Toth PD, Burgess L, et al. A 52-week placebo-controlled trial of evolocumab in hyperlipidemia. N Engl J Med. 2014;370(19):1809-19.
12. Rader DJ, deGoma EM. Future of cholesteryl ester transfer protein inhibitors. Annu Rev Med. 2014;65:385-403.
13. Cannon CP, Shah S, Dansky HM, Davidson M, Brinton EA, Gotto AM, et al. Safety of anacetrapib in patients with or at high risk for coronary heart disease. N Engl J Med. 2010;363(25):2406-15.
14. Nicholls SJ, Brewer HB, Kastelein JJ, Krueger KA, Wang MD, Shao M, et al. Effects of the CETP inhibitor evacetrapib administered as monotherapy or in combination with statins on HDL and LDL cholesterol: a randomized controlled trial. JAMA. 2011;306(19):2099-109.
15. Yamamoto T, Wada F, Harada-Shiba M. Development of Antisense Drugs for Dyslipidemia. J Atheroscler Thromb. 2016.

16. Lorenzatti AJ, Retzlaff BM. Unmet needs in the management of atherosclerotic cardiovascular disease: Is there a role for emerging anti-inflammatory interventions? Int J Cardiol. 2016;221:581-6.
17. Ridker PM, Danielson E, Fonseca FA, Genest J, Gotto AM, Jr., Kastelein JJ, et al. Rosuvastatin to prevent vascular events in men and women with elevated C-reactive protein. N Engl J Med. 2008;359(21):2195-207.
18. Home PD, Pocock SJ, Beck-Nielsen H, Curtis PS, Gomis R, Hanefeld M, et al. Rosiglitazone evaluated for cardiovascular outcomes in oral agent combination therapy for type 2 diabetes (RECORD): a multicentre, randomised, open-label trial. Lancet. 2009;373(9681):2125-35.
19. Dormandy JA, Charbonnel B, Eckland DJ, Erdmann E, Massi-Benedetti M, Moules IK, et al. Secondary prevention of macrovascular events in patients with type 2 diabetes in the PROactive Study (PROspective pioglitAzone Clinical Trial In macroVascular Events): a randomised controlled trial. Lancet. 2005;366(9493): 1279-89.
20. Ridker PM, Thuren T, Zalewski A, Libby P. Interleukin-1beta inhibition and the prevention of recurrent cardiovascular events: rationale and design of the Canakinumab Anti-inflammatory Thrombosis Outcomes Study (CANTOS). Am Heart J. 2011;162(4):597-605.
21. Everett BM, Pradhan AD, Solomon DH, Paynter N, Macfadyen J, Zaharris E, et al. Rationale and design of the cardiovascular inflammation reduction trial: a test of the inflammatory hypothesis of atherothrombosis. Am Heart J. 2013;166(2):199-207 e15.
22. Ghosh R, Walsh SR, Tang TY, Noorani A, Hayes PD. Gene therapy as a novel therapeutic option in the treatment of peripheral vascular disease: systematic review and meta-analysis. Int J Clin Pract. 2008;62(9):1383-90.
23. Rajagopalan S, Mohler ER, 3rd, Lederman RJ, Mendelsohn FO, Saucedo JF, Goldman CK, et al. Regional angiogenesis with vascular endothelial growth factor in peripheral arterial disease: a phase II randomized, double-blind, controlled study of adenoviral delivery of vascular endothelial growth factor 121 in patients with disabling intermittent claudication. Circulation. 2003;108(16):1933-8.
24. Kusumanto YH, van Weel V, Mulder NH, Smit AJ, van den Dungen JJ, Hooymans JM, et al. Treatment with intramuscular vascular endothelial growth factor gene compared with placebo for patients with diabetes mellitus and critical limb ischemia: a double-blind randomized trial. Hum Gene Ther. 2006;17(6):683-91.
25. Nikol S, Baumgartner I, Van Belle E, Diehm C, Visona A, Capogrossi MC, et al. Therapeutic angiogenesis with intramuscular NV1FGF improves amputation-free survival in patients with critical limb ischemia. Mol Ther. 2008;16(5):972-8.
26. Belch J, Hiatt WR, Baumgartner I, Driver IV, Nikol S, Norgren L, et al. Effect of fibroblast growth factor NV1FGF on amputation and death: a randomised placebo-controlled trial of gene therapy in critical limb ischaemia. Lancet. 2011;377(9781):1929-37.
27. Morishita R, Makino H, Aoki M, Hashiya N, Yamasaki K, Azuma J, et al. Phase I/IIa clinical trial of therapeutic angiogenesis using hepatocyte growth factor gene transfer to treat critical limb ischemia. Arterioscler Thromb Vasc Biol. 2011;31(3):713-20.

28. Creager MA, Olin JW, Belch JJ, Moneta GL, Henry TD, Rajagopalan S, et al. Effect of hypoxia-inducible factor-1alpha gene therapy on walking performance in patients with intermittent claudication. Circulation. 2011;124(16):1765-73.
29. Grossman PM, Mendelsohn F, Henry TD, Hermiller JB, Litt M, Saucedo JF, et al. Results from a phase II multicenter, double-blind placebo-controlled study of Del-1 (VLTS-589) for intermittent claudication in subjects with peripheral arterial disease. Am Heart J. 2007;153(5):874-80.
30. Asahara T, Murohara T, Sullivan A, Silver M, van der Zee R, Li T, et al. Isolation of putative progenitor endothelial cells for angiogenesis. Science. 1997;275:964-7.
31. Tateishi-Yuyama E, Matsubara H, Murohara T, Ikeda U, Shintani S, Masaki H, et al. Therapeutic Angiogenesis using Cell Transplantation (TACT) Study Investigators. Therapeutic angiogenesis for patients with limb ischaemia by autologous transplantation of bone-marrow cells: a pilot study and a randomised controlled trial. Lancet. 2002;360(9331):427-35.
32. Walter DH, Krankenberg H, Balzer JO, Kalka C, Baumgartner I, Schlüter M, et al. PROVASA Investigators. Intraarterial administration of bone marrow mononuclear cells in patients with critical limb ischemia: a randomized-start, placebo-controlled pilot trial (PROVASA). Circ Cardiovasc Interv. 2011;4(1):26-37.
33. Teraa M, Sprengers RW, van der Graaf Y, Peters CE, Moll FL, Verhaar MC. Autologous bone marrow-derived cell therapy in patients with critical limb ischemia: a meta-analysis of randomized controlled clinical trials. Ann Surg. 2013;258(6):922-9.
34. Huang P, Li S, Han M, Xiao Z, Yang R, Han ZC. Autologous transplantation of granulocyte colony-stimulating factor-mobilized peripheral blood mononuclear cells improves critical limb ischemia in diabetes. Diabetes Care. 2005;28(9):2155-60.
35. Ozturk A, Kucukardali Y, Tangi F, Erikci A, Uzun G, Bashekim C, et al. Therapeutical potential of autologous peripheral blood mononuclear cell transplantation in patients with type 2 diabetic critical limb ischemia. J Diabetes Complications. 2012;26(1):29-33.
36. Mohammadzadeh L, Samedanifard SH, Keshavarzi A, Alimoghaddam K, Larijani B, Ghavamzadeh A, et al. Therapeutic outcomes of transplanting autologous granulocyte colony-stimulating factor-mobilised peripheral mononuclear cells in diabetic patients with critical limb ischaemia. Exp Clin Endocrinol Diabetes. 2013;121(1):48-53.
37. Matoba S, Tatsumi T, Murohara T, Imaizumi T, Katsuda Y, Ito M, et al. Long-term clinical outcome after intramuscular implantation of bone marrow mononuclear cells (Therapeutic Angiogenesis by Cell Transplantation [TACT] trial) in patients with chronic limb ischemia. Am Heart J. 2008;156(5):1010-8.
38. Huang PP, Yang XF, Li SZ, Wen JC, Zhang Y, Han ZC. Randomised comparison of G-CSF-mobilized peripheral blood mononuclear cells versus bone marrow-mononuclear cells for the treatment of patients with lower limb arteriosclerosis obliterans. Thromb Haemost. 2007;98(6):1335-42.
39. Kamata Y, Takahashi Y, Iwamoto M, Matsui K, Murakami Y, Muroi K, et al. Local implantation of autologous mononuclear cells from bone marrow and peripheral blood for treatment of ischaemic digits in patients with connective tissue diseases. Rheumatology (Oxford). 2007;46(5):882-4.

40. Lee KB, Choi J, Cho SB, Chung JY, Moon ES, Kim NS, et al. Topical embryonic stem cells enhance wound healing in diabetic rats. J Orthop Res, 2011;29(10):1554-62.
41. Kataoka K, Medina RJ, Kageyama T, Miyazaki M, Yoshino T, Makino T, Huh NH. Participation of adult mouse bone marrow cells in reconstitution of skin. Am J Pathol. 2003;163(4):1227-31.
42. Kwon DS, Gao X, Liu YB, et al. "Treatment with bone marrow-derived stromal cells accelerates wound healing in diabetic rats," International Wound Journal. 2008;5(3):453-63.
43. Falanga V, Iwamoto S, Chartier M, Yufit T, Butmarc J, Kouttab N, et al. Autologous bone marrow-derived cultured mesenchymal stem cells delivered in a fibrin spray accelerate healing in murine and human cutaneous wounds. Tissue Eng. 2007;13 (6), 1299-1312.
44. Pedroso DC, Tellechea A, Moura L, Fidalgo-Carvalho I, Duarte J, Carvalho E, et al. Improved survival, vascular differentiation and wound healing potential of stem cells co-cultured with endothelial cells. PloS one. 2011;6(1):e16114.
45. Fraser JK, Wulur I, Alfonso Z, Hedrick MH. Fat tissue: an underappreciated source of stem cells for biotechnology. Trends Biotechnol. 2006;24(4):150-4.
46. Toyserkani NM, Christensen ML, Sheikh SP, Sørensen JA. Adipose-derived stem cells: new treatment for wound healing? Ann Plast Surg. 2015;75(1):117-23.
47. Bensaid W, Triffitt JT, Blanchat C, Oudina K, Sedel L, Petite H. A biodegradable fibrin scaffold for mesenchymal stem cell transplantation Biomaterials. 2003;24 (14):2497-2502.
48. Blumberg SN, Berger A, Hwang L, Pastar I, Warren SM, Chen W. The role of stem cells in the treatment of diabetic foot ulcers. Diabetes Res Clin Pract. 2012;96(1):1-9.
49. Rustad KC, Wong VW, Sorkin M, Glotzbach JP, Major MR, Rajadas J, et al. Enhancement of mesenchymal stem cell angiogenic capacity and stemness by a biomimetic hydrogel scaffold. Biomaterials. 2012;33(1):80-90.
50. Mulder G, Lee DK. A retrospective clinical review of extracellular matrices for tissue reconstruction: equine pericardium as a biological covering to assist with wound closure. Wounds. 2009;21(9):254-61.
51. Heimbach DM, Warden GD, Luterman A, Jordan MH, Ozobia N, Ryan CM, et al. Multicenter postapproval clinical trial of Integra dermal regeneration template for burn treatment. J Burn Care Rehabil. 2003;24(1):42-8.
52. Driver VR, Lavery LA, Reyzelman AM, Dutra TG, Dove CR, Kotsis SV. A clinical trial of Integra Template for diabetic foot ulcer treatment. Wound Repair Regen. 2015;23(6):891-900.
53. Powell JT, Brown LC, Forbes JF, Fowkes FG, Greenhalgh RM, Ruckley CV, et al. Final 12-year follow-up of surgery versus surveillance in the UK Small Aneurysm Trial. Br J Surg. 2007;94(6):702-8.
54. Ashton HA, Buxton MJ, Day NE, Kim LG, Marteau TM, Scott RA, et al. Multicentre Aneurysm Screening Study Group. The Multicentre Aneurysm Screening Study (MASS) into the effect of abdominal aortic aneurysm screening on mortality in men: a randomised controlled trial. Lancet. 2002;360(9345):1531-9.
55. Brown LC, Powell JT, Thompson SG, Epstein DM, Sculpher MJ, Greenhalgh RM. The UK EndoVascular Aneurysm Repair (EVAR) trials: randomised trials of EVAR versus standard therapy. Health Technol Assess. 2012;16(9):1-218.

56. Abraham PA, Perejda AJ, Carnes WH, Uitto J. Marfan syndrome. Demonstration of abnormal elastin in aorta. Journal of Clinical Investigation. 1982;70(6):1245-52.
57. Tsamis A, Krawiec JT, Vorp DA. Elastin and collagen fibre microstructure of the human aorta in ageing and disease: a review. Journal of the Royal Society Interface. 2013;10(83):20121004. doi:10.1098/rsif.2012.1004.
58. Campa JS, Greenhalgh RM, Powell JT. Elastin degradation in abdominal aortic aneurysms. Atherosclerosis. 1987;65(1-2):13-21.
59. Bode MK, Soini Y, Melkko J, Satta J, Risteli L, Risteli J. Increased amount of type III pN-collagen in human abdominal aortic aneurysms: evidence for impaired type III collagen fibrillogenesis. J Vasc Surg. 2000;32(6):1201-7.
60. Satta J, Juvonen T, Haukipuro K, Juvonen M, Kairaluoma MI. Increased turnover of collagen in abdominal aortic aneurysms, demonstrated by measuring the concentration of the aminoterminal propeptide of type III procollagen in peripheral and aortal blood samples. J Vasc Surg. 1995;22(2):155-60.
61. Treska V, Topolcan O. Plasma and tissue levels of collagen types I and III markers in patients with abdominal aortic aneurysms. Int Angiol. 2000;19(1):64-8.
62. Vandenbroucke RE, Libert C. Is there new hope for therapeutic matrix metalloproteinase inhibition? Nat Rev Drug Discov. 2014;13(12):904-27.
63. Sparano JA, Bernardo P, Stephenson P, Gradishar WJ, Ingle JN, Zucker S, et al. Randomized phase III trial of marimastat versus placebo in patients with metastatic breast cancer who have responding or stable disease after first-line chemotherapy: Eastern Cooperative Oncology Group trial E2196. J Clin Oncol. 2004;22(23):4683-90. Erratum in: J Clin Oncol. 2005;23(1):248.
64. Leighl NB, Paz-Ares L, Douillard JY, Peschel C, Arnold A, Depierre A, et al. Randomized phase III study of matrix metalloproteinase inhibitor BMS-275291 in combination with paclitaxel and carboplatin in advanced non-small-cell lung cancer: National Cancer Institute of Canada-Clinical Trials Group Study BR.18. J Clin Oncol. 2005;23(12):2831-9.
65. Preshaw PM, Hefti AF, Jepsen S, Etienne D, Walker C, Bradshaw MH. Subantimicrobial dose doxycycline as adjunctive treatment for periodontitis. A review. J Clin Periodontol. 2004;31(9):697-707.
66. Petrinec D, Liao S, Holmes DR, Reilly JM, Parks WC, Thompson RW. Doxycycline inhibition of aneurysmal degeneration in an elastase-induced rat model of abdominal aortic aneurysm: preservation of aortic elastin associated with suppressed production of 92 kD gelatinase. J Vasc Surg. 1996;23(2):336-46.
67. Prall AK, Longo GM, Mayhan WG, Waltke EA, Fleckten B, Thompson RW, et al. Doxycycline in patients with abdominal aortic aneurysms and in mice: comparison of serum levels and effect on aneurysm growth in mice. J Vasc Surg. 2002;35(5):923-9.
68. Mosorin M, Juvonen J, Biancari F, Satta J, Surcel HM, Leinonen M. Use of doxycycline to decrease the growth rate of abdominal aortic aneurysms: a randomized, double-blind, placebo-controlled pilot study. J Vasc Surg. 2001;34(4):606-10.
69. Dodd BR, Spence RA. Doxycycline inhibition of abdominal aortic aneurysm growth: a systematic review of the literature. Curr Vasc Pharmacol. 2011;9(4):471-8.
70. Meijer CA, Stijnen T, Wasser MN, Hamming JF, van Bockel JH, Lindeman JH, Pharmaceutical Aneurysm Stabilization Trial Study Group. Doxycycline for

stabilization of abdominal aortic aneurysms: a randomized trial. Ann Intern Med. 2013;159(12):815-23.
71. Anidjar S, Salzmann JL, Gentric D, Lagneau P, Camilleri JP, Michel JB. Elastase-induced experimental aneurysms in rats. Circulation. 1990;82(3):973-81.
72. Fujie K, Shinguh Y, Yamazaki A, Hatanaka H, Okamoto M, Okuhara M. Inhibition of elastase-induced acute inflammation and pulmonary emphysema in hamsters by a novel neutrophil elastase inhibitor FR901277. Inflamm Res. 1999;48(3):160-7.
73. Lee SK, Lee SS, Song IS, Kim YS, Park YW, Joo JY, et. al. Paradoxical effects of elastase inhibitor guamerin on the tissue repair of two different wound models: sealed cutaneous and exposed tongue wounds. Exp Mol Med. 2004;36(3):259-67.
74. Delbosc S, Rouer M, Alsac JM, Louedec L, Philippe M, Meilhac O, et. al. Elastase inhibitor AZD9668 treatment prevented progression of experimental abdominal aortic aneurysms. J Vasc Surg. 2016;63(2):486-92.e1.

CHAPTER 2

Newer Oral Anticoagulants

Sameer Tulpule

INTRODUCTION

For more than half a century, warfarin, a vitamin K antagonist (VKA), has been the cornerstone for the prevention and treatment of thromboembolic disease. Although being cheap and readily available, its narrow therapeutic index and multiple drug and diet interactions meant that it affected compliance questioning its safety and efficacy. A meta-analysis revealed that 44% of bleeding complications with warfarin were associated with supra-therapeutic international normalised ratios (INRs) and that 48% of thromboembolic events occurred with sub-therapeutic readings.[1]

Options for anticoagulation have been expanding steadily over the past few decades, providing a greater number of agents for prevention and management of thromboembolic disease. In the last 5 years, oral anticoagulant therapy is now witnessing a revolution after the completion of large phase III clinical trials on the commonly termed the new oral anticoagulants (NOACs) that target key coagulation factors, such as factors Xa and IIa (thrombin). Advantages of these new agents include the use of fixed-dosing with no need for monitoring, few interactions, and a wider therapeutic window. However, the lack of an effective antidote, their cost, and reservations in patients with kidney disease means that careful consideration should be given to patient selection before offering these drugs to patients.

This review discusses the newer oral anticoagulants, their indications, precautions, monitoring and management of bleeds.

NEWER ORAL ANTICOAGULANTS

Mechanism of Action

Thrombin: Thrombin (factor IIa) is the final enzyme of the clotting cascade that produces fibrin; it is formed by the proteolytic cleavage of prothrombin

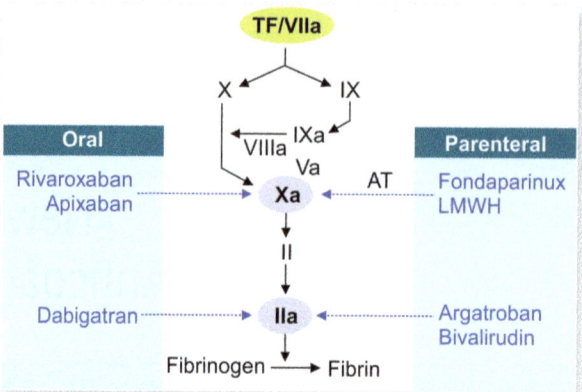

Figure 1: Intrinsic and extrinsic coagulation pathways

(factor II) by factor Xa. Thrombin has a central role in coagulation: it cleaves fibrinogen to fibrin; activates other procoagulant factors including factors V, VIII, XI, and XIII; and activates platelets.[2]

Direct thrombin inhibitors (DTIs) can bind to the active site of the thrombin enzyme (univalent DTIs) or to two sites: the active site and "exosite I," a positively charged region of the thrombin molecule that is physically separated from the active site (divalent DTIs).[3,4] Exosite I is also the site of interaction of many physiologic thrombin substrates, including fibrinogen, factor V, protein C, thrombomodulin (a thrombin receptor on endothelial cells), and thrombin receptors (PAR1 and PAR4) on platelets.[3-7]

Thrombin is active in both circulating and clot-bound forms. Direct thrombin inhibitors are able to block the action of both forms of thrombin because their site of binding to thrombin is not masked by fibrin (or binding is not obstructed). In contrast, heparins are only able to inactivate thrombin in the fluid phase, via antithrombin (previously called antithrombin III).[8-11]

Factor Xa: Factor Xa acts immediately upstream of thrombin in the clotting cascade, at the convergence point of the intrinsic and extrinsic coagulation pathways (Fig. 1), it is formed by the proteolytic cleavage of factor X by one of two X-ase (ten-ase) complexes, which are made up of other procoagulant factors. Inhibition of factor Xa can prevent amplified thrombin generation because one molecule of factor Xa can cleave over 1000 molecules of prothrombin to thrombin.[12] Direct factor Xa inhibitors bind to the active site of factor Xa and inhibit factor Xa activity without a requirement for cofactors.

PHARMACOLOGY

Direct Xa Inhibitors

Several oral agents are available, including *rivaroxaban* (Xarelto), *apixaban* (Eliquis), and *edoxaban* (Lixiana, Savaysa). There are no parenteral direct factor Xa inhibitors in clinical use.[13-16]

Rivaroxaban is a highly selective and competitive reversible inhibitor of both free and clot bound factor Xa (FXa). Being a selective inhibitor of FXa it can terminate the amplified burst of thrombin generation. Rivaroxaban attains peak plasma concentration in 2-4 hours and has a half-life of approximately 9 hours. It has excellent oral bioavailability of 80-100% with two-thirds of the administered dose undergoing metabolic degradation, with half then being eliminated renally and the other half eliminated by the fecal route. Approximately, one-third of the drug is excreted as unchanged active substance in urine.[14]

Rivaroxaban is currently approved by the EMA and FDA for the prevention of stroke and systemic embolism in patients with non-valvular atrial fibrillation at a single oral dose of 20 mg. A prospectively evaluated reduced dose of 15 mg is recommended in patients with a creatinine clearance of <50–30 ml/min. Its use is not recommended in patients with a creatinine clearance of <15 ml/min and in severe hepatic impairment. Rivaroxaban is also approved for the prevention of VTE after elective hip or knee surgery, at the dose of 10 mg OD, starting 6–10 hours after surgery and for 5 weeks for hip and 2 weeks for knee surgery and also acute and long-term therapy of VTE [including deep vein thrombosis (DVT) or pulmonary embolism (PE)], with the initial dose of 15 mg BID for the first 21 days in all the patients, followed by a maintenance dose of 20 mg OD, that can be reduced to 15 mg OD in subjects with renal function impairment in relation to the individual risk of bleeding.[15,16]

Apixaban is a direct, reversible, competitive, and selective inhibitor of factor Xa and the last NOAC approved by the FDA and EMA for the prevention of stroke and embolism in non-valvular AF. It has excellent oral bioavailability and a half-life of approximately eight hours.[17-19]

Current recommended dosing is 5 mg BID daily for patients with normal renal function and 2.5 mg BID for patients with two of the following characteristics: age >80 years, body weight <60 kg, and serum creatinine >1.5 mg/dl. It is primarily metabolised by the liver. Its use is not recommended in those with a creatinine clearance <15 ml/min or in those with severe hepatic impairment.

Similar to rivaroxaban, apixaban is contraindicated in concomitant use with drugs capable of inducing or inhibiting cytochrome P450 enzymes.

Edoxaban is another reversible factor Xa inhibitor. It is rapidly absorbed and reaches peak plasma concentration within 1–2 hours. Up to 50% of edoxaban is eliminated by the kidneys. Since it is a substrate for P-glycoprotein, concomitant administration with quinidine, amiodarone, and verapamil will result in a significant increase of plasma levels of edoxaban.[20-23] Therefore, in patients under concomitant use of potent glycoprotein inhibitors (verapamil or quinidine), body weight <60 kg, or moderate to severe renal impairment (CrCl <50 ml/min), edoxaban dose should be reduced by 50%.

Direct Thrombin (IIa) Inhibitors

Direct thrombin inhibitors (DTIs) prevent thrombin from cleaving fibrinogen to fibrin. They bind to thrombin directly, rather than by enhancing the activity of antithrombin, as is done by heparin.

Dabigatran is an orally absorbed pro-drug with approximately 5% bioavailability. It is converted to the active agent, which has a half-life of approximately eight hours after a single dose and 17 hours after multiple doses. Dabigatran is a direct thrombin inhibitor that is active against both free and clot-bound thrombin. The activity of dabigatran is directed against the conversion of fibrinogen to fibrin, but it also inhibits platelet activation by thrombin and the activation of clotting factors V, VIII, and XI by thrombin. It has an 80% renal excretion.

In contrast to VKAs, dabigatran has no major drug–food interactions and few drug–drug interactions. However, concurrent administration with P-glycoprotein inhibitors or P- glycoprotein inducers is contraindicated. Although concomitant administration of dabigatran and pantoprazole may reduce the anticoagulant effect, dose adjustment is not considered necessary.[24,25]

The usual dose for dabigatran is 150 mg twice daily (BD), which has been approved by the FDA and the EMA. A lower dose of 110 mg BD, only approved by the EMA, is recommended for patients over age 80 or at high risk of bleeding. The FDA, but not the EMA, approved 75 mg BID for patients with creatinine clearance (CrCl) of 15–30 ml/min based on pharmacokinetic models, but that dose has not been studied in the pivotal study of dabigatran.

PREVENTION OF VENOUS THROMBOEMBOLISM IN SURGICAL PATIENTS

Rivaroxaban

Two studies were carried out in patients undergoing total hip replacement.

The first compared rivaroxaban 10 mg orally once daily with enoxaparin 40 mg once daily subcutaneously starting 12 hours preoperatively, both for 35 ± 4 days (RECORD 1)[26] Rivaroxaban showed superiority to enoxaparin for the reduction of total VTE, major VTE (i.e. a composite of proximal DVT, non-fatal PE, or VTE related death), with no difference in major bleeding events.

The second (RECORD 2) compared oral rivaroxaban 10 mg once daily for 35 ± 4 days with enoxaparin 40 mg once daily starting 12 hours preoperatively for 12 ± 2 days.[27] Rivaroxaban showed superiority in the incidence of total VTE, major VTE, and proximal or distal DVT, and notably in the incidence of symptomatic VTE.

Two studies were carried out in patients undergoing total knee replacement.

In the first study, (RECORD 3), rivaroxaban 10 mg orally once daily was compared with enoxaparin 40 mg subcutaneously daily starting 12 hours preoperatively, with either agent continued for 12 ± 2 days.[28] In this study, rivaroxaban was superior to enoxaparin in the reduction of total VTE, major VTE and distal DVT, and significantly reduced the incidence of symptomatic VTE.

In the second study, (RECORD 4), patients undergoing total knee replacement were randomly assigned to receive either rivaroxaban 10 mg daily PO or enoxaparin 30 mg twice daily starting 12 to 24 hours postoperatively, with both given for 12 ± 4 days.[29,30] There was a significant decrease in total

VTE with rivaroxaban, but the difference in the incidence of major VTE and symptomatic VTE did not reach statistical significance.

A pooled analysis of four phase III studies was performed comparing rivaroxaban 10 mg/day with enoxaparin (either 40 mg/day or 30 mg twice per day) for thromboprophylaxis after total hip or knee replacement surgery.[30] The following results were obtained:
- Compared with enoxaparin, thromboprophylaxis with rivaroxaban was associated with significantly fewer symptomatic VTE events and all-cause mortality (odds ratio 0.48; 95% CI 0.30–0.76) during the treatment period.
- The composite of major and non-major clinically relevant bleeding during the treatment period was 2.8% with rivaroxaban versus 2.5% with enoxaparin (odds ratio 1.17; 95% CI 0.93–1.46).
- In all studies with rivaroxaban there was no significant elevation of liver enzymes or increase in thrombotic events during the treatment period.
- Can incorporate XAMOS data as follows:
  Rivaroxaban has also been evaluated for effectiveness and safety in a International, Non-Interventional study compared with standard-of-care after major orthopaedic surgery of the hip or knee. A total of 17,701 patients were enrolled from 252 centres in 37 countries. Patients receiving rivaroxaban had a significantly lower incidence of symptomatic venous thromboembolic events compared with the standard-of-care group (0.65% vs 1.02%). The incidences of treatment-emergent bleeding events in the safety and adjusted safety populations were similar. The results from the XAMOS study show that the data from the RECORD program were reflected in routine clinical practice.[31]

A similar retrospective cohort study from the ORTHO-TEP registry evaluated the relative efficacy and safety of rivaroxaban versus low molecular weight heparin thromboprophylaxis in 5061 unselected consecutive patients undergoing hip and knee replacement surgery. Results included the following:[32]
- Rates of symptomatic VTE were significantly lower for rivaroxaban (2.1 versus 4.1%)
- Rates of major bleeding were significantly lower for rivaroxaban (2.9 versus 7.0%)
- The mean length of hospitalisation was significantly shorter in the rivaroxaban group (8.3 versus 11.1 days).

DABIGATRAN

For the prevention of VTE, dabigatran has been studied in patients undergoing total hip or total knee replacement surgery. Based on a phase II dose-finding study in patients undergoing total hip or knee replacement surgery, a safe and effective daily dosing of dabigatran etexilate was suggested to be in the range between 100 mg and 300 mg/day.[33,34] A meta-analysis of available efficacy and safety data from three trials has concluded that dabigatran, at the recommended dose of 220 mg once daily, was non-inferior to enoxaparin (40 mg/day) for VTE prophylaxis after total knee or total hip arthroplasty, with a similar toxicity profile.[34-37]

In patients undergoing total knee replacement surgery (the REMODEL study) oral dabigatran 150 mg or 220 mg daily was compared with enoxaparin 40 mg daily starting 12 hours preoperatively, with mandatory venography at day 6 to 10 and follow up for 10 to 14 weeks.[34] In the dabigatran 150 mg/day group the first dose was given one to four hours postoperatively at a dose of 75 mg, and thereafter 150 mg once/day, and in the 220 mg/day dabigatran group the initial dose was 110 mg, followed by 220 mg/day.

This trial was designed as a non-inferiority study and achieved non-inferiority compared with enoxaparin for the prevention of total VTE and reduction of all-cause mortality. There was no difference in the incidence of symptomatic VTE. Bleeding rates were low and comparable in both groups, with 89% of major bleeding events being noted at the surgical site.

The RENOVATE trial in patients undergoing total hip replacement surgery compared oral dabigatran 150 mg/day or 220 mg/day starting within one to four hours postoperatively with enoxaparin 40 mg once daily starting 12 hours preoperatively.[35] All treatment continued for 28 to 35 days, at which time venography was done.[35] For the composite endpoint of total VTE and all-cause mortality, both arms of the dabigatran study showed non-inferiority to enoxaparin, with similar bleeding rates and with most major bleeding events being at the surgical site.

The REMOBILIZE trial was carried out in patients undergoing total knee replacement surgery. In this study, dabigatran etexilate 150 mg/day or 220 mg/day starting with a dose of either 75 or 110 mg 6–12 hours postoperatively, respectively in the two groups, was compared with enoxaparin 30 mg twice daily, starting 12-24 hours postoperatively.[37] Venography was performed at day 12-15. Dabigatran failed to meet the predefined criteria for non-inferiority against enoxaparin in terms of the composite endpoint. Rates for major VTE or death were similar and major bleeding events were comparable. As with fondaparinux and rivaroxaban, dabigatran was not as effective against the North American regimen of enoxaparin (i.e. 30 mg twice daily) as it was against the dosing favoured in Europe (i.e. 40 mg once daily).

In all three studies with dabigatran there was no significant elevation of liver enzymes or in thrombotic events following the treatment period.[34-37]

Apixaban

In a double-blind randomised study comparing apixaban to enoxaparin for thromboprophylaxis after knee replacement, apixaban did not meet the prespecified criteria for noninferiority, but its use was associated with lower rates of clinically relevant bleeding and it had a similar adverse event profile to enoxaparin.[38] Other phase II and III trials have shown that apixaban compared favourably to both enoxaparin and warfarin as VTE prophylaxis in total knee replacement surgery.[38-41] and that thromboprophylaxis with apixaban, as compared with enoxaparin, was associated with significantly lower rates of venous thromboembolism without increased bleeding in patients undergoing total hip replacement.[42] Dose reduction is not required if the creatinine clearance is ≥30 ml/min.[43]

A randomised, dose-ranging study compared three different schedules of apixaban (oral daily doses of 5 mg twice daily, 10 mg twice daily, or 20 mg once daily) or LMWH followed by a vitamin K antagonist (VKA), all given for a total of 84–91 days, in 520 patients with symptomatic DVT. Results were as follows:[44]

- The primary efficacy end-point, a composite of symptomatic recurrent VTE and asymptomatic deterioration of bilateral compression ultrasound or perfusion lung scan obtained at the end of treatment, occurred in 4.7 and 4.2% of those treated with apixaban and LMWH/VKA, respectively.
- The primary safety end-point, a composite of major and clinically relevant, non-major bleeding was noted in 7.3 and 7.9% of those treated with apixaban and LMW heparin/VKA, respectively.
- There was no evidence for a dose-response relationship with apixaban for either the efficacy or safety end-points. Routine liver function testing revealed no evidence of liver toxicity.

Edoxaban: Data regarding the use of edoxaban, a factor Xa inhibitor, for the prevention of VTE come from two randomised trials in Japanese patients undergoing total knee replacement or total hip replacement. These trials (STARS E-3 and STARS J-5) compared edoxaban with the low molecular weight heparin enoxaparin.[45] A pooled analysis of the results showed that when compared with enoxaparin, edoxaban was associated with a lower incidence of DVT and PE (5.1 versus 10.7%) and a similar safety profile.[46]

Numerous randomised trials and meta-analyses have compared the efficacy and safety of factor Xa and direct thrombin inhibitors to conventional VTE prophylaxis in patients following total hip and knee replacement.[47-51] The most commonly studied agents are the direct thrombin inhibitor, dabigatran, and the orally active factor Xa inhibitors rivaroxaban, apixaban, and edoxaban. These agents have been compared to LMW heparin (enoxaparin, dalteparin). They have not been compared with warfarin, aspirin, or UFH

While data from randomised trials, systematic reviews and meta-analyses report favourable effects on all outcomes (symptomatic DVT, nonfatal pulmonary embolism and mortality), others report unchanged or improved rates of symptomatic DVT only.[47-51] Similarly, while some analyses report no difference in rates of bleeding others report increased bleeding risk with these agents. Conflicting results may be due to differences among the studies in the agent used, dosing, timing of initiation, duration of prophylaxis. Despite conflicting data, meta-analyses suggest that, on balance, the benefits of direct thrombin inhibitors and factor Xa inhibitors for the prevention of VTE are marginal and may be offset by an increased risk of bleeding:

One 2012 meta-analysis of 22 randomised trials (32,159 patients) compared the factor Xa inhibitors (rivaroxaban, apixaban, edoxaban) with LMW heparin in adults for VTE prevention following hip or knee replacement.[47] The efficacy and safety of the direct thrombin inhibitor was not examined in this analysis. Factor Xa inhibitors were associated with a reduced risk of symptomatic DVT (4 fewer events per 1000) without an effect on nonfatal pulmonary embolism or death. However, high doses of factor Xa inhibitors, but not lower doses, increased the risk of bleeding more than the LMW heparins (2 more bleeding events per 1000). Major limitations of this analysis were that many included studies reported bleeding as a composite outcome and the outcomes were missing in 3 to 41%

of patients. In addition, the enoxaparin dosing in most of the included studies was the lower dose of 40 mg daily, whereas in North America the usual dose of enoxaparin is 30 mg twice-daily. Thus, use of a 40 mg dose as a comparator may favour efficacy while increase bleeding events in this analysis.

Additional systematic reviews and meta-analyses report no difference between LMW heparin and the direct thrombin inhibitor, dabigatran, in the rates of VTE prevention [relative risk (RR) 0.71, 95% CI 0.23–2.12] or bleeding (RR 1.12, 95% CI 0.94–1.35).[48,49] In addition, indirect comparison of the newer orally active agents with each other suggested that rivaroxaban was more efficacious at preventing symptomatic DVT (RR 0.50, 95% CI 0.37–0.68) than dabigatran or apixaban but was associated with excess bleeding risk (RR 1.14; 95% CI 0.80–1.64).[48,49]

Additional trials will be required to establish the optimal agent, dosing, overall relative safety, and efficacy of these new anticoagulants compared to conventional VTE prophylaxis.

Management of Venous Thromboembolism

Rivaroxaban and apixaban are the only direct oral anticoagulants that have been studied and approved by regulatory agencies as monotherapy (i.e. no pre-treatment with heparin is necessary) for the treatment of patients with VTE. They may be preferred in those who wish to avoid the burden of injections in whom convenience or oral medication is a personal preference.

Large randomised trials and one meta-analysis have reported the safety and efficacy of these agents for the treatment and prevention of recurrent VTE [deep vein thrombosis (DVT) and/or pulmonary embolism (PE)].[53-59] Most of these trials were performed in stable patients and were designed as noninferiority trials that compare the newer agent with standard anticoagulation (i.e. heparin followed by warfarin) and showed comparable safety and efficacy.

Rivaroxaban demonstrated similar efficacy to conventional therapy (heparin followed by warfarin) for the treatment of acute VTE in a large, prospective, randomised controlled trial. For most patients receiving rivaroxaban, no parenteral anticoagulation was administered, and rivaroxaban was the initial anticoagulant used. EINSTEIN-DVT and EINSTEIN-PE were open-label randomised trials that enrolled a total of 8281 patients with acute DVT or PE and demonstrated the noninferiority of rivaroxaban (15 mg twice daily for three weeks followed by 20 mg once daily) to conventional therapy (enoxaparin followed by warfarin) for a treatment period of 3, 6, or 12 months. In key subgroups, including fragile patients, cancer patients, patients presenting with large clots, and those with a history of recurrent VTE, the efficacy and safety of rivaroxaban were similar compared with conventional therapy.[53,54]

AMPLIFY was a prospective, randomised, double-blind trial that compared apixaban (10 mg twice daily for seven days for initial anticoagulation followed by 5 mg twice daily for six months) with conventional anticoagulation (subcutaneous enoxaparin for five days followed by warfarin for six months) in 5395 patients for the treatment of acute VTE (DVT and/or PE).[55] There was no difference in the rates of recurrent symptomatic VTE or VTE-related death (2.3 versus 2.7%) between the groups, and fewer bleeding events were reported in the apixaban group (4.3 versus 9.7%). Subgroup analysis suggested that the efficacy of apixaban for the prevention of VTE or VTE-related deaths occurred in all patient groups (e.g. DVT, PE, unprovoked VTE, extensive PE).

Edoxaban has been shown to have a similar efficacy and superior safety profile when compared with warfarin for the treatment of acute VTE. In one trial, 4921 patients with acute VTE (DVT and/or PE) were randomised to receive 3 to 12 months of edoxaban or warfarin following initial therapy for five days with unfractionated or LMW heparin.[56] Edoxaban was administered orally at 60 mg once daily. A lower dose (30 mg once daily) was used for patients with a CrCl of 30 to 50 ml per minute or low body weight ≤60 kg. Compared with warfarin, edoxaban had a similar rate of recurrent symptomatic VTE or VTE-related death (3.2 versus 3.5%) and fewer bleeding events (8.5 versus 10.3%).

Of potential clinical interest was the superior efficacy in the prespecified subgroup of patients with PE that had right ventricular (RV) dysfunction as assessed by elevated brain natriuretic peptide (BNP) or increased RV dimensions on computed tomography (CT). However BNP is a nonspecific biomarker of RV dysfunction, and echocardiography is a more accurate test than CT for the assessment of RV dysfunction. Further study of this agent in this population of patients with severe PE and RV dysfunction by echocardiogram is warranted to validate these findings.

A large, randomised controlled trial suggested that dabigatran has similar efficacy to warfarin for the prevention of recurrent VTE. However, concerns have been raised about its efficacy and risk of thrombosis given the broad inferiority margin set in one of the trials (RE-COVER), and its safety and risk of bleeding events given the irreversibility of this drug. In a randomised, double-blind trial (RE-COVER I), 2539 patients with acute VTE were treated for six months with either dabigatran (150 mg by mouth twice per day) or warfarin, each after seven days of initial parenteral anticoagulation.[57] Compared with warfarin, dabigatran had a similar incidence of recurrent VTE (2.4 versus 2.1%), VTE-related deaths (0.1 versus 0.2%), major bleeding events (1.6 versus 1.9 %), and any bleeding event (16.1 versus 21.9%). These results suggest that the efficacy and safety profile of dabigatran is similar to that of warfarin for the treatment of acute VTE. Similar results were reported in an identically designed trial of 2589 patients with acute DVT (RECOVER II).[58]

ATRIAL FIBRILLATION

Dabigatran

The RE-LY (Randomised Evaluation of Long-term anticoagulant therapy with dabigatran etexilate) phase III trial was a prospective, randomised, open-label, phase III trial comparing two blinded doses of dabigatran etexilate (110 or 150 mg BID) with warfarin in 18,113 patients with AF and at least one additional risk factor (a mean CHADS score of 2.1).[2] Patients with severely impaired renal function (CrCl <30 ml/min), active liver disease, stroke within 14 days, or at a high risk of bleeding were excluded.

For the primary efficacy endpoint of stroke and systemic embolism, dabigatran 150 mg BID was superior to warfarin with no significant differences in major bleedings. Gastrointestinal (GI) bleeding was more frequent with dabigatran 150 mg BD. Dabigatran 110 mg BD was non-inferior to warfarin for the primary endpoint, with a reduction of 20% in major bleedings. In thewarfarin group, international normalised ratio (INR) was within the the rapeutic range 64% of the study period beyond the first week. A post hoc analysis of 1989 electrical cardioversions in 1270 patients did not show significant differences in the rate of stroke within 30 days after the procedure between warfarin and dabigatran 110 or 150. About 25% of the patients underwent a transoesophageal study before cardioversion. There was no significant difference in the incidence rate of left atrial thrombus (1.1% for warfarin, 1.2% for dabigatran 150 mg BD, and 1.8% for 110 mg BD).

The subsequent Long-term Multicenter Extension of Dabigatran Treatment in Patients with Atrial Fibrillation (RELY-ABLE) study provided additional information on the long-term effects of the two doses of dabigatran in patients completing RE-LY by extending the follow-up of patients on dabigatran from a mean of 2 years at the end of RE-LY by an additional 2.3 years.[60] No patients on warfarin were enrolled in this study. RELY-ABLE confirmed the results reported in RE-LY. Moreover, there were no significant differences in stroke or mortality between dabigatran 110 and 150 mg BD, but a higher rate of major bleeding was observed with the higher dose of dabigatran.

Recently, the safety profile of dabigatran (150 and 75 mg BD) in real US clinical practice has been reported in an elderly Medicare cohort with non-valvular AF.[61] Compared with warfarin, dabigatran was associated with a reduced risk of ischaemic stroke, intracranial haemorrhage and mortality, but with an increased risk of major GI bleeding. These results were stronger in the subgroup treated with dabigatran 150 mg BD. Around 16% of patients received dabigatran 75 mg BD and among these, none of the study outcomes were statistically significantly different from warfarin except for a lower risk of intracranial haemorrhage with dabigatran. Unfortunately, known severe renal impairment was only present in up to 7% of the subgroup of dabigatran 75 mg BD and results must be interpreted carefully.

RIVAROXABAN

The ROCKET AF was a double-blinded study in which 14,264 patients with non-valvular AF were randomly assigned to rivaroxaban 20 mg once daily or dose adjusted warfarin; patients with CrCl of 30–49 ml/min received 15 mg of rivaroxaban. ROCKET AF enrolled patients with AF and multiple co-morbidities at moderate to high risk of stroke (mean CHADS = 3.5). The patients had substantial rates of coexisting illnesses, 60% had heart failure, 40% had diabetes; 55 % of the patients had had a previous stroke, systemic embolism, or transient ischemic attack. Those with CrCl of <30 ml/min, significant liver disease, any stroke within 14 days (or severe strokes within 3 months), high risk of bleeding were excluded from the study. After a median follow-up of 1.93 years, rivaroxaban was noninferior to warfarin for the prevention of stroke or systemic embolism (hazard ratio in the rivaroxaban group, 0.79; 95% confidence interval (CI), 0.66 to 0.96; P<0.001 for noninferiority). The rates of major and non-major clinically relevant bleeding were similar in the rivaroxaban and warfarin groups with more frequent GI bleeding in the rivaroxaban arm. However, there was significant reduction in critical organ, intracranial and fatal bleeding in the rivaroxaban arm as compared to warfarin.[16]

The safety and effectiveness of rivaroxaban has also been evaluated in unselected NVAF patients from everyday practice. XANTUS is the first international, prospective, observational study for any NOAC to describe effectiveness across a broad NVAF patient population. There were 6784 patients treated with rivaroxaban at 311 centres in Europe, Israel, and Canada. The mean patient age was 71.5 years with a mean CHADS2 score of 2.0. The mean treatment duration was 329 days. In total, 6522 (96.1%) patients did not experience any of the outcomes of treatment-emergent all-cause death, major bleeding or stroke/SE. In XANTUS, rivaroxaban demonstrated low rates of stroke/SE(0.7 events per 100 patient-years vs 1.7 events per 100 patient years in ROCKET AF), major bleeding (2.1 events per 100 patient-years vs 3.6 events per 100 patient years) and GI bleeding (0.9 events per 100 patient-years) than that seen in ROCKET AF (2.0 events per 100 patient-years). The incidence rates of fatal bleeding, critical organ bleeding, and intracranial haemorrhage were similar to those observed in ROCKET AF.[62]

APIXABAN

The Apixaban for Reduction In STroke and Other ThromboemboLic Events in AF (ARISTOTLE) was a randomised, double-blinded, double-dummy, phase III trial comparing apixaban (5 mg BID) with dose-adjusted warfarin in 18,201 patients with non-valvular AF (a mean CHADS2 score of 2.1).[4] Apixaban 2.5 mg BID was used among patients with two or more of the following conditions: >80 years of age, weight, 60 kg, or a serum creatinine level >1.5 mg/dl. After a mean follow-up of 1.8 years, apixaban was significantly better than warfarin, with fewer primary outcomes (overall strokes—both ischaemic and haemorrhagic—and systemic emboli), but with no significant differences in rates of ischaemic strokes. Patients treated with apixaban had significantly lesser intracranial bleeds, but GI bleedings were similar between both groups. All-cause mortality was found to be significantly lower in the apixaban group.

Apixaban was also compared with aspirin alone in the AVERROES study, a double-blinded study of 5599 patients who were not suitable candidates for VKA treatment (mean CHADS2 score of 2).[63] After a mean follow-up of 1.1 years, the study was prematurely stopped due to a clear benefit in favour of apixaban. The primary outcome of stroke or systemic embolism was significantly lower in the apixaban group versus aspirin, whereas bleeding risk (major bleeding and intracranial bleeding) between two groups was similar. Patients with severe renal impairment (serum creatinine >2.5 mg/dl or CrCl <25 ml/min) were excluded from the ARISTOTLE and AVERROES trials.[4,30] Additional exclusion criteria were stroke within the previous 7 days, and concomitant treatment with aspirin at a dose of >165 mg a day or for both aspirin and clopidogrel.

Edoxaban

The Effective Anticoagulation with Factor Xa Next Generation in Atrial Fibrillation–Thrombolysis in Myocardial Infarction 48 (ENGAGE AF-TIMI 48) was a three-group, randomised, double blinded, double-dummy phase III trial, which compared the two dose regimens of edoxaban (30 and 60 mg once daily) with warfarin 35 in a total of 21,026 patients with non-valvular AF. For patients in either group of edoxaban, the dose was halved in any of the following characteristics: CrCl of 30–50 mL/min, body weight of 60 kg or less, or concomitant use of verapamil or quinidine. After a follow-up of 2.8 years, both regimens of edoxaban were non-inferior to warfarin with respect to the prevention of stroke or systemic embolism; however, the lower dose trended toward inferiority, with a hazard ratio of 1.13 vs. Warfarin, and was inferior to specifically prevent ischaemic stroke. Edoxaban was associated with lower, dose-related rates of bleeding, including major bleeding, intracranial bleeding, and life-threatening bleeding. An exception was GI bleeding, which occurred more frequently with high-dose edoxaban but less frequently with low-dose edoxaban compared with warfarin. Finally, the incidence rate of haemorrhagic stroke and the rate of death from cardiovascular causes were significantly lower with both edoxaban regimens. Patients with severe renal dysfunction (CrCl <30 ml/min), high risk of bleeding, use of dual antiplatelet, acute coronary syndromes or coronary revascularisation, and strokes within 30 days were excluded.

PRACTICAL MANAGEMENT

Monitoring

A clinical advantage of NOACs is their predictable anticoagulant effect enabling the administration of fixed doses without the need of routine monitoring. However, the lack of a reliable method or a clear marker of anticoagulant activity makes ensuring compliance very difficult. In addition, estimation of anticoagulation level might be useful in particular scenarios such as during acute bleeding, or stroke or when patients need an urgent surgery.

Although quantitative tests for NOAC assessment exist, such as DTIs and FXa inhibitors, they are not commonly available in most hospitals. Nevertheless, other more common tests may assess qualitatively NOAC activity. When interpreting these results, it is essential to take into account when the last dose of NOAC was administered since its maximum effect will be reached at its maximal plasma concentration. Furthermore, the estimated elimination half-life will depend on patient characteristics, and particularly important, on renal function, especially for those NOAC with a high renal clearance.

For dabigatran, diluted thrombin time (dTT), activated partial thromboplastin time (aPTT), and ecarin clotting time (ECT) can be useful; an aPTT level (i.e. 12–24 hours after ingestion) of ≥2 the upper limit of normal or ECT ≥3 times elevated may be associated with a higher risk of bleeding.[64,65] A dTT with appropriate calibrators for dabigatran is also available (Hemoclot) and that with the Hemoclot >200 ng/ml after 12 hours of the last dose is associated with a higher risk of bleeding as well. Each factor Xa inhibitor (rivaroxaban, apixaban, and edoxaban) affects the PT and aPTT to a different extent, and any of these tests is ideal to assess anticoagulant effect. Activated partial thromboplastin time has a weak prolongation under theseNOACs and suffers of variability of assays, and paradoxical response at low concentrations. On the other side, PT is prolonged in a concentration-dependent manner for factor Xa inhibitors; however, its effect depend on the assay and on the particular factor Xa inhibitor. It could be useful for rivaroxaban, although sensitivity depends very much on the PT reagents. In particular, Neoplastin Plus has a close correlation to plasma concentrations of rivaroxaban. There are currently no much data available for edoxaban and apixaban. Finally, plasma concentrations of factor Xa inhibitors can be estimated by the commercially available Anti-FXa 'chromogenic assays' with good inter laboratory precision. Unfortunately, practical data to associate a coagulation parameter or level with bleeding risk are not yet available.

ELECTIVE SURGERY

Standard Bleeding Risk Procedure

Standard bleeding risk procedures include colonoscopy, uncomplicated laparoscopic procedures, and any aspirations not involving the spinal canal.

In patients with normal CrCl (>50 ml/min per 1.73 m^2), dabigatran use should be stopped at least 48 hours before the procedure. Rivaroxaban and apixaban use should be stopped at least 24 hours before the procedure.

In patients with impaired CrCl (<50 ml/min per 1.73 m^2), dabigatran therapy should be stopped at least 72 hours before the procedure if CrCl is 30 to <50 ml/min per 1.73 m^2 and at least 4 days earlier if CrCl is <30 ml/min per 1.73 m^2. Rivaroxaban and apixaban administration should be stopped at least 48 hours before the procedure.

High Bleeding Risk Procedures

High bleeding risk procedures include major cardiac surgery, insertion of pacemakers or defibrillators, neurosurgery, major cancer/urologic/vascular surgery, spinal puncture, etc.

In patients with normal CrCl (50 ml/min per 1.73 m^2), dabigatran, rivaroxaban, and apixaban administration should be stopped at least 48 hours before the procedure.

In patients with impaired CrCl (<50 ml/min per 1.73 m^2), dabigatran use should be stopped at least 4 days before the procedure if CrCl is 30 to <50 ml/min per 1.73 m^2 and at least 6 days earlier if CrCl is <30 ml/min per 1.73 m^2. Rivaroxaban and apixaban administration should be stopped at least 2 days before the procedure.[65]

Emergency Surgery

Ideally, surgical intervention should be delayed for the estimated time that the drugs are cleared. If available, assays may provide information on the presence or absence of residual drug. However, if urgent surgery is needed within a few hours after the last dose, clinicians should anticipate bleeding complications.

Reinitiation of NOACs After the Procedure

This process depends on the nature of the surgery, the urgency for restarting thromboprophylaxis therapy, and the haemostatic state of the patient.[65] Given the rapid clearance of the NOACs from the circulation and the rapid onset of action when reintroduced, no bridging therapy with LMWH or unfractionated heparin is necessary. For procedures in which good hemostasis is achieved, anticoagulation may be resumed the same evening, at least 4 to 6 hours after surgery with a reduced dose (dabigatran, 75 mg; rivaroxaban, 10 mg; or apixaban, 2.5 mg) for the first dose and, thereafter, the usual maintenance dose.[65] For major abdominal surgery or urologic surgery with incomplete haemostasis, resumption should be delayed until there is adequate haemostasis.[65]

COMPLEX CLINICAL SCENARIOS

Acute Stroke Requiring Thrombolytics

The safety of administration of thrombolytics in patients receiving concurrent NOAs is not established and poses a very high risk of bleeding. Anecdotal reports have documented the successful use of thrombolytics in patients taking dabigatran who were at least 7 hours past their last dose.[66,67] Similar anecdotal reports have also been documented for rivaroxaban however there is an urgent need for further studies on the safety of thrombolysis in stroke patients taking NOACs.[68]

Cardioversion

For patients with AF of more than 48 hours' duration, therapeutic anticoagulation for at least 3 weeks before and 4 weeks after cardioversion is recommended.[65] In the RE-LY trial, the stroke and systemic embolism rates within 30 days of this procedure were 0.8% and 0.3% for the dabigatran, 150 and 110 mg doses, respectively, vs 0.6% with the warfarin; major bleeding rates were similar between the groups.[66] Hence, patients may continue taking dabigatran for cardioversion. The ROCKET-AF (rivaroxaban) and ARISTOTLE (apixaban) also suggest that that electrical cardioversion in patients treated with NOACs has a similar (and very low) thrombo-embolic risk as under warfarin. Also additional evidence from the X-VERT trial which is the first prospective randomized trial of a novel oral anticoagulant in patients with atrial fibrillation undergoing elective cardioversion has confirmed the low peri-cardioversion stroke risk in patients treated with rivaroxaban (0.51%) compared with warfarin (1.02%).[70]

Mechanical Heart Valves

Currently, the use of NOACs in patients with mechanical heart valves cannot be recommended owing to the lack of clinical evidence. A phase 2 study (the

RE-ALIGN trial) investigated the use of dabigatran in patients with mechanical heart valves;[71] however, it was terminated early owing to excess thrombotic complications in the dabigatran group. This has led the FDA and EMA to consider mechanical heart valves as a contraindication for dabigatran therapy.[72]

Heparin-Induced Thrombocytopaenia (HIT)

Parenteral direct thrombin inhibitors have been used as an alternative anticoagulant in patients with HIT. However regarding oral agents, Krauel et al. demonstrated that neither dabigatran nor rivaroxaban had any effect on the interaction of PF4 or anti-PF4/heparin antibodies with platelets, thus making them potential options for anticoagulation in patients with HIT and possibly even for the treatment of HIT-induced thrombosis.[73] However, there are neither randomised controlled trials nor anecdotal case reports describing the off-label use of NOACs in the treatment of HIT-induced thrombosis; hence, its use cannot be recommended until more evidence is available.

Cancer-associated VTE

The LMWH is superior to VKAs in treating cancer-associated VTE,[74] but studies evaluating NOACs for acute VTE were compared only with VKAs. Nevertheless, the RE-COVER study[75] found that dabigatran use was noninferior to VKA use (3.1% vs 5.3%) in preventing recurrent symptomatic VTE/death in patients with cancer (9.5% of the study population). In the EINSTEIN DVT and PE studies,[76,77] patients with cancer (12% and <5%, respectively, of the study population) were included in the analysis. Compared with long term VKA, rivaroxaban showed similar efficacy in prevention recurrent venous thromboembolism [(HR) 0·67, 95% CI 0·35 to 1·30] with less risk of bleeding (HR 0·80, 95% CI 0·54 to 1·20) in patients with a variety of active cancers.[78] Given the small number of patients with cancer in these studies, future trials testing the efficacy and safety of NOAs in patients with cancer are needed before they can be recommended.[79]

MANAGEMENT OF BLEEDING COMPLICATIONS/OVERDOSE

Lack of specific agents that reverse the anticoagulant effect complicates the management of NOAC-associated bleeding events or the periprocedural reversal of anticoagulation. Management of minor bleeding, e.g. epistaxis, consists of addressing the potential anatomical defects, e.g. cauterisation or nasal packing. The decision to hold the next dose of drug will hinge on the comorbidities and assessment of risks of drug discontinuation. Given the relatively short half-lives of the NOACs in patients with normal renal function, most of the anticoagulant effects should dissipate within 48 hours.[79] Administration of oral activated charcoal retards absorption of recently ingested drug, e.g. within a couple hours of presentation.[79,80] Given that only 35% of dabigatran is bound to plasma proteins, hemodialysis typically removes 60% of dabigatran and should be considered, especially in patients with impaired renal function. However, given the extensive volume of distribution

(50-70 L) of dabigatran, a "rebound" increase in dabigatran plasma levels may occur after haemodialysis. Although there are no data, dialysis is unlikely to be effective for rivaroxaban and apixaban as they are more than 85-90% protein bound.

Recombinant Factor VIIa

This agent has been used in clinical practice to help reverse life-threatening bleeds caused by NOACs. It decreases the bleeding time in animal models but does not reverse the anticoagulation effect on most other laboratory coagulation tests.[81,82] Other than anecdotal case reports, there are no randomised controlled studies confirming its benefit in these situations. One must keep in mind the potential serious adverse effects of recombinant factor VIIa, including disseminated intravascular coagulation and systemic thrombosis.

Prothrombin Complex Concentrates

There are 2 types of PCCs available. 3-factor prothrombin complex concentrates (PCCs) [Bebulin (Baxter), and Profilnine SD (Grifols)] are available with relatively similar concentrations of nonactivated factors II, IX, and X but low concentrations of non activated factor VII.[83,84] Then there is an "activated" 4-factor PCC (FEIBA NF, Baxter) that contains relatively similar concentrations of nonactivated factors II, IX, and X and activated factor VII. The use of either PCC may increase the risk of thrombosis, there are norandomised controlled studies confirming its benefit in these situations. One must keep in mind the potential serious adverse effects of recombinant factor VIIa, including disseminated intravascular coagulation and systemic thrombosis.

REVERSAL AGENTS

Idarucizumab (Praxbind)[85,86]

Based on studies in healthy volunteers as well as results from an interim analysis of the RE-VERSE AD™ trial.[2,3,7,8] the reversal effects of Praxbind® were evident immediately, within minutes after administration of 5 g of Praxbind®.[2,3,7,8] No procoagulant effect was observed after the administration of Praxbind.

REFERENCES

1. Kirchhof P, Ammentorp B, Darius H, et al. Management of atrial fibrillation in seven European countries after the publication of the 2010 ESC guidelines on atrial fibrillation. Primary results of the PREFER in AF Registry. Europace. 2014; 16: 6-14. DOI:10.1093/europace/eut263
2. Rydel TJ, Ravichandran KG, Tulinsky A, Bode W, Huber R, Roitsch C, et al. The structure of a complex of recombinant hirudin and human a-thrombin. Science. 1990;249(4966):277-80.

3. Di Nisio M, Middeldorp S, Büller HR. Direct thrombin inhibitors. New England Journal of Medicine. 2005;353(10):1028-40.
4. Grütter MG, Priestle JP, Rahuel J, Grossenbacher H, Bode W, Hofsteenge J, et al. Crystal structure of the thrombin-hirudin complex: a novel mode of serine protease inhibition. The EMBO journal. 1990;9(8):2361.
5. Hirsh J, Weitz JI. New antithrombotic agents. The Lancet. 1999;353(9162):1431-6.
6. Hall SW, Nagashima M, Zhao L, Morser J, Leung LL. Thrombin interacts with thrombomodulin, protein C, and thrombin-activatable fibrinolysis inhibitor via specific and distinct domains. Journal of Biological Chemistry. 1999;274(36):25510-6.
7. Sheehan JP, Sadler JE. Molecular mapping of the heparin-binding exosite of thrombin. Proceedings of the National Academy of Sciences. 1994;91(12):5518-22.
8. Weitz JI, Hudoba M, Massel D, Maraganore J, Hirsh J. Clot-bound thrombin is protected from inhibition by heparin-antithrombin III but is susceptible to inactivation by antithrombin III-independent inhibitors. Journal of Clinical Investigation. 1990;86(2):385.
9. Turpie AG. New oral anticoagulants in atrial fibrillation. European heart journal. 2007.
10. Berry CN, Girardot C, Lecoffre C, Lunven C. Effects of the synthetic thrombin inhibitor argatroban on fibrin-or clot-incorporated thrombin: comparison with heparin and recombinant Hirudin. Thrombosis and haemostasis. 1994;72(3):381-6.
11. Lefkovits J, Topol EJ. Direct thrombin inhibitors in cardiovascular medicine. Circulation. 1994;90(3):1522-36.
12. Laux V, Perzborn E, Heitmeier S, von Degenfeld G, Dittrich-Wengenroth E, Buchmuller A. Inhibitors of coagulation proteins-the end of the heparin and low-molecular-weight heparin era for anticoagulant therapy. Thromb Haemost. 2009;102(5):892-9.
13. Ansell J, Crowther M, Burnett A, Garcia D, Kaatz S, Lopes RD, et al. Comment on: Editorial by Husted et al."Non-vitamin K antagonist oral anticoagulants (NOACs): No longer new or novel". Thrombosis and Haemostasis. 2014;112(4):841.
14. Palareti G, Ageno W, Ferrari A, Filippi A, Imberti D, Pengo V, et al. Clinical management of rivaroxaban-treated patients. Expert Opin Pharmacother. 2013;14(5):655-67.
15. Summary of Product Characteristics;EMA. Available from: http://www.ema.europa.eu/ema/index.jsp?curl=pages/medicines/human/medicines/000944/human_med_001155.jsp&mid=WC0b01ac058001d124.
16. Patel MR, Mahaffey KW, Garg J, et al. Rivaroxaban versus warfarin in nonvalvular atrial fibrillation. N Engl J Med. 2011;365:883-91.
17. Luettgen JM, Bozarth TA, Bozarth JM, Barbera FA, Lam PY, Quan ML, et al. In Vitro evaluation of apixaban, a novel, potent, selective and orally bioavailable factor Xa inhibitor. Blood. 2006;108(11):4130.
18. Pinto DJ, Orwat MJ, Koch S, Rossi KA, Alexander RS, Smallwood A, et al. Discovery of 1-(4-methoxyphenyl)-7-oxo-6-(4-(2-oxopiperidin-1-yl) phenyl)-4, 5, 6, 7-tetrahydro-1 H-pyrazolo [3, 4-c] pyridine-3-carboxamide (Apixaban, BMS-562247), a highly potent, selective, efficacious, and orally bioavailable inhibitor of blood coagulation factor Xa. Journal of Medicinal Chemistry. 2007;50(22): 5339-56.
19. He K, He B, Grace JE, Xin B, Zhang D, Pinto DJ, et al. Preclinical pharmacokinetic and metabolism of apixaban, a potent and selective factor Xa inhibitor. Blood. 2006;108(11):910.

20. Ogata K, Mendell-Harary J, Tachibana M, Masumoto H, Oguma T, Kojima M, et al. Clinical safety, tolerability, pharmacokinetics, and pharmacodynamics of the novel factor Xa inhibitor edoxaban in healthy volunteers. The Journal of Clinical Pharmacology. 2010;50(7):743-53.
21. Matsushima N, Lee F, Sato T, Weiss D, Mendell J. Bioavailability and safety of the factor Xa inhibitor edoxaban and the effects of quinidine in healthy subjects. Clinical pharmacology in Drug Development. 2013;2(4):358-66.
22. Matsushima N, Lee F, Sato T, Weiss D, Mendell J. Absolute bioavailability of edoxaban in healthy subjects. AAPS J. 2011;13(Suppl 2):T2362.
23. Salazar DE, Mendell J, Kastrissios H, Green M, Carrothers TJ, Song S, et al. Modelling and simulation of edoxaban exposure and response relationships in patients with atrial fibrillation. Thrombosis and Haemostasis. 2012;107(5):925-34.
24. Stangier J. Clinical pharmacokinetics and pharmacodynamics of the oral direct thrombin inhibitor dabigatran etexilate. Clinical Pharmacokinetics. 2008;47(5):285-95.
25. Stangier J, Stähle H, Rathgen K, Fuhr R. Pharmacokinetics and pharmacodynamics of the direct oral thrombin inhibitor dabigatran in healthy elderly subjects. Clinical Pharmacokinetics. 2008;47(1):47-59.
26. Kim SM, Moon YW, Lim SJ, Kim DW, Park YS. Effect of oral factor Xa inhibitor and low-molecular-weight heparin on surgical complications following total hip arthroplasty. Thrombosis and Haemostasis. 2016;115(3):600-7.
27. Eriksson BI, Borris LC, Friedman RJ, Haas S, Huisman MV, Kakkar AK, et al. Rivaroxaban versus enoxaparin for thromboprophylaxis after hip arthroplasty. New England Journal of Medicine. 2008;358(26):2765-75.
28. Kakkar AK, Brenner B, Dahl OE, Eriksson BI, Mouret P, Muntz J, et al, RECORD2 Investigators. Extended duration rivaroxaban versus short-term enoxaparin for the prevention of venous thromboembolism after total hip arthroplasty: a double-blind, randomised controlled trial. The Lancet. 2008;372(9632):31-9.
29. Lassen MR, Ageno W, Borris LC, Lieberman JR, Rosencher N, Bandel TJ, et al. Rivaroxaban versus enoxaparin for thromboprophylaxis after total knee arthroplasty. New England Journal of Medicine. 2008;358(26):2776-86.
30. Turpie AG, Lassen MR, Davidson BL, Bauer KA, Gent M, Kwong LM, et al. Rivaroxaban versus enoxaparin for thromboprophylaxis after total knee arthroplasty (RECORD4): a randomised trial. The Lancet. 2009;373(9676):1673-80.
31. Turpie AGG, Haas S, Kreutz R, Mantovani LG, Pattanayak CW, Holberg G, et al. A non-interventional comparison of rivaroxaban with standard of care for thromboprophylaxis after major orthopaedic surgery in 17,701 patients with propensity score adjustment. Thromb Haemost. 2013.
32. Beyer-Westendorf J, Lützner J, Donath L, Radke OC, Kuhlisch E, Hartmann A, et al. Efficacy and safety of rivaroxaban or fondaparinux thromboprophylaxis in major Newer Oral Anticoagulants orthopedic surgery: findings from the ORTHO-TEP registry. Journal of Thrombosis and Haemostasis. 2012;10(10):2045-52.
33. Eriksson BI, Dahl OE, Ahnfelt L, Kälebo P, Stangier J, Nehmiz G, et al. Dose escalating safety study of a new oral direct thrombin inhibitor, dabigatran etexilate, in patients undergoing total hip replacement: BISTRO I. Journal of Thrombosis and Haemostasis. 2004;2(9):1573-80.
34. Eriksson BI, Dahl OE, Rosencher N, Kurth AA, van Dijk CN, Frostick SP, et al. Oral dabigatran etexilate vs. subcutaneous enoxaparin for the prevention of venous

thromboembolism after total knee replacement: the RE-MODEL randomized trial. Journal of Thrombosis and Haemostasis. 2007;5(11):2178-85.
35. Eriksson BI, Dahl OE, Rosencher N, Kurth AA, van Dijk CN, Frostick SP, et al. Dabigatran etexilate versus enoxaparin for prevention of venous thromboembolism after total hip replacement: a randomised, double-blind, non-inferiority trial. The Lancet. 2007;370(9591):949-56.
36. Wolowacz SE, Roskell NS, Plumb JM, Caprini JA, Eriksson BI. Efficacy and safety of dabigatran etexilate for the prevention of venous thromboembolism following total hip or knee arthroplasty-A meta-analysis. Thrombosis and Haemostasis. 2009;101(1):77-85.
37. Ginsberg JS, Davidson BL, Comp PC, Francis CW, Friedman RJ, Huo MH, et al. RE-MOBILIZE Writing Committee: Oral thrombin inhibitor dabigatran etexilate vs North American enoxaparin regimen for prevention of venous thromboembolism after knee arthroplasty surgery. J Arthroplasty. 2009;24(1):1-9.
38. Lassen MR, Raskob GE, Gallus A, Pineo G, Chen D, Portman RJ. Apixaban or enoxaparin for thromboprophylaxis after knee replacement. New England Journal of Medicine. 2009;361(6):594-604.
39. Garcia D, Libby E, Crowther MA. The new oral anticoagulants. Blood. 2010; 115(1):15-20.
40. Lassen MR, Davidson BL, Gallus A, Pineo G, Ansell J, Deitchman D. The efficacy and safety of apixaban, an oral, direct factor Xa inhibitor, as thromboprophylaxis in patients following total knee replacement1. Journal of Thrombosis and Haemostasis. 2007;5(12):2368-75.
41. Lassen MR, Raskob GE, Gallus A, Pineo G, Chen D, Hornick P. Apixaban versus enoxaparin for thromboprophylaxis after knee replacement (ADVANCE-2): a randomised double-blind trial. The Lancet. 2010;375(9717):807-15.
42. Lassen MR, Gallus A, Raskob GE, Pineo G, Chen D, Ramirez LM. Apixaban versus enoxaparin for thromboprophylaxis after hip replacement. New England Journal of Medicine. 2010;363(26):2487-98.
43. Poulsen BK, Grove EL, Husted SE. New oral anticoagulants. Drugs. 2012;72(13):1739-53.
44. Buller H, Deitchman D, Prins M, Segers A. Efficacy and safety of the oral direct factor Xa inhibitor apixaban for symptomatic deep vein thrombosis. The Botticelli DVT dose-ranging study. Journal of Thrombosis and Haemostasis. 2008;6(8):1313-8.
45. Fuji T, Wang CJ, Fujita S, Kawai Y, Nakamura M, Kimura T, Ibusuki K, Ushida H, Abe K, Tachibana S1. Safety and efficacy of edoxaban, an oral factor Xa inhibitor, versus enoxaparin for thromboprophylaxis after total knee arthroplasty: the STARS E-3 trial. Thromb Res. 2014 Dec;134(6):1198-204
46. Fuji T, Fujita S, Tachibana S, Kawai Y, Koretsune Y, Yamashita T, Nakamura M. Efficacy and safety of edoxaban versus enoxaparin for the prevention of venous thromboembolism following total hip arthroplasty STARS J V trial. Blood [52nd Annu Meet Am Soc Hematol (Dec 4-7, Orlando). 2010] 2010, 116(21): Abst 3320.
47. Sobieraj DM, Coleman CI, Tongbram V, Lee S, Colby J, Chen WT, et al. Venous thromboembolism prophylaxis in orthopedic surgery (Internet). Rockville (MD): Agency for Healthcare Research and Quality (US);2012 Mar. Report No. 12-EHC02O-EF.
48. Gómez-Outes A, Terleira-Fernández AI, Suárez-Gea ML, Vargas-Castrillón E. Dabigatran, rivaroxaban, or apixaban versus enoxaparin for thromboprophylaxis

after total hip or knee replacement: systematic review, meta-analysis, and indirect treatment comparisons. BMJ. 2012.
49. Loke YK, Kwok CS. Dabigatran and rivaroxaban for prevention of venous thromboembolism–systematic review and adjusted indirect comparison. Journal of Clinical Pharmacy and Therapeutics. 2011;36(1):111-24.
50. Adam SS, McDuffie JR, Lachiewicz PF, Ortel TL, Williams JW. Comparative effectiveness of new oral anticoagulants and standard thromboprophylaxis in patients having total hip or knee replacement: a systematic review. Annals of Internal Medicine. 2013;159(4):275-84.
51. Hull RD, Liang J, Bergqvist D, Yusen RD. Benefit-to-harm ratio of thromboprophylaxis for patients undergoing major orthopaedic surgery. Thrombosis and haemostasis. 2014;111(2):199-212.
52. www.discoverymedicine.com/Ingo-Ahrens/2012/06/23/developmenta-andclinical-applications-of-novel-oral-anticoagulants-part-i-clinically-approved-drugs/
53. Einstein Investigators. Oral rivaroxaban for symptomatic venous thromboembolism. N Engl J Med. 2010;2010(363):2499-510.
54. Einstein-PE Investigators. Oral rivaroxaban for the treatment of symptomatic pulmonary embolism. N Engl J Med. 2012;2012(366):1287-97.
55. Agnelli G, Buller HR, Cohen A, Curto M, Gallus AS, Johnson M, et al. Oral apixaban for the treatment of acute venous thromboembolism. N Engl J Med. 2013;2013(369):799-808.
56. Hokusai-VTE Investigators. Edoxaban versus warfarin for the treatment of symptomatic venous thromboembolism. N Engl J Med. 2013;2013(369):1406-15.
57. Schulman S, Kearon C, Kakkar AK, Mismetti P, Schellong S, Eriksson H, et al. Dabigatran versus warfarin in the treatment of acute venous thromboembolism. New England Journal of Medicine. 2009;361(24):2342-52.
58. Schulman S, Kakkar AK, Goldhaber SZ, Schellong S, Eriksson H, Mismetti P, et al. Treatment of acute venous thromboembolism with dabigatran or warfarin and pooled analysis. Circulation. 2013:CIRCULATIONAHA-113.
59. Robertson L, Kesteven P, McCaslin JE. Oral direct thrombin inhibitors or oral factor Xa inhibitors for the treatment of deep vein thrombosis. The Cochrane Library. 2015.
60. Connolly SJ, Wallentin L, Ezekowitz MD, Eikelboom JW, Oldgren J, Reilly PA, et al. The long-term multi-center observational study of dabigatran treatment in patients with atrial fibrillation:(RELY-ABLE) study. Circulation. 2013:CIRCULATIONAHA-113.
61. Graham DJ, Reichman ME, Wernecke M, Zhang R, Southworth MR, Levenson M, et al. Cardiovascular, bleeding, and mortality risks in elderly Medicare patients Newer Oral Anticoagulants treated with dabigatran or warfarin for non-valvular atrial fibrillation. Circulation. 2014:CIRCULATIONAHA-114.
62. Camm AJ, Amarenco P, Haas S, Hess S, Kirchhof, Kuhls S, Eickels MV et al. XANTUS: a real-world, prospective, observational study of patients treated with rivaroxaban for stroke prevention in atrial fibrillation. Eur Heart J. 2016;37(14):1145-53.
63. Connolly SJ, Eikelboom J, Joyner C, Diener HC, Hart R, Golitsyn S, et al. Apixaban in patients with atrial fibrillation. New England Journal of Medicine. 2011;364(9):806-17.
64. Van Ryn J, Stangier J, Haertter S, Liesenfeld KH, Wienen W, Feuring M, et al. Dabigatran etexilate-a novel, reversible, oral direct thrombin inhibitor:

interpretation of coagulation assays and reversal of anticoagulant activity. Thrombosis and Haemostasis. 2010;103(6):1116.
65. Heidbuchel H, Verhamme P, Alings M, Antz M, Hacke W, Oldgren J, et al. European Heart Rhythm Association Practical Guide on the use of new oral anticoagulants in patients with non-valvular atrial fibrillation. Europace. 2013;15(5):625-51.
66. De Smedt A, De Raedt S, Nieboer K, De Keyser J, Brouns R. Intravenous thrombolysis with recombinant tissue plasminogen activator in a stroke patient treated with dabigatran. Cerebrovascular diseases. 2010;30(5):533-4.
67. Matute MC, Guillán M, Garcia-Caldentey J, Buisan J, Aparicio M, Masjuan J, et al. Thrombolysis treatment for acute ischaemic stroke in a patient on treatment with dabigatran. Thrombosis and haemostasis. 2011;106(1):178-9.
68. Fluri F, Heinen F, Kleinschnitz C. Intravenous Thrombolysis in a Stroke Patient Receiving Rivaroxaban. Cerebrovasc Dis Extra. 2013 Jan-Dec; 3(1): 153–155. Nagarakanti R, Ezekowitz MD, Oldgren J, Yang S, Chernick M, Aikens TH, et al.
69. Dabigatran versus warfarin in patients with atrial fibrillation an analysis of patients undergoing cardioversion. Circulation. 2011;123(2):131-6.
70. Cappato R, Ezekowitz MD, Klein AL, Camm AJ, Ma CS, Le Heuzey JY. Rivaroxaban vs. vitamin K antagonists for cardioversion in atrial fibrillation. Eur Heart J. 2014;35(47):3346-55.
71. Dabigatran etexilate in patients with mechanical heart valves. http://www.clinicaltrials.gov/ct2/show/NCT01452347?term1/4NCT01452347&rank1/4. Last accessed on 2/25/2013.
72. US Food and Drug Administration. FDA Drug Safety Communication: Pradaxa (dabigatran etexilate mesylate) should not be used in patients with mechanical prosthetic heart valves. US Department of Health and Human Services. www.fda.gov/ Drugs/ DrugSafety/ ucm332912. htm. Accessed. 2013;10.
73. Krauel K, Hackbarth C, Fürll B, Greinacher A. Heparin-induced thrombocytopenia: in vitro studies on the interaction of dabigatran, rivaroxaban, and low-sulfated heparin, with platelet factor 4 and anti-PF4/heparin antibodies. Blood. 2012;119(5):1248-55.
74. Kearon C, Akl EA, Comerota AJ, Prandoni P, Bounameaux H, Goldhaber SZ, et al. Antithrombotic therapy for VTE disease: antithrombotic therapy and prevention of thrombosis: American College of Chest Physicians evidence-based clinical practice guidelines. Chest Journal. 2012;141(2 suppl):e419S-94S.
75. Schulman S, Kearon C, Kakkar AK, Mismetti P, Schellong S, Eriksson H, et al. Dabigatran versus warfarin in the treatment of acute venous thromboembolism. New England Journal of Medicine. 2009;361(24):2342-52.
76. Bauersachs R, Berkowitz SD, Brenner B, Buller HR, Decousus H, Gallus AS, et al. Oral rivaroxaban for symptomatic venous thromboembolism. New England Journal of Medicine. 2010;363(26):2499-510.
77. Büller HR, Prins MH, Lensin AW, Decousus H, Jacobson BF, Minar E, et al. Oral rivaroxaban for the treatment of symptomatic pulmonary embolism. The New England Journal of Medicine. 2012;366(14):1287-97.
78. Siegal DM, Garcia D. Anticoagulants in cancer. Journal of Thrombosis and Haemostasis. 2012;10(11):2230-41.
79. Kaatz S, Kouides PA, Garcia DA, Spyropolous AC, Crowther M, Douketis JD, et al. Guidance on the emergent reversal of oral thrombin and factor Xa inhibitors. American Journal of Hematology. 2012;87(S1):S141-5.

80. Van Ryn J, Sieger P, Kink-Eiband M, Gansser D, Clemens A. Adsorption of Dabigatran Etexilate in Water or Dabigatran in Pooled Human Plasma by Activated Charcoal in Vitro. Blood. 2009;114(22):1065.
81. Van Ryn J, Ruehl D, Priepke H, Hauel N, Wienen W. Reversibility of the anticoagulant effect of high doses of the direct thrombin inhibitor dabigatran, by recombinant factor VIIa or activated prothrombin complex concentrate. In Haematologica-The Hematology Journal 2008;(Vol. 93, pp. 148-148). Via Giuseppe Belli 4, 27100 Pavia, Italy: Ferrata Storti Foundation.
82. Tinel H, Huetter J, Perzborn E. Recombinant factor VIIa partially reverses the anticoagulant effect of high-dose rivaroxaban: a novel, oral factor Xa inhibitor in rats. J Thromb Haemost. 2007;5(suppl 2):W652.
83. Dentali F, Marchesi C, Pierfranceschi MG, Crowther M, Garcia D, Hylek E, et al. Safety of prothrombin complex concentrates for rapid anticoagulation reversal of vitamin K antagonists. Thromb Haemost. 2011;106(3):429-38.
84. Eerenberg ES, Kamphuisen PW, Sijpkens MK, Meijers JC, Buller HR, Levi M. Reversal of rivaroxaban and dabigatran by prothrombin complex concentrate a randomized, placebo-controlled, crossover study in healthy subjects. Circulation. 2011;124(14):1573-9.
85. Pollack Jr CV, Reilly PA, Eikelboom J, Glund S, Verhamme P, Bernstein RA, et.al. Idarucizumab for dabigatran reversal. New England Journal of Medicine. 2015;373(6):511-20.
86. Pollack CV, Reilly PA, Bernstein R, Dubiel R, Eikelboom J, Glund S, et al. Design and rationale for RE-VERSE AD: A phase 3 study of idarucizumab, a specific reversal agent for dabigatran. Thromb Haemost. 2015;114(1):198-205.

CHAPTER

3

Statins in Peripheral Vascular Disease

Siddharth Rajput

INTRODUCTION—LIPIDS, FATTY STREAKS, SIMPLE AND COMPLEX PLAQUES

Over the last 50 years or so, the relationship between dyslipidaemia and atherosclerosis has been an area of active research as the prevalence of atherosclerosis and associated cardiovascular complications increases in the developed and the developing world alike. Atherosclerosis is the sequelae of chronic arterial inflammation secondary to prolonged exposure to oxidative stressors and involves multiple cell types and cellular mediators. Circulating blood is in constant contact with endothelial cells (ECs) that separate circulating platelets, monocytes, and coagulation factors from the highly thrombogenic internal elastic lamina and basement membrane. Vascular ECs also separate vascular smooth muscle cells (VSMCs) in the media from circulating growth factors. Production of reactive oxygen species, such as those secondary to cigarette smoking or exposure to glycation end products, for example, damage the ECs, resulting in decreased nitric oxide (NO) production and activation of both platelets and circulating monocytes. The expression of inflammatory mediators induces monocyte adhesion and migration to the area of injury where oxidized low-density lipid particles (oxLDLs) are engulfed, changing the morphology of each macrophage to a lipid-filled foam cell. Vascular smooth muscle cells are also affected and change from a contractile to a proliferative and secretory phenotype. In areas of vessel injury, VSMCs migrate from the media across the internal elastic lamina to the intima, where they proliferate and deposit a collagen-rich extracellular matrix forming a vascular lesion, known as a fatty streak. The cycle of inflammatory factor release and the subsequent cellular response results in the development of an "atherosclerotic plaque".[1] This fibroatheroma contains a complex network of proliferating VSMCs, extracellular matrix proteins, and macrophages. Larger lesions contain a milieu of cells, matrix metalloproteinases, and inflammatory factors as well as alter luminal haemodynamics. A plaque may remain stable for many years, however, as the atheroma grows, the size of the lesion may preclude perfusion by the vasa vasorum, compromising the delivery of nutrients to the plaque. The increased demand for oxygen and nutrients in the plaque leads to a relatively hypoxic environment, resulting in VSMC death, thinning the protective fibrous cap, and increasing the likelihood of rupture. Dyslipidaemia has long been recognized as an independent risk factor for atherosclerosis-related coronary artery and peripheral vascular disease and is the target for numerous interventions to attenuate the associated large disease burden. High levels of low-density lipoproteins (LDLs) and by products of oxidation reactions with LDL (i.e. oxLDL) injure ECs and promote monocyte adhesion, VSMC migration, and platelet activation—events that initiate the development of atherosclerotic plaque. In contrast, high levels of high-density lipoproteins (HDLs) have been independently shown to be atheroprotective, by providing an opposing effect to LDL. While LDL and HDL remain the 2 most studied lipoproteins with regard to atherosclerotic disease, very low-density lipoproteins (VLDLs) and triglycerides have also gained attention as potential targets for therapy in the cholesterol metabolism pathways.

STATINS: 3-HYDROXY-3-METHYLGLUTARYL-COENZYME A REDUCTASE INHIBITORS

The 3-hydroxy-3-methylglutaryl-coenzyme A (HMG-CoA) reductase inhibitors, more commonly known as statins, are the single most effective cholesterol reducing medications available today. Statins competitively inhibit HMG-CoA reductase, the key enzyme of cholesterol synthesis in the liver. Statins decrease levels of LDL production as well as remove existing LDL from circulation by increasing serum LDL uptake by the liver. Statins also increase uptake of very low-density lipoproteins (VLDLs) as well as decrease total cholesterol and triglycerides by the liver. Statins were first discovered in 1971 by Japanese biochemist Akira Endo when he isolated the agent mevastatin from the fungus *Penicillium citrinum*.[2] However, the first clinical application of a statin was by Merck & Co (Kenilworth, New Jersey) who isolated lovastatin from the *Aspergillus terreus* in 1976 and marketed the first commercially available statin in 1987 as Mevacor.[3] Since then, several other both synthetic and naturally occurring statins were created and/or isolated by competing pharmaceutical companies for therapeutic use. Statins have also been combined with other agents, including niacin and ezetimibe to create combination therapy in efforts to further decrease cholesterol levels in the circulation. Today, the Joint Task Force on Practice Guidelines[4] for the treatment of blood cholesterol to reduce atherosclerotic cardiovascular disease (ASCVD) risk in adults from the American College of Cardiology (ACC) and the American Heart Association (AHA) support the use of statins for the prevention of ASCVD in many higher risk primary and all secondary prevention individuals without heart failure. Moreover, their review of the literature shows that statin therapy reduces ASCVD events in individuals with LDL levels as low as 70 mg/dl, suggesting that statins are beneficial irrespective of initial LDL levels. To date, there has been no specific validated LDL target in the peripheral arterial disease (PAD) population. Furthermore, ethical issues preclude conducting prospective randomized placebo controlled trials of statins in patients with PAD. Despite these challenges, the Society of Vascular Surgery (SVS) recently published guidelines[5] for management of asymptomatic PAD, claudication, and cerebrovascular disease (CBD). They derive their recommendations from the ACC/AHA guidelines, which recommend that statins should be considered in all individuals with an estimated 10- year risk of major cardiovascular events >7.5%. Therefore, the SVS recommends their use in both symptomatic and asymptomatic noncoronary ASCVD. As a whole, most vascular surgeons and vascular medicine clinicians agree statin therapy is an essential component in the management of patients with atherosclerotic disease. The use of statins to modify lipid profiles in patients with noncoronary ASVCD is summarised subsequently.

Statins and Aortic Aneurysms

Atherosclerosis of the aorta results in subsequent aneurysmal degeneration and also has a pathophysiological role in dissections as well as other aortic degenerative disease. In a retrospective review of over 600 patients with thoracic aortic aneurysms, performed by the Yale group using multivariate analysis (after adjusting for age, gender, chronic obstructive pulmonary disease, cardiovascular disease, family history, aneurysm location, and aneurysm size), patients on statins had a decreased rate of rupture, dissection, repair, or death (mean follow-up of 3.5 years).[6] A subsequent study by the same group on a larger cohort of patients further supported the protective effects of statins on long-term outcomes for patients with thoracic aortic aneurysms; however, patients with aneurysms of the aortic root were still at risk, despite treatment with a statin.[7] Several other observational studies document nearly a 50% reduction in growth rates of abdominal aortic aneurysms in patients on statin therapy.[8-10] These studies also noted reduced mortality in outcomes of patients undergoing surgical intervention for their abdominal aneurysms, even when ruptured.[10,11] In summary, statins are associated with a slower progression of aortic atherosclerotic disease and aneurysm expansion; however, it should be noted that these studies are retrospective with a relatively smaller sample size.

Statins and PAD

Approximately 8-12 million people in the United States have PAD, ranging from claudication to critical limb ischemia (CLI).[12] PAD is also recognized as a sensitive marker for coronary artery disease (CAD), cerebrovascular disease (CBD), and cardiovascular mortality.[4] Patients with PAD have a relative risk of cardiovascular mortality ranging from 1.4 to 5.9 compared to patients without PAD.[13-15] These numbers stress the importance of identifying best medical therapies that modify the systemic effects of PAD. The benefit of statin therapy to attenuate or stabilise aortic atherosclerosis was known even in the 1990s.[16,17] More recently, 3 small clinical trials have evaluated the effects of statins and other pharmaceuticals on aortic atherosclerosis monitoring progression of disease with novel noninvasive imaging techniques.[18-20] In Japan, 108 patients with hypercholesterolaemia were randomized to atorvastatin, etidronate (a bisphosphonate used in treatment of osteoporosis), or both drugs daily.[20] Using magnetic resonance imaging (MRI), they found that atorvastatin monotherapy significantly reduced the amount of thoracic aortic plaque, while etidronate monotherapy reduced only abdominal aortic plaque.[20] Combination therapy of atorvastatin plus etidronate for 12 months significantly reduced both thoracic and abdominal aortic plaques.[20] A second US study found a dose-related relationship between statin therapy and reduction in atherosclerotic inflammation, as a rapid dose-dependent reduction in radiotracer uptake on positron emission tomography in the aorta occurred in patients on high-dose atorvastatin compared to lower doses.[19] The same dose-dependent effect was noted in patients taking rosuvastatin.[18]

The Heart Protection Study (HPS) from 2002 was the first large multicentre randomised controlled trial (RCT) of a statin (simvastatin 40 mg daily vs placebo) that included a large enough number of patients with PAD (6748 patients) to draw conclusions on the effects of statins in this population.[21] HPS found that patients with PAD allocated to simvastatin had a 22% relative reduction in the rate of first major vascular events (coronary events, strokes, or revascularisation) and that all (20,536) patients of the study had a 16% relative reduction. Furthermore, this effect was seen across all subgroups included in the study, irrespective of their pretreatment LDL cholesterol levels. Post-hoc analysis of the 1990s Scandinavian Simvastatin Survival Study (4S), performed on 4444 patients with CAD also showed that effective cholesterol lowering slows the progression of atherosclerosis in the periphery and results in less signs and symptoms of PAD.[22] Patients treated with statins had significantly lower relative risks of intermittent claudication, carotid bruit, femoral bruit, and angina pectoris than the placebo group. Newer prospective observational studies, such as the REduction of Atherothrombosis for Continued Health (REACH) Registry,[23] report the same findings. A total of 5861 patients with PAD were included in the registry, and only 62% of these patients were on a statin. The REACH Registry observed a significantly greater incidence of worsening claudication, new revascularization procedures (open or endovascular), and amputations in the nonstatin-treated group. They concluded that patients with PAD on statins have ~18% lower long-term risk of adverse limb outcomes when compared to those not on statin therapy.[23] These and many other studies support the use of statins in patients with PAD for primary and secondary prevention of ASCVD and adverse limb outcomes.[24-27]

In the early 2000s, 3 small prospective placebo-controlled randomized clinical trials were performed in patients with claudication to evaluate the effect of simvastatin[28,29] and atorvastatin[30] on exercise performance. At 3- to 6-month follow-up, patients in the statin therapy group were noted to have longer pain-free walking distance, increased total walking distance, and significantly improved ankle–brachial indexes (ABIs) both at rest and after exercise.[28-30] However, more recently, another small observational study shows that although ABIs improved in the statin treatment group, there was no difference in muscle perfusion, metabolism, nor exercise parameters over time in these patients.[31]

Further evidence is emerging regarding the effects of statins on patients undergoing infrainguinal bypass surgery for treatment of CLI. This group of patients is located on the opposite end of the spectrum of PAD, with severe atherosclerosis causing ischaemic rest pain, tissue loss, and limb loss. The studies showed that statin therapy was independently associated with fewer combined ASCVD complications, shorter hospital length of stay, improved long-term survival at 5.5 years,[32] increased graft patency and limb salvage rates.[33,34] Almost 10 years later, 2 more retrospective studies were published on the effects of statin therapy in patients with CLI undergoing infrainguinal bypass surgery and endovascular intervention.[35,36] Both studies found improved rates of survival in patients treated with statins. In the endovascular therapy observational cohort study, statins were associated with improved target lesion patency rates as well as decreased rates of stroke and MI.[35,36]

In summary, the scarce literature supporting the use of statin therapy in patients with claudication and CLI implies a strong association with increased primary prevention of ASCVD events, secondary prevention of adverse lower extremity events, and overall reduced mortality; however, these studies do not show that statins have any significant effect on the patency of infrainguinal bypasses.

Statins and Cerebrovascular Disease

About 87% of all strokes in the United States are ischaemic-type infarcts.[37] A major preventable cause of ischaemic stroke is atherosclerotic occlusive disease of the extracranial carotid artery. Initial studies only recruited patients with elevated LDL profiles, while later studies were all inclusive regarding the initial LDL levels, and measured early carotid atherosclerosis by B-mode ultrasonography of mean maximum intimal-medial thickness (IMT) of carotid artery walls.[38-43] The agents tested included lovastatin, pravastatin, atorvastatin, and simvastatin. All 6 studies showed significant reductions in IMT in patients with hypercholesterolaemia and asymptomatic early carotid atherosclerosis. Once established that statins had beneficial effect on patients with all types of ASCVD, not just coronary heart disease, further studies emerged assessing the impact of statins on stroke incidence. The first of these studies to include stroke as a prescribed end point was the Cholesterol and Recurrent Events (CARE) trial. The CARE investigators found a 32% reduction in all-cause strokes and a 27% reduction in stroke or TIA in patients with a recent MI (within the past 10 months of study enrolment) when treated with pravastatin.[44] Pravastatin was studied in 2 other international multicentre trials. The first of these was a secondary prevention trial of pravastatin known as LIPID (Long-term Intervention with Pravastatin in Ischemic Disease) that included over 9000 patients.[45] The other was a primary prevention trial in >6500 males with hypercholesterolemia known as WOSCOPS (West of Scotland Prevention Coronary Prevention Study).[46] Pooled data from the CARE, LIPID, and WOSCOPS trials showed that pravastatin reduced the risk of stroke over a wide range of lipid values, including those with LDL <100 mg/dl prior to treatment initiation among patients with documented coronary disease.[47] Larger scale prospective data demonstrating that cholesterol lowering statin therapy reduces the risk of stroke was elicited from the landmark HPS.[21] Results of the HPS trial were similar to the CARE trial with a

25% overall stroke reduction, including fatal stroke. Interestingly, this study also showed a 50% reduction in intervention with carotid endarterectomy or carotid artery stenting.

Once the safety and efficacy of statins in secondary prevention were established, clinical trials began to focus on primary prevention of major cardiovascular events in patients at risk of stroke without previous coronary events. The WOSCOPS mentioned previously, was the first of the primary prevention studies to show a trend toward reduction in incidence of all strokes in 1995. By the end of the 2000s, over 10 RCTs including Anglo-Scandinavian Cardiac Outcomes Trial (ASCOT) in 2004; all concluded that statins reduce the 5-year incidence of major coronary events, coronary revascularisation, and stroke by 20% per 18 mg/dl reduction in LDL cholesterol.[48,49] Of note, this finding holds true irrespective of initial LDL levels. Furthermore, the dose of statin has also been studied by The Treating to New Targets (TNT) study where it was found that higher dose statin therapy reduced both stroke and all cerebrovascular events by an additional 20–25% compared to the lower dose.[50]

In 2006, the Stroke Prevention by Aggressive Reduction in Cholesterol Levels (SPARCL) investigators studied the effectiveness of high-dose atorvastatin in prevention of fatal or nonfatal stroke in patients who had suffered either a stroke or TIA within 6 months of study enrolment. This secondary prevention study found that statins reduced the overall incidence of strokes as well as all cardiovascular events in patients with previous stroke.[51] However, these effects were marginal, with only a 5-year absolute risk reduction of 2.2%[51] and contrasted with results of the HPS study, which found no reduction in the risk of stroke among patients with prior CBD.[21] Analysis of the studies would later show that patients in the HPS study with a prior stroke or TIA were enrolled at a time point greater than 4 years after their stroke, despite the fact that most recurrent strokes usually occur within the first year after the index event. These findings imply that initiation of statin therapy in the immediate post-stroke period may be effective secondary prevention of another stroke but that statins have little to no effect when initiated later.

Finally, the JUPITER (Justification for the Use of Statins in Prevention: an Intervention Trial Evaluating Rosuvastatin) trial looked at patients on rosuvastatin with normal LDL levels but known elevated C-reactive protein levels and also found a 51% reduction in ischaemic strokes (P ¼ .004), again suggesting that statins are protective against stroke, despite a normal LDL profile.[52] An important adverse event associated with the statin treatment group in the SPARCL trial was the increased incidence of haemorrhagic stroke.[51] This effect was also noted in the HPS study. In 2011, a meta-analysis and systematic review of 23 randomised trials and 19 observational studies of statins and stroke comprising a total of 248,391 patients and 14,784 intracerebral haemorrhages was published. The authors found no evidence that statins were actually associated with intracerebral haemorrhage.[53]

In summary, statin therapy is effective for the primary and secondary prevention of stroke and TIAs in patients with and without coronary manifestations of ASCVD, without increased risk of haemorrhagic stroke.

Statins and Atherosclerotic Renovascular and Chronic Kidney Disease

Atherosclerotic renovascular hypertension is a form of secondary hypertension due to renal artery stenosis and the introduction of statins and angiotensin receptor blocking agents (ARBs) has converted this pathology into a slowly progressive disease.[54] Small retrospective studies on the effects of statins in patients with atherosclerotic renal artery disease have been published with little to no long-term follow-up data.[54,55] One study showed an improvement in overall mortality as well as a slower rate of progression of renal insufficiency.[56] Three large-scale RCTs, the Stent Placement and Blood Pressure and Lipid-Lowering for the Prevention of Progression of Renal Dysfunction Caused by Atherosclerotic Ostial Stenosis of the Renal Artery (STAR), the Angioplasty and Stenting for Renal Artery Stenosis (ASTRAL), and the Cardiovascular Outcomes in Renal Atherosclerotic Lesions (CORAL), performed in the 2000s all compared endovascular surgical intervention to best medical therapy for atherosclerotic renal artery disease.[57-59] An angiotensin receptor blocker (ARB), a statin, and an antiplatelet agent comprised thee medical regimen. All 3 studies showed no evidence of clinical benefit from revascularisation in patients with renovascular disease compared to best medical therapy alone.[57-59] Since then, statins have been studied in select subgroups of patients with renovascular disease. In Canada, in a cohort study on elderly patients with renovascular disease, statins were associated with improved overall prognosis.[60] Despite having a larger burden of both cardiovascular and renal comorbidity, the group of patients treated with a statin had a significantly lower incidence of MI, stroke, heart failure, acute renal failure, dialysis, and death compared to those not on statin therapy.[41] These beneficial effects were not similarly observed in patients with chronic kidney disease (CKD), although CKD is considered to be an independent risk factor for recurrent cardiovascular events, and patients with end-stage renal disease (ESRD) have the highest incidence of ASCVD.[37,61,62] The Kidney Disease Outcomes Quality Initiative (KDOQI) has established guidelines for the management of dyslipidaemia in patients with CKD because of this population's increased risk of both symptomatic and asymptomatic ASCVD. Since then, 2 randomised placebo-controlled trials have been published evaluating the safety and efficacy of statins in patients with ESRD. The first of these trials, the Deutsche Diabetes Dialyse Studie (4D), was performed in Germany solely on diabetic patients with ESRD. Despite the cholesterol-lowering effects of atorvastatin, no difference occurred in the incidence of the individual or combined end point of cardiac death, nonfatal MI, or stroke.[63] Surprisingly, they found a 2-fold increase in the incidence of fatal stroke in the treatment group. The second trial performed in the United States, a Study to Evaluate the Use of Rosuvastatin in Subjects On Regular Hemodialysis: an Assessment of Survival and Cardiovascular Events (AURORA), was conducted on varied patients with ESRD on haemodialysis.[64] With almost 4 years of follow-up, no difference was found between rosuvastatin-treated groups and controls with respect to nonfatal MI, nonfatal stroke, or death from cardiovascular sources. The negative outcomes of the 4D and AURORA trials left many questions unanswered, specifically about the effectiveness and safety of statins in patients with early-stage CKD. In 2011, the Study of Heart and Renal Protection (SHARP) looked exclusively at patients with CKD, including patients with ESRD and treated them with a statin in combination with ezetimibe.[65] The end point was a composite of nonfatal MI, cardiac death, stroke, and any revascularization procedure. The SHARP trial found a 17% reduction in the composite end point for those in the treatment arm.[65] When subgroup analysis was performed on the different stages of CKD, the ESRD group showed no difference in the rate of primary outcome further proving that targeting a reduction in mortality with statins in this group of patients may be futile.[65] In summary, statin therapy is beneficial and should be prescribed for primary and secondary prevention of cardiovascular events in the CKD population; however, patients with ESRD may not share the same benefits of therapy.

REFERENCES

1. Helkin A, Patel S, Gahtan V. Atherosclerosis. In: Valentine RJ EJ (ed). Scientific American vascular and endovascular surgery. Hamilton, ON: Decker Intellectual Properties; June 2015. DOI: 10.2310/7900.3003. Available at: http://www.sciamvascsurg.com
2. Endo A. The discovery and development of HMG-CoA reductase inhibitors. J Lipid Res. 1992; 33(11):1569-82.
3. Alberts AW. Lovastatin and simvastatin—inhibitors of HMG CoA reductase and cholesterol biosynthesis. Cardiology. 1990; 77(suppl 4):14-21.
4. Stone NJ, Robinson JG, Lichtenstein AH, et al. 2013 ACC/AHA guideline on the treatment of blood cholesterol to reduce atherosclerotic cardiovascular risk in adults: a report of the American College of Cardiology/American Heart Association Task Force on Practice Guidelines. Circulation. 2014;129(25 suppl 2): S1-S45.
5. O'Donnell TF Jr, Passman MA. Clinical practice guidelines of the Society for Vascular Surgery (SVS) and the American Venous Forum (AVF)—Management of venous leg ulcers. Introduction. J Vasc Surg. 2014;60(2 suppl):1S-2S.
6. Jovin IS, Duggal M, Ebisu K, et al. Comparison of the effect on long-term outcomes in patients with thoracic aortic aneurysms of taking versus not taking a statin drug. Am J Cardiol. 2012; 109(7):1050-4.
7. Stein LH, Berger J, Tranquilli M, Elefteraides JA. Effect of statin drugs on thoracic aortic aneurysms. Am J Cardiol. 2013; 112(8):1240-5.
8. Periard D, Guessous I, Mazzolai L, Haesler E, Monney P, Hayoz D. Reduction of small infrarenal abdominal aortic aneurysm expansion rate by statins. VASA. 2012;41(1):35-42.
9. Schouten O, van Laanen JH, Boersma E, et al. Statins are associated with a reduced infrarenal abdominal aortic aneurysm growth. Eur J Vasc Endovasc Surg. 2006;32(1):21-26.
10. Sukhija R, Aronow WS, Sandhu R, Kakar P, Babu S. Mortality and size of abdominal aortic aneurysm at long-term follow-up of patients not treated surgically and treated with and without statins. Am J Cardiol. 2006;97(2):279-80.
11. Feeney JM, Burns K, Staff I, et al. Prehospital HMG Co-A reductase inhibitor use and reduced mortality in ruptured abdominal aortic aneurysm. J Am Coll Surg. 2009;209(1): 41-6.

12. Hirsch AT, Hartman L, Town RJ, Virnig BA. National health care costs of peripheral arterial disease in the Medicare population. Vasc Med. 2008;13(3):209-15.
13. Criqui MH, Langer RD, Fronek A, et al. Mortality over a period of 10 years in patients with peripheral arterial disease. N Engl J Med. 1992;326(6):381-6.
14. Criqui MH, Ninomiya JK, Wingard DL, Ji M, Fronek A. Progression of peripheral arterial disease predicts cardiovascular disease morbidity and mortality. J Am Coll Cardiol. 2008; 52(21):1736-42.
15. Parikh SV, Saya S, Divanji P, et al. Risk of death and myocardial infarction in patients with peripheral arterial disease undergoing percutaneous coronary intervention (from the National Heart, Lung and Blood Institute Dynamic Registry). Am J Cardiol. 2011;107(7):959-64.
16. Tomochika Y, Okuda F, Tanaka N, et al. Improvement of atherosclerosis and stiffness of the thoracic descending aorta with cholesterol-lowering therapies in familial hypercholesterolemia. Arterioscler Thromb Vasc Biol. 1996;16(8): 955-62.
17. Pitsavos CE, Aggeli KI, Barbetseas JD, et al. Effects of pravastatin on thoracic aortic atherosclerosis in patients with heterozygous familial hypercholesterolemia. Am J Cardiol. 1998; 82(12):1484-8.
18. Yogo M, Sasaki M, Ayaori M, et al. Intensive lipid lowering therapy with titrated rosuvastatin yields greater atherosclerotic aortic plaque regression: serial magnetic resonance imaging observations from RAPID study. Atherosclerosis. 2014;232(1): 31-9.
19. Tawakol A, Fayad ZA, Mogg R, et al. Intensification of statin therapy results in a rapid reduction in atherosclerotic inflammation: results of a multicenter fluorodeoxyglucose-positron emission tomography/computed tomography feasibility study. J Am Coll Cardiol. 2013;62(10):909-17.
20. Kawahara T, Suzuki G, et al. Atorvastatin, etidronate, or both in patients at high risk for atherosclerotic aortic plaques: a randomized, controlled trial. Circulation. 2013;127(23):2327-35.
21. Heart Protection Study Collaborative G. MRC/BHF Heart Protection Study of cholesterol lowering with simvastatin in 20,536 high-risk individuals: a randomised placebo-controlled trial. Lancet. 2002;360(9326):7-22.
22. Randomised trial of cholesterol lowering in 4444 patients with coronary heart disease: the Scandinavian Simvastatin Survival Study (4 S). Lancet. 1994;344(8934):1383-9.
23. Ohman EM, Bhatt DL, Steg PG, et al. The REduction of Atherothrombosis for Continued Health (REACH) Registry: an international, prospective, observational investigation in subjects at risk for atherothrombotic events-study design. Am Heart J. 2006;151(4):786. e1-e10.
24. Armstrong EJ, Chen DC, Westin GG, et al. Adherence to guideline-recommended therapy is associated with decreased major adverse cardiovascular events and major adverse limb events among patients with peripheral arterial disease. J Am Heart Assoc. 2014;3(2):e000697.
25. Feringa HH, Karagiannis SE, van Waning VH, et al. The effect of intensified lipid-lowering therapy on long-term prognosis in patients with peripheral arterial disease. J Vasc Surg. 2007; 45(5):936-43.
26. Feringa HH, van Waning VH, Bax JJ, et al. Cardioprotective medication is associated with improved survival in patients with peripheral arterial disease. J Am Coll Cardiol. 2006;47(6): 1182-7.

27. Schillinger M, Exner M, Mlekusch W, et al. Statin therapy improves cardiovascular outcome of patients with peripheral artery disease. Eur Heart J. 2004;25(9):742-8.
28. Aronow WS, Nayak D, Woodworth S, Ahn C. Effect of simvastatin versus placebo on treadmill exercise time until the onset of intermittent claudication in older patients with peripheral arterial disease at six months and at one year after treatment. Am J Cardiol. 2003;92(6):711-2.
29. Mondillo S, Ballo P, Barbati R, et al. Effects of simvastatin on walking performance and symptoms of intermittent claudication in hypercholesterolemic patients with peripheral vascular disease. Am J Med. 2003;114(5):359-64.
30. Mohler ER III, Hiatt WR, Creager MA. Cholesterol reduction with atorvastatin improves walking distance in patients with peripheral arterial disease. Circulation. 2003;108(12):1481-6.
31. McDermott MM, Guralnik JM, Greenland P, et al. Statin use and leg functioning in patients with and without lower-extremity peripheral arterial disease. Circulation. 2003;107(5):757-61.
32. Ward RP, Leeper NJ, Kirkpatrick JN, Lang RM, Sorrentino MJ, Williams KA. The effect of preoperative statin therapy on cardiovascular outcomes in patients undergoing infrainguinal vascular surgery. Int J Cardiol. 2005;104(3):264-8.
33. Abbruzzese TA, Havens J, Belkin M, et al. Statin therapy is associated with improved patency of autogenous infrainguinal bypass grafts. J Vasc Surg. 2004;39(6):1178-85.
34. Henke PK, Blackburn S, Proctor MC, et al. Patients undergoing infrainguinal bypass to treat atherosclerotic vascular disease are underprescribed cardioprotective medications: effect on graft patency, limb salvage, and mortality. J Vasc Surg. 2004;39(2): 357-65.
35. Suckow BD, Kraiss LW, Schanzer A, et al. Statin therapy after infrainguinal bypass surgery for critical limb ischemia is associated with improved 5-year survival. J Vasc Surg. 2015;61(1):126-33.
36. Westin GG, Armstrong EJ[2], Bang H[3], et al. Association between statin medications and mortality, major adverse cardiovascular event, and amputation-free survival in patients with critical limb ischemia. J Am Coll Cardiol. 2014;63(7):682-90.
37. Mozaffarian D, Benjamin EJ, Go AS, et al. Heart disease and stroke statistics–2015 update: a report from the American Heart Association. Circulation. 2015;131(4):e29-e322.
38. Byington RP, Furberg CD, Crouse JR III, Espeland MA, Bond MG. Pravastatin, Lipids, and Atherosclerosis in the Carotid Arteries (PLAC-II). Am J Cardiol. 1995;76(9):54C-9C.
39. Furberg CD, Adams HP Jr, Applegate WB, et al. Effect of lovastatin on early carotid atherosclerosis and cardiovascular events. Asymptomatic Carotid Artery Progression Study (ACAPS) Research Group. Circulation. 1994;90(4):1679-87.
40. Hodis HN, Mack WJ, LaBree L, et al. Reduction in carotid arterial wall thickness using lovastatin and dietary therapy: a randomized controlled clinical trial. Ann Intern Med. 1996;124(6):548-56.
41. Kroon AA, van Asten WN, Stalenhoef AF. Effect of apheresis of low-density lipoprotein on peripheral vascular disease in hypercholesterolemic patients with coronary artery disease. Ann Intern Med. 1996;125(12):945-54.
42. MacMahon S, Sharpe N, Gamble G, et al. Effects of lowering average of below-average cholesterol levels on the progression of carotid atherosclerosis: results

of the LIPID Atherosclerosis Substudy. LIPID Trial Research Group. Circulation. 1998; 97(18):1784-90.
43. Mercuri M, Bond MG, Sirtori CR, et al. Pravastatin reduces carotid intima-media thickness progression in an asymptomatic hypercholesterolemic mediterranean population: the Carotid Atherosclerosis Italian Ultrasound Study. Am J Med. 1996; 101(6):627-34.
44. Plehn JF, Davis BR, Sacks FM, et al. Reduction of stroke incidence after myocardial infarction with pravastatin: the Cholesterol and Recurrent Events (CARE) study. The Care Investigators. Circulation. 1999;99(2):216-23.
45. Prevention of cardiovascular events and death with pravastatin in patients with coronary heart disease and a broad range of initial cholesterol levels. The Long-Term Intervention with Pravastatin in Ischaemic Disease (LIPID) Study Group. N Engl J Med. 1998;339(19):1349-57.
46. Shepherd J, Cobbe SM, Ford I, et al. Prevention of coronary heart disease with pravastatin in men with hypercholesterolemia. West of Scotland Coronary Prevention Study Group. N Engl J Med. 1995;333(20):1301-7.
47. Byington RP, Davis BR, Plehn JF, et al. Reduction of stroke events with pravastatin: the Prospective Pravastatin Pooling (PPP) Project. Circulation. 2001;103(3):387-92.
48. Sever PS, Dahlo¨f B, Poulter NR, et al. Prevention of coronary and stroke events with atorvastatin in hypertensive patients who have average or lower-than-average cholesterol concentrations, in the Anglo-Scandinavian Cardiac Outcomes Trial–Lipid Lowering Arm (ASCOT-LLA): a multicentre randomised controlled trial. Drugs. 2004;64(suppl 2): 43-60.
49. Baigent C, Keech A, Kearney PM, et al. Efficacy and safety of cholesterol-lowering treatment: prospective meta-analysis of data from 90,056 participants in 14 randomised trials of statins. Lancet. 2005;366(9493):1267-78.
50. Waters DD, LaRosa JC, Barter P, et al. Effects of high-dose atorvastatin on cerebrovascular events in patients with stable coronary disease in the TNT (treating to new targets) study. J Am Coll Cardiol. 2006;48(9):1793-99.
51. Amarenco P, Bogousslavsky J, Callahan A III, et al. High-dose atorvastatin after stroke or transient ischemic attack. N Engl J Med. 2006;355(6):549-59.
52. Everett BM, Glynn RJ, MacFadyen JG, Ridker PM. Rosuvastatin in the prevention of stroke among men and women with elevated levels of C-reactive protein: Justification for the Use of Statins in Prevention: an Intervention Trial Evaluating Rosuvastatin (JUPITER). Circulation. 2010;121(1): 143-50.
53. Hackam DG, Woodward M, Newby LK, et al. Statins and intracerebral hemorrhage: collaborative systematic review and metaanalysis. Circulation. 2011;124(20):2233-42.
54. Ritchie J, Green D, Kalra PA. Current views on the management of atherosclerotic renovascular disease. Ann Med. 2012; 44(suppl 1):S98-S110.
55. Cheung CM, Shurrab AE, Buckley DL, et al. MR-derived renal morphology and renal function in patients with atherosclerotic renovascular disease. Kidney Int. 2006;69(4):715-22.
56. Silva VS, Martin LC, Franco RJ, et al. Pleiotropic effects of statins may improve outcomes in atherosclerotic renovascular disease. Am J Hypertens. 2008;21(10):1163-8.

57. Bax L, Woittiez AJ, Kouwenberg HJ, et al. Stent placement in patients with atherosclerotic renal artery stenosis and impaired renal function: a randomized trial. Ann Intern Med. 2009; 150(12):840-8, W150-W151.
58. Cooper CJ, Murphy TP, Matsumoto A, et al. Stent revascularization for the prevention of cardiovascular and renal events among patients with renal artery stenosis and systolic hypertension: rationale and design of the CORAL trial. Am Heart J. 2006;152(1):59-66.
59. ASTRAL Investigators, Wheatley K, Ives N, Gray R, et al. Revascularization versus medical therapy for renal-artery stenosis. N Engl J Med. 2009;361(20):1953-62.
60. Hackam DG, Wu F, Li P, et al. Statins and renovascular disease in the elderly: a population-based cohort study. Eur Heart J. 2011;32(5):598-610.
61. Parfrey PS, Foley RN. The clinical epidemiology of cardiac disease in chronic renal failure. J Am Soc Nephrol. 1999; 0(7):1606-15.
62. Sarnak MJ, Levey AS, Schoolwerth AC, et al. Kidney disease as a risk factor for development of cardiovascular disease: a statement from the American Heart Association Councils on Kidney in Cardiovascular Disease, High Blood Pressure Research, Clinical Cardiology, and Epidemiology and Prevention. Circulation. 2003;108(17):2154-69.
63. Wanner C, Krane V, Ma"rz W, et al. Atorvastatin in patients with type 2 diabetes mellitus undergoing hemodialysis. N Engl J Med. 2005;353(3):238-48.
64. Fellstro"m BC, Jardine AG, Schmieder RE, et al. Rosuvastatin and cardiovascular events in patients undergoing hemodialysis. N Engl J Med. 2009;360(14):1395-1407.
65. Baigent C, Landray MJ, Reith C, et al. The effects of lowering LDL cholesterol with simvastatin plus ezetimibe in patients with chronic kidney disease (Study of Heart and Renal Protection): a randomised placebo-controlled trial. Lancet. 2011;377(9784):2181-92.

CHAPTER

4

Endovascular Management of Abdominal Aortic Aneurysms: Devices Available and Evidence for Use

Riza Ibrahim

INTRODUCTION

Since Juan Parodi,[1] performed the first endovascular aneurysm repair (EVAR) more than two decades ago, there has been continuous attempts to work towards developing an ideal stent graft. This is evidenced by the regular releases of new devices as well as updated older devices on to the market. Unfortunately, no device at present has all the characteristics that would make it an ideal stent graft.[2]

An ideal stent graft should:
1. Be easy to deploy
   - Low profile
   - Easy to cannulate contralateral gate or do away with the need to
   - Have excellent marker visibility
2. Be able to adapt to adverse aortic anatomy (angulated neck, tortuous iliacs, thrombus etc.)
3. Be able to reduce the risk of endoleaks and thus guarantee prevention of rupture and eliminate the need for secondary re-interventions.
4. Be inexpensive.

Most current stent grafts do not fulfil one or more of the above characteristics. The search for the holy grail thus continues![3]

Most large volume vascular units adopt either a 'horses for courses' approach, where a device that suits the patient's aortic anatomy is chosen or use the units favoured 'work horse' on most occasions accepting the fact that on many occasions the usage is outside the manufacturer's instructions for use.

The devices that have been included in this chapter are all CE marked,[4] FDA approved[5] or both. The list is thus not comprehensive as several locally manufactured devices in countries like China, South Korea, Brazil and the Czech Republic are not CE marked or FDA approved and are not widely available for use outside their countries of manufacture.

BASIC DESIGN AND PRINCIPLES OF ENDOVASCULAR STENT GRAFTS FOR ABDOMINAL AORTIC ANEURYSM (AAA) REPAIR

While details of the instruction for use of every stent graft is beyond the scope of this chapter, there are some basics that most, if not all, stent grafts used for treating AAAs adhere to.
- All AAA stent grafts have a metal skeleton of either Nitinol or stainless steel.
- All AAA stent grafts have a covering of either Dacron, Polyester or ePTFE.
- All stent grafts come in a delivery system that can be retrieved after deployment of the graft.
- All stent grafts used to treat AAAs need good access vessels, i.e. the common femoral and iliac arteries should be of reasonable caliber (between 5 and 8 mm), depending on the size of the delivery system.
- All stent grafts need good proximal (from 7 to 15 mm of good quality aorta below the lowest renal artery) and distal landing zones.
- All stent grafts (especially the ones without hook or barb fixation), work better when there is minimal thrombus in the landing zones.
- All stent grafts (except the uni-iliac variety), need adequate space at the aortic bifurcation, to avoid compression and potential for limb occlusion.
- Severe aortic neck angulation and iliac vessel tortuosity are predictors of stent graft failure to prevent AAA rupture.[6]
- All stent grafts need to be oversized (between 10 and 15%), compared to the diameter of the aortic landing zones.
- All stent graft repairs need adequate follow up to pick up potential problems before they escalate into aneurysm rupture.

Commonly Used AAA Repair Stent Grafts

As mentioned above there are a large number of stent grafts that are commercially available. Some (or their previous iterations) have been around for more than 10-15 years while some have only recently been commercially available. This means that there is potentially a larger body of evidence around the older grafts. The author makes no attempt to pick one over the other, as all have their strengths and weaknesses.

Most Commonly Used Modular Bifurcated Grafts

The Zenith® and Zenith flex® (Cook Medical), the Endurant®, Endurant 11s(Medtronic) and the Gore® Excluder (W L Gore) have been in use for much longer than most other stent grafts. The Zenith® grafts have supra renal fixation and an excellent track record.[7,8] There seems to be a reduction in number of secondary re-interventions over the years[9] with increasing experience with the Zenith. The Zenith® platform also comes with and iliac branched device which can be used to address the issues surrounding ectatic or aneurysmal common iliac arteries (Fig. 1).[10]

The Endurant® and Endurant 11s® from Medtronic,[11] are arguably the most widely used endografts round the world. Its ease of use and 'physician friendly'

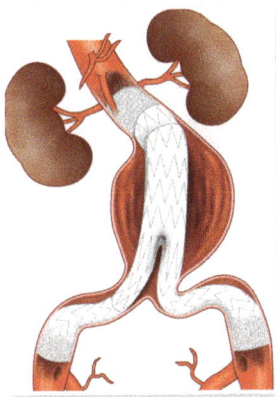

Figure 1: Zenith® stent graft

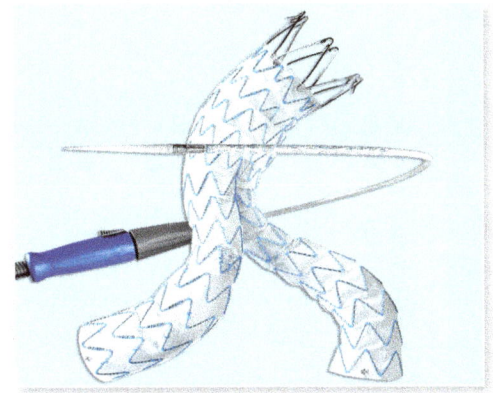

Figure 2: Endurant® Stent graft

delivery system has led to this being used with excellent results.[12,13] Although, unlike the Cook device it does not have an iliac branched or fenestrated iteration, the Endurant® has been used to repair perirenal aneurysms using the chimney or snorkel technique with reasonable success (Fig. 2).[14]

The Gore Excluder®,[15] is another in this series of modular bifurcated grafts that has a large volume of evidence behind it.[16,17] It differs from the Endurant® and Zenith® in that it has a covering of ePTFE rather than Polyester or Dacron. Its C3 variant is repositionable and an iliac-branched device is available.[18,19]

The E-tegra® (Jotec GmbH), stent graft is similar to the grafts from Cook and Medtronic and performs very well within its instructions for use. The E-tegra® can be used along with Jotec's E-iliac® iliac branched device to treat aorto-iliac aneurysms. The Treovance® (Bolton Medical) is very similar in design to the above grafts and has a reasonable body of evidence regarding its performance (Fig. 3 and Table 1).[20,21]

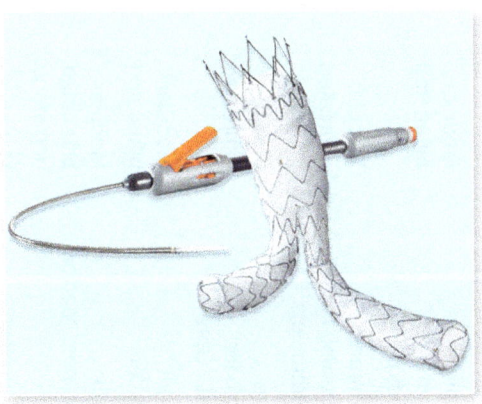

Figure 3: Jotec E-Tegra® stent

Table 1: Endovascular stent grafts used to repair abdominal aortic aneurysms and their main characteristics

Device name	Type of graft	French size main body	Max proximal diameter of stent (millimeters)	Largest available flared limb diameter (millimeters)	Ilia branch available	IFU neck length (millimeters)	IFU aortic neck angle (degrees)
Zenith® Zenith Flex® (Cook)	Modular bifurcated	18–22	36	24	Yes	15	Up to 60
Endurant® Endurant 11s® (Medtronic)	Modular bifurcated	14–20	36	28	No	10	Up to 60
Gore Excluder® (W. L. Gore)	Modular bifurcated	16–18	35	27	Yes	15	Up to 60
Incraft® (Cordis)	Modular bifurcated	14–16	34	24	No	15	Up to 60
Aorfix® (Lombard Medical)	Modular bifurcated ring stent	22	31	20	No	15	Up to 90
Anaconda® (Vascutek Terumo)	Modular bifurcated ring stent	20–22	34	23	No	15	Up to 90

Contd...

Contd...

Device name	Type of graft	French size main body	Max proximal diameter of stent (millimeters)	Largest available flared limb diameter (millimeters)	Ilia branch available	IFU neck length (millimeters)	IFU aortic neck angle (degrees)
Ovation® (Endologix)	Modular bifurcated polymer ring seal.	14–15	34	28	No	7	Up to 60
E-tegra® (Jotec GmbH)	Modular bifurcated	18–20	36	25	Yes	15	Up to 60
Treovance® (Bolton Medical)	Modular bifurcated	18–19	36	24	No	10	Up to 60
AFX® (Endologix)	Non-modular bifurcated	19	34	25	No	15	Up to 60
Nellix® (Endologix)	Parallel stents polymer filled endobags	17	Parallel 10 mm stents. Can treat up to 32 mm aortic neck	Endobags fill the iliac artery	No	10	Up to 60
Altura® (Lombard Medical)	Parallel double D stents	14	30	21	No	15	Up to 60

Other Modular Bifurcated Stent Grafts

The Aorfix™ (Lombard Medical) and Anaconda™ (Vascutek Terumo), stent grafts have ring stents as opposed to Z stents and this makes them able to confirm to tortuous anatomy much better. The Aorfix™ was the first to get CE marked and FDA approved for use in angulated aortic necks up to 90 degrees.[22-25] It has also proven itself in adapting to tortuous iliac anatomy.[26] The Aorfix™ has no suprarenal fixation but has a fish-mouth appearance proximally. If the renal arteries are placed in the trough of the fish mouth some amount of the covered portion will extend to the supra renal region of the aorta. The superior mesenteric artery thus needs to be at least 10 mm above the lowest renal artery (Fig. 4).

The Anaconda™ is very similar in design to the Aorfix™, but comes with suprarenal fixation and a magnetic wire to aid cannulation of the contralateral gate. Given its ring stent design it also performs well in tortuous anatomy.[27,28] In addition the Anaconda™ is available with an 'off the shelf' fenestrated cuff. The Anaconda™ is also licensed for use in aortic neck angulation up to 90 degrees.

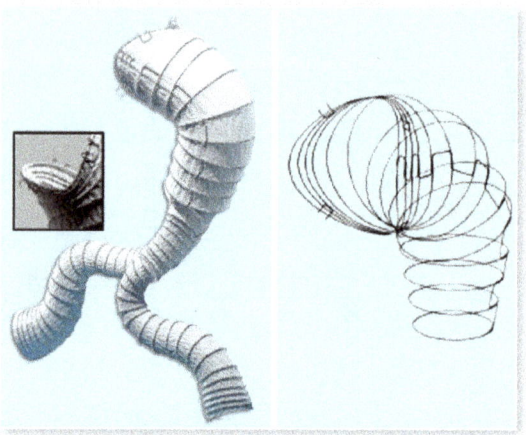

Figure 4: Aorfix™ stent graft

Low Profile Modular Bifurcated Stent Grafts

The Incraft® (Cordis), is a bifurcated modular stent graft with an ultra-low profile delivery system (14F). It lends itself well to pre-cutaneous use. It is also very useful in patients with a narrow aortic bifurcation and small access vessels as often seen in females.[29-31]

The Ovation® (Endologix) stent graft is another ultra-low profile graft.[32] Its instructions for use (IFU) lends itself to be used in short (no less than 7 mm) and conical aortic necks.[33] It has two proximal sealing rings that are filled with polymer and this along with its long suprarenal fixation allows short necks to be treated. The low profile is also useful when a per-cutaneous approach is used.[34] There have however been some reports regarding anaphylaxis due to polymer leakage.[35] There has been some work regarding aortic neck evolution following endovascular stent grafting[36,37] and in short conical necks where a fenestrated repair is not feasible the Ovation® could be considered (Fig. 5).

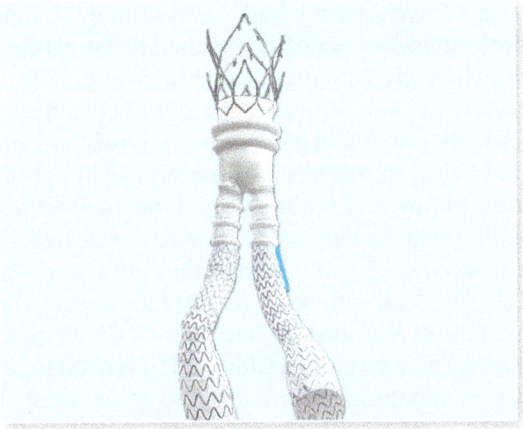

Figure 5: Ovation® stent graft

Non-modular Bifurcated Device

The AFX® (Endologix) is a bifurcated device which is non-modular, i.e. both limbs of the bifurcated graft go up one of the iliac arteries and the bifurcation of the graft is made to sit on the aortic bifurcation. Once the main body is deployed an infra-renal cuff is then deployed, (if needed), to complete the procedure and get a seal in the infra-renal position. The cuffs come with and without suprarenal fixation. This device is made of stainless steel and Endologix's proprietary ePTFE (Strata®), which is draped outside the steel skeleton. The flaring out of the Strata provides an element to the seal at the aortic neck.[38,39] Endologix has made improvements with the top cuff by introducing the Vela® variant. The instructions for use of this states that it can be used in narrow aortic bifurcations (up to 17 mm) (Fig. 6).

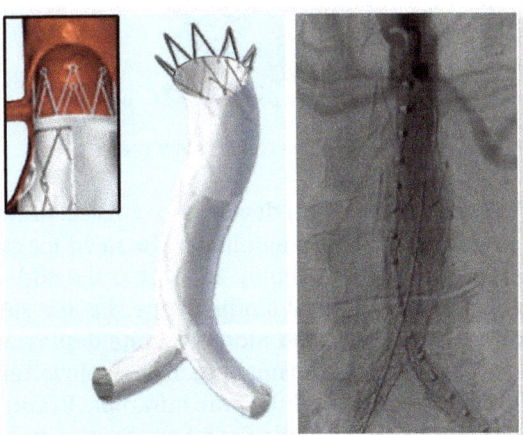

Figure 6: The AFX® stent graft

Parallel Stent Grafts

The Nellix® (Endologix) device provides endovascular aneurysm sealing (EVAS). It consists of two parallel, balloon mounted, 10 mm covered stent grafts. Each stent graft has an endobag attached to it and these are filled with polymer (polyethylene glycol) and allowed to cure during the deployment process. This leads to the aneurysm sac being completely filled by the endobags, which in theory should prevent any flow of blood into the aneurysm sac. Planning and sizing for this device is slightly different from other devices in that the volume of polymer required to fill the aneurysm sac needs to be calculated, in addition to the lengths that need to be treated. So far the results of this device are encouraging.[40-42] Some other advantages are that an iliac aneurysm can also be dealt with when treating the aorta as the endobags fill the space in an ectatic or aneurysmal iliac artery.[43] Given the simplicity of the deployment process (no gate cannulation), it lends itself to being used in the ruptured aneurysm situation.[44] There are also good results being reported when the chimney or snorkel technique is used with the Nellix® to treat perirenal aneurysms.[45]

The concerns regarding the Nellix® center around how to deal with a type 1 endoleaks[46,47] and reports regarding caudal migration of the graft,[48] possibly due to continuing dilatation of the aortic neck. More data are needed to clearly understand these processes (Fig. 7).

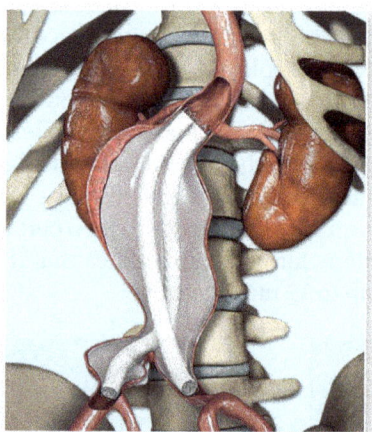

Figure 7: The Nellix® stent graft

The Altura™ (Lombard Medical) device also consists of two parallel self-expandable stent grafts. This again eliminates the need for cannulation of a contralateral gate and is quick to deploy. It also has the added advantage of retrograde deployment at the distal landing zone (i.e. the stent opens from bottom upwards), thus helping with more accurate deployment at the iliac artery bifurcation. The two stents do not have to be deployed at the same level at the top and this may help gain a little more infrarenal fixation. The Altura™ has only been commercially available for a few months and long-term real world experience is lacking (Fig. 8).

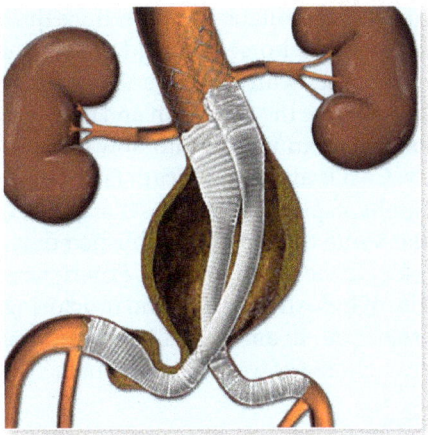

Figure 8: The Altura™ stent graft

Uni-iliac Devices

The uni-iliac device, where only a single stent graft is passed up one iliac and deployed, followed by occlusion of the contralateral iliac and a fem-fem crossover bypass is done, is rarely used. Some indications for employing this technique include (a) an occluded iliac artery, (b) a very narrow aortic bifurcation and (c) as an emergency to treat a ruptured aneurysm. Most of modular bifurcated devices mentioned above have a uni-iliac version of the graft or provide a converter whereby the bifurcated device can be converted to a uni-iliac devise (Fig. 9).

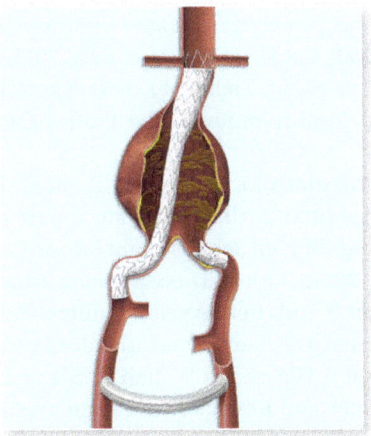

Figure 9: Uni-iliac procedure

CONCLUSION

With a myriad of devices available, choosing a device can be quite confusing to those starting out to do endovascular aneurysm repairs. Although a 'horses for courses' approach seems reasonable, it may reduce the experience that could be gained from using a 'work horse'. It would be reasonable to start with and gain considerable experience with any of the above devices that have long-term real world data. This will give the physician and the team, experience with the procedure itself, as well as an insight into how to troubleshoot or bail out if this were necessary. Cost is also a significant factor in device selection. Some of the newer stent grafts, especially the ones that use polymer are significantly more expensive that some of the well-established devices. At the end of the day there is no perfect device and personal experience, cost, patient's aortic anatomy, availability of industry support and proctoring, etc. will be the main drivers for device selection. In amongst all this one would be well advised to consider the patient's choice as well as open repair.

REFERENCES

1. Veith FJ, Marin ML, Cynamon J, et. al. 1992: Parodi, montefiore, and the first abdominal aortic aneurysm stent graft in the United States. Annals of Vascular Surgery. 2005;749-51.
2. Buckley CJ, Buckley SD. Limitations of Current EVAR Endografts and Potential Solutions for Their Deficiencies. Semin Vasc Surg. 2012;25(3):136-7.
3. Donas KP, Torsello G. Complications and reinterventions after EVAR: Are they decreasing in incidence? Journal of Cardiovascular Surgery. 2011;189-92.
4. Durand M, Seris E. Le marquage CE. IRBM. 2010;31(1):30-5.
5. Zuckerman DM, Brown P, Nissen SE. Medical device recalls and the FDA approval process. Arch Intern Med [Internet]. 2011;171(11):1006-11. Available from: http://www.ncbi.nlm.nih.gov/pubmed/21321283.
6. Bastos Goncalves F, Hoeks SE, Teijink JA, Moll FL, Castro JA, Stolker RJ, et al. Risk factors for proximal neck complications after endovascular aneurysm repair using the endurant stentgraft. Eur J Vasc Endovasc Surg. 2015;49(2):156-62.
7. Verhoeven ELG, Bos WTGJ, Tielliu IFJ, Zeebregts CJAM, Prins TR, Oranen BI, et al. The Cook Zenith endovascular graft. J Cardiovasc Surg (Torino). 2006;47(3):261-8.
8. Verhoeven BAN, Waasdorp EJ, Gorrepati ML, et al. Long-term results after endovascular abdominal aortic aneurysm repair using the Cook Zenith endograft. J Vasc Surg Off Publ Soc Vasc Surg Int Soc Cardiovasc Surg North Am Chapter [Internet]. 2011;53(2):48-57.e2. Available from: http://www.ncbi.nlm.nih.gov/sites/entrez/?cmd=Retrieve&db=pubmed&dopt=AbstractPlus&query_hl=4&itool=pubmed_DocSum&myncbishare=antonius&list_uids=21055897.
9. Iwakoshi S, Ichihashi S, Higashiura W, Itoh H, Sakaguchi S, Tabayashi N, et al. A decade of outcomes and predictors of sac enlargement after endovascular abdominal aortic aneurysm repair using zenith endografts in a Japanese population. J Vasc Interv Radiol. 2014;25(5):694-701.
10. Gray D, Shahverdyan R, Jakobs C, et. al. Endovascular aneurysm repair of aortoiliac aneurysms with an iliac side-branched stent graft: Studying the morphological applicability of the cook device. Eur J Vasc Endovasc Surg. 2015;49(3):283-8.
11. Medtronic. The Endurant Stent Graft. IFU. 2013;6(May 2012):1-6.

12. Bisdas T, Weiss K, Eisenack M, Austermann M, Torsello G, Donas KP. Durability of the Endurant stent graft in patients undergoing endovascular abdominal aortic aneurysm repair. J Vasc Surg. 2014;60(5):1125-31.
13. Donas KP, Torsello G, Weiss K, Bisdas T, Eisenack M, Austermann M. Performance of the Endurant stent graft in patients with abdominal aortic aneurysms independent of their morphologic suitability for endovascular aneurysm repair based on instructions for use. J Vasc Surg. 2015;62(4):848-54.
14. Donas KP, Torsello GB, Piccoli G, Pitoulias GA, Torsello GF, Bisdas T, et al. The PROTAGORAS study to evaluate the performance of the Endurant stent graft for patients with pararenal pathologic processes treated by the chimney/snorkel endovascular technique. Journal of Vascular Surgery. 2016;1-7.
15. W.L. Gore & Associates. GORE® EXCLUDER® AAA Endoprosthesis ANNUAL CLINICAL UPDATE. The Journal of medicine and philosophy. 2013.
16. Pratesi C, Piffaretti G, Pratesi G, Castelli P. ITalian Excluder Registry and results of Gore Excluder endograft for the treatment of elective infrarenal abdominal aortic aneurysms. J Vasc Surg. 2014;59(1).
17. Krajcer Z. The Gore Excluder AAA endoprosthesis with C3 delivery system: Results in high-volume centers. J Cardiovasc Surg (Torino). 2014;55(1):41-9.
18. Katsargyris A, Botos B, Oikonomou K, Pedraza De Leistl M, Ritter W, Verhoeven ELG. The new C3 gore excluder stent-graft: Single-center experience with 100 patients. Eur J Vasc Endovasc Surg. 2014;47(4):342-8.
19. Millon A, Della Schiava N, Arsicot M, De Lambert A, Feugier P, Magne JL, et al. Preliminary experience with the GORE® EXCLUDER® Iliac Branch Endoprosthesis for common iliac aneurysm endovascular treatment. Ann Vasc Surg [Internet]. 2016;1-7. Available from: http://linkinghub.elsevier.com/retrieve/pii/S0890509616300152
20. Kahlberg A, Mascia D, Marone EM, Logaldo D, Tshomba Y, Chiesa R. The Bolton Treovance endograft: Single center experience. J Cardiovasc Surg (Torino). 2014;55(1):77-84.
21. Chiesa R, Riambau V, Coppi G, Zipfel B, Llagostera S, Marone EM, et al. The Bolton Treovance abdominal stent-graft: European clinical trial design. Journal of Cardiovascular Surgery. 2012;595-604.
22. Fillinger MF. The Pythagoras U.S. Clinical Trial of the Aorfix Endograft for Endovascular AAA Repair (EVAR) With Highly-angulated Aortic Necks [Internet]. VascularWeb > Education and Meetings > 2012 Vascular Annual Meeting > Program and Abstracts >. 2012. Available from: http://www.vascularweb.org/educationandmeetings/2012 Vascular Annual Meeting/programindetail/Pages/Saturday, June 9 Abstracts/LB1.aspx
23. John Hardman, Kajendran Balasubramaniam, A Weale MH. Endovascular treatment of morphologically challenging abdominal aortic aneurysms using flexible endograft. Interv Cardiol. 2010;2(3):275-80.
24. Sbarzaglia P, Grattoni C, Oshoala K, Castriota F, Dalessandro G, Cremonesi A. Aorfix??? device for abdominal aortic aneurysm with challenging anatomy. J Cardiovasc Surg (Torino). 2014;55(1):61-70.
25. Malas MB, Jordan WD, Cooper MA, Qazi U, Beck AW, Belkin M, et al. Performance of the Aorfix endograft in severely angulated proximal necks in the PYTHAGORAS United States clinical trial. J Vasc Surg. 2015;62(5):1108-17.

26. Weale AR, Balasubramaniam K, Hardman J, et. al. Use of the Aorfix stent graft in patients with tortuous iliac anatomy. J Cardiovasc Surg (Torino). 2010;51(4):461-6.
27. Karkos CD, Kapetanios DM, Anastasiadis PT, Grigoropoulou FS, Kalogirou TE, Giagtzidis IT, et al. Endovascular Repair of Abdominal Aortic Aneurysms with the AnacondaTM Stent Graft: Mid-term Results from a Single Center. Cardiovasc Intervent Radiol. 2015;38(6):1416-24.
28. R??del SGJ, Zeebregts CJ, Huisman AB, Geelkerken RH. Results of the Anaconda endovascular graft in abdominal aortic aneurysm with a severe angulated infrarenal neck. J Vasc Surg. 2014;59(6).
29. Coppi G, Njila M, Coppi G, Saitta G, Silingardi R, Pratesi C, et al. INCRAFT Stent-Graft System: One-year outcome of the INNOVATION trial. J Cardiovasc Surg (Torino). 2014;55(1):51-9.
30. Bertoglio L, Logaldo D, Marone EM, Rinaldi E, Chiesa R. Technical features of the INCRAFT AAA Stent Graft System. J Cardiovasc Surg (Torino). 2014;55(5):705-15.
31. Torsello G, Scheinert D, Brunkwall JS, Chiesa R, Coppi G, Pratesi C. Safety and effectiveness of the INCRAFT AAA Stent Graft for endovascular repair of abdominal aortic aneurysms. J Vasc Surg. 2015;61(1):1-8.
32. Ierardi AM, Tsetis D, Ioannou C, Laganà D, Floridi C, Petrillo M, et al. Ultra-low profile polymer-filled stent graft for abdominal aortic aneurysm treatment: a two-year follow-up. Radiol Med [Internet]. 2015;1-7. Available from: http://link.springer.com/article/10.1007/s11547-015-0499-z\nhttp://link.springer.com/article/10.1007/s11547-015-0499-z#page-1
33. Sirignano P, Menna D, Capoccia L, Mansour W, Speziale F. Not only the Proximal Neck. Comment on "initial Single-center Experience with the Ovation Stent-graft System in the Treatment of Abdominal Aortic Aneurysms: Application to Challenging Iliac Access Anatomies." Annals of Vascular Surgery. 2015. p. 1480-2.
34. Georgakarakos E, Trellopoulos G, Pelekas D, Ioannou C V., Kontopodis N, Tsetis D. Regarding "one-year outcomes from an international study of the Ovation abdominal stent graft system for endovascular aneurysm repair." Journal of Vascular Surgery. 2014;877.
35. Sfyroeras GS, Moulakakis KG, Antonopoulos CN, Manikis D, Vasdekis SN. Anaphylactic Reaction During Implantation of the Ovation Stent-Graft System in a Patient With Abdominal Aortic Aneurysm. J Endovasc Ther [Internet]. 2015;22(4):620-2. Available from: http://jet.sagepub.com/lookup/doi/10.1177/1526602815593489
36. Nano G, Mazzaccaro D, Stegher S, Occhiuto MT, Malacrida G, Tealdi DG, et al. Early experience with Ovation endograft system in abdominal aortic disease. J Cardiothorac Surg [Internet]. 2014;9(1):48. Available from: http://www.pubmedcentral.nih.gov/articlerender.fcgi?artid=3995648&tool=pmcentrez&rendertype=abstract
37. De Donato G, Setacci F, Bresadola L, Castelli P, Chiesa R, Mangialardi N, et al. Aortic neck evolution after endovascular repair with TriVascular Ovation stent graft. Journal of Vascular Surgery. 2016;8-15.
38. Diethrich EB. Novel sealing concept in the Endologix AFX unibody stent-graft. Journal of Cardiovascular Surgery. 2014;93-102.
39. Melas N, Stavridis K, Saratzis A, Lazarides J, Gitas C, Saratzis N. Active Proximal Sealing in the Endovascular Repair of Abdominal Aortic Aneurysms Early Results

With a New Stent-Graft. J Endovasc Ther [Internet]. 2015;22(2):174-8. Available from: http://jet.sagepub.com/content/22/2/174\nhttp://jet.sagepub.com/content/22/2/174.abstract\nhttp://jet.sagepub.com/content/22/2/174.full.pdf\nhttp://www.ncbi.nlm.nih.gov/pubmed/25809356
40. Holden A. Endovascular sac sealing concept: Will the Endologix Nellix??? device solve the deficiencies? J Cardiovasc Surg (Torino). 2015;56(3):339-53.
41. B??ckler D, Holden A, Thompson M, Hayes P, Krievins D, De Vries JPPM, et al. Multicenter Nellix EndoVascular Aneurysm Sealing system experience in aneurysm sac sealing. J Vasc Surg. 2015;62(2):290-8.
42. Carpenter JP, Cuff R, Buckley C, Healey C, Hussain S, Reijnen MMPJ, et al. Results of the Nellix system investigational device exemption pivotal trial for endovascular aneurysm sealing. Journal of Vascular Surgery. 2016;23-31e1.
43. Youssef M, Nurzai Z, Zerwes S, Jakob R, Dunschede F, Dorweiler B, et al. Initial Experience in the Treatment of Extensive Iliac Artery Aneurysms With the Nellix Aneurysm Sealing System. J Endovasc Ther [Internet]. 2016;23(2):290-6. Available from: http://www.ncbi.nlm.nih.gov/pubmed/26802611
44. Reijnen MMPJ, de Bruin JL, Mathijssen EGE, Zimmermann E, Holden A, Hayes P, et al. Global Experience With the Nellix Endosystem for Ruptured and Symptomatic Abdominal Aortic Aneurysms. J Endovasc Ther [Internet]. 2016;23(1):21-8. Available from: http://www.ncbi.nlm.nih.gov/pubmed/26620398
45. Torella F, Chan TY, Shaikh U, England A, Fisher RK, McWilliams RG. ChEVAS: Combining Suprarenal EVAS with Chimney Technique. Cardiovasc Intervent Radiol. 2015;38(5):1294-8.
46. Hughes CO, de Bruin JL, Karthikesalingam A, Holt PJ, Loftus IM, Thompson MM. Management of a Type Ia Endoleak With the Nellix Endovascular Aneurysm Sealing System. J Endovasc Ther [Internet]. 2015;22(3):309-11. Available from: http://jet.sagepub.com/lookup/doi/10.1177/1526602815579254
47. Ameli-Renani S, Morgan RA. Transcatheter Embolisation of Proximal Type 1 Endoleaks Following Endovascular Aneurysm Sealing (EVAS) Using the Nellix Device: Technique and Outcomes. Cardiovasc Intervent Radiol. 2015;38(5):1137-42.
48. England A, Torella F, Fisher RK, McWilliams RG. Migration of the Nellix endoprosthesis. Journal of Vascular Surgery. 2015.

CHAPTER 5

Current Concepts in the Management of Type B Aortic Dissections

Raghuram Lakshminarayan, Paul M Scott

INTRODUCTION

Type B aortic dissection (AD) presents most commonly with abrupt onset, severe chest pain. This can variously be anterior (62.9%), posterior (44.1%) and sharp (68.3%) or tearing (48.3%) in nature. Nonspecific features of myocardial ischaemia or ST elevation are present in over 50% of cases.[1]

Given the relative incidences of aortic dissection (6/100,000)[2] and myocardial infarction (MI; 200–600/100,000),[3] the clinical difficulty in reliably distinguishing between aortic dissection and MI, the rapid fatality of type A dissection, and the increased incidence of haemorrhagic complications in those treated with antithrombotics or fibrinolytics[4] a reliable and rapidly available test is required when these patients present acutely.

Furthermore, such a test should ideally be able to help distinguish between those with type A dissection necessitating emergency surgical intervention, and between those with type B dissection best managed either conservatively or, with stent grafting.

Chest radiographs are routinely obtained but the findings are nonspecific or indeed normal in 15.8%, severely limiting utility in aortic dissection. Computed tomography (CT) is now rapid, accurate and widely available. Crucially, there is widespread expertise in the interpretation of CT which when combined with its co-location within or adjacent to many emergency departments makes it the most widely utilised modality.[5]

Because of the relative rarity of aortic dissection, use of aortic dissection risk scores have been advocated in an attempt to improve pickup of AD and allow targeted imaging based on the presence of a higher score. Data from the IRAD registry was analysed retrospectively, to produce such a scoring system.[6]

In the presence of 2 or more high-risk features from the 3 categories listed below in Table 1, aortic imaging is expedited. In cases with a single high-risk feature, alternative diagnoses are considered. If not found again imaging for dissection is undertaken. Although the sensitivity of the score based on IRAD[6] data was good at 95.7%, the prospective sensitivity and specificity have not

Table 1: High-risk conditions, pain features and exam features.[6]

High-risk conditions	High-risk pain features	High-risk exam features
• Marfans syndrome • Family history of aortic disease • Known aortic valve disease • Recent aortic catheterisation • Known thoracic aneurysm	• Chest back or abdominal pain • Abrupt in onset • Severe in intensity • Ripping or tearing	• Evidence of perfusion deficit • Pulse deficit/Systolic BP differential/Focal neurology • Murmur of aortic insufficiency • Hypertension or shock state

been validated, and given the frequency of the pain features described in other conditions, the increased pickup rate is likely to be at the cost of increased rate of scanning.

Biomarkers may have a role in the diagnosis and stratification of patients with possible or confirmed dissection. D-dimer assay represents the most widely used and available assay at present. At a level of 500-ng/ml within 24-hour onset of symptoms the sensitivity and specificity of D-dimer for acute aortic dissection was 96.6% and 46.6% respectively in the IRAD-Bio study.[7] The low specificity reflects the elevation of D-dimer in other conditions, such as pulmonary thromboembolism, trauma, recent surgery, etc. However, levels below this in the 1st 24 hour place the patient in a lower risk group for classical dissection with flowing blood in both lumens.

In intramural haematoma, because circulating blood does not come in contact with thrombotic non-intimal aortic surface, the coagulation cascade may not be activated. In the absence of production of fibrin, the fibrinolytic pathway producing D-Dimer is not activated making D-Dimer assay less useful in this subgroup of patients. Similarly, lumen thrombosis in type B dissection is may be associated with lower D-dimer concentrations.

Smooth muscle myosin heavy chain (sm-MHC) is released into the circulation during damage to smooth muscle cells.[8] This occurs in aortic dissection induced damage to medial smooth muscle cells. Its presence in uterine and small intestine will rarely confound its use due to limited symptom overlap. However, although sensitive and specific in the 1st 3 hours (90% sensitivity, 97% specificity), the short useful timescale and absence of wide availability mean this remains largely an academic tool at the present time.

Calponin, common in smooth muscle, Soluble elastin fragments and transforming growth factor β all display elevation in acute aortic dissection but are limited by their availability which is rare outside the research field.

IMAGING OF TYPE B AORTIC DISSECTION (TYPE B AD)

Transthoracic echocardiography (TTE), transoesophageal echocardiography (TOE) and magnetic resonance imaging (MRI) are all similarly reliable[5] but require experienced operators (echocardiography) or access to a relatively scarce resource in many centres (MRI). MRI is also hampered by practical issues relating to establishing safety of previous implants in the acute setting and limited acute access, both in terms of location and out of hours staffing. Catheter angiography is very rarely used as a primary diagnostic modality. Consequently, these modalities are either reserved as "problem solving" tools or utilised in centres with an established history of their usage.

Computed Tomography in Type B Aortic Dissection

Technical considerations: Mortality from aortic dissection significantly outweighs any risks related to the radiation dose or contrast load. Coverage of the whole aorta with is useful in identifying branch vessel compromise and in allowing identification of true and false lumens via continuity of the true lumen with un-dissected segment of the aorta.[9] Precontrast and portal venous delayed phase images help identify intramural haematoma,[10] calcification and organ malperfusion. ECG gating reduces motion artefact significantly in the arterial scan.

The Stanford classification was proposed in 1970 and is the most widely used anatomical classification system.[11] In the Stanford system; Type A (Fig. 1) involves the ascending aorta (regardless of the site of any intimal tear) and type B (Fig. 2) does not involve the ascending aorta.

The principal advantage of the Stanford system is in driving management decisions. Type A dissection represents a surgical emergency with a non-surgically managed mortality of 20% at 24 hours, 30% at 48 hours and 40% at 7 days. With surgical repair these fall to 10%, 12% and 20%[1] respectively. Conversely medically treated *uncomplicated* type B AD patients have a mortality of 10% at 30 days. This underpins the classic management paradigm for type A versus type B aortic dissection.

Similarly, in Type B AD, uncomplicated dissection has in hospital mortality of 13%,[12] whereas the presence of shock (encompassing patients with rupture)

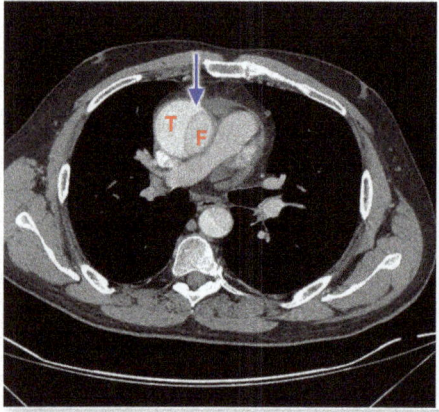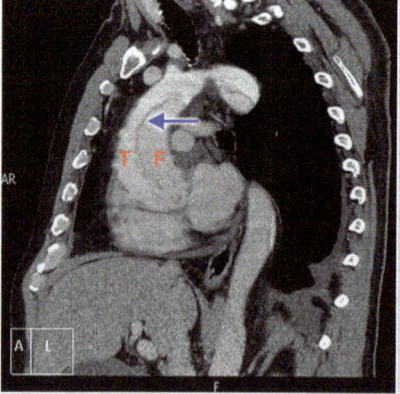

Figure 1: Axial and sagittal images of a Stanford type A aortic dissection. The ascending aorta is involved. The images showed the presence of true (T) and false (F) lumens as well as the intimal flap (blue arrows)

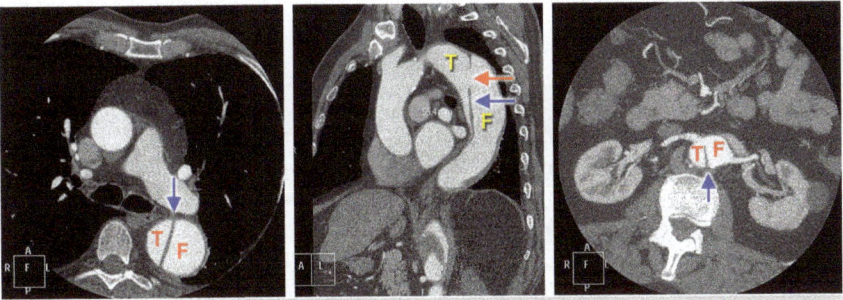

Figure 2: Axial and sagittal images of a Stanford type B aortic dissection. The role of MDCT is to identify the presence of intimal flap (blue arrows), entry point (red arrow), true (T) and false (F) lumens, the extend of the dissection and end organ perfusion

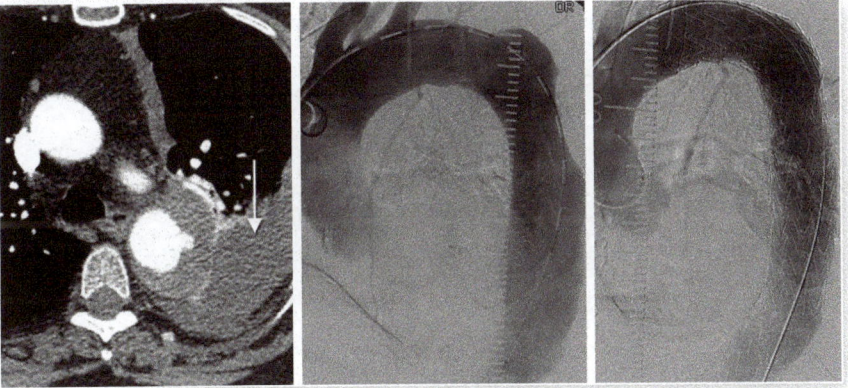

Figure 3: Aortic rupture following a type B dissection treated with a stent graft

(Fig. 3) or branch vessel compromise (Fig. 4) greatly increases the likelihood of death with odds ratio for death in shock or branch vessel compromise of 23.8 or 2.9, respectively.[10]

Univariate analysis within the same study identified aneurysm size over 6 cm (Fig. 5) and periaortic haematoma (Fig. 6) as independent predictors of in-hospital death.[10] Consequently, these are important findings within the acute type B AD population on imaging and need to be actively sought on imaging. Treatment of these patients by stent grafting likely represents the best option in these higher risk patients.

ESTABLISHED INDICATIONS FOR TREATMENT OF TYPE B DISSECTIONS

- Aortic rupture
- Branch vessel malperfusion
- Rapid false lumen dilatation or overall trans-aortic enlargement more than 10 mm in the first two weeks.
- Uncontrolled hypertension and/or pain.

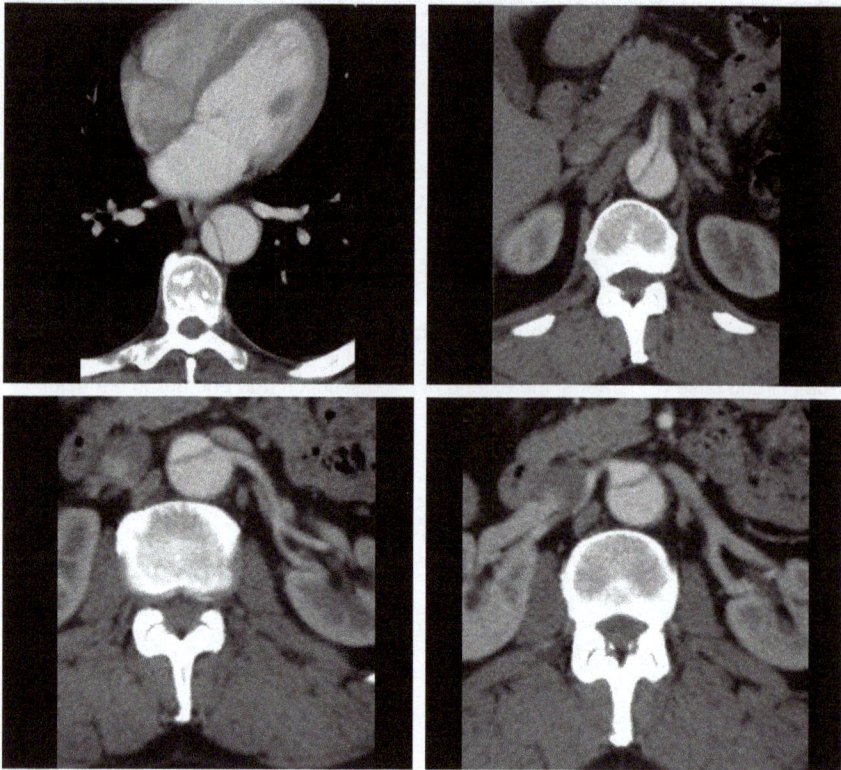

Figure 4: Acute type B dissection involving the superior mesenteric artery causing malperfusion with the true lumen supplying the right renal artery and false lumen supplying the left renal artery

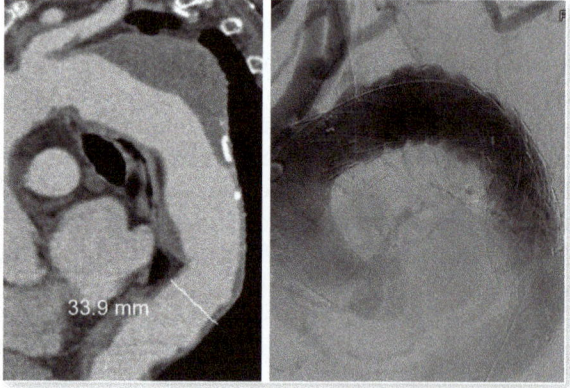

Figure 5: Late aneurysm formation treated with a stent graft along with a carotid subclavian bypass

Since treatment of contained rupture and malperfusion are almost exclusively undertaken by stent graft placement within the descending thoracic aorta, signs which differentiate the two lumens are useful.

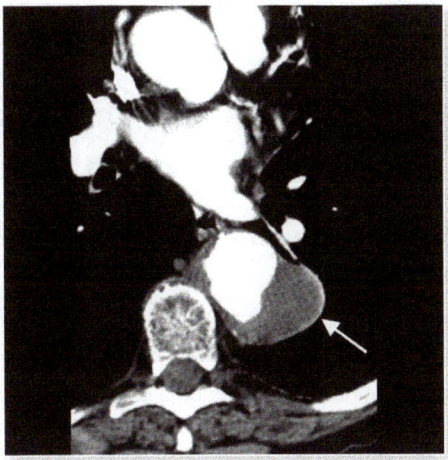

Figure 6: Periaortic haematoma (arrow)

Continuity of the undissected portion of the aorta with the true lumen represents a logical means of determining true from false lumen. Similarly, blind ending lumens represent the false lumen. If craniocaudal coverage of the dissected segment of aorta is incomplete, then size of the lumens is useful with the false lumen representing the larger lumen (Fig. 2) in the majority of cases.

Acute angle with the outer wall or "beak sign" is also a reliable indicator of the false lumen.[9] The presence of thrombus in the beak can make this more difficult to appreciate. Thrombus is commoner in the false lumen and intimal calcification will tend to only (by definition) occur on the true lumen side of the dissection flap in acute dissections.[9]

In 2013 the DISSECT classification was proposed.[13] This system represents a mnemonic attempting aid decision making and description in the stent graft era.

- **D**-Duration. Acute: <2 weeks. Subacute: 2 weeks to 3 months. Chronic: 3 months or greater.
- **I**-Intimal flap location: Ascending aorta, aortic arch, descending aorta, abdominal aorta, unknown.
- **S**-Size of aorta. Based on maximal trans-axial diameter orthogonal to the long axis of the aorta.
- **SE**-Segmental extent of involvement. Reflecting the realisation that in type A aortic dissection significant complications acutely and chronically can be a feature of the distal dissection which may require endovascular therapy.
- **C**-Clinical. Documentation of aortic valve involvement, cardiac tamponade, rupture, branch vessel malperfusion, progression of aortic involvement, Other—uncontrolled hypertension or clinical symptoms, rapid false lumen expansion or transaortic lumen enlargement of >10 mm in 1st 2-week period.

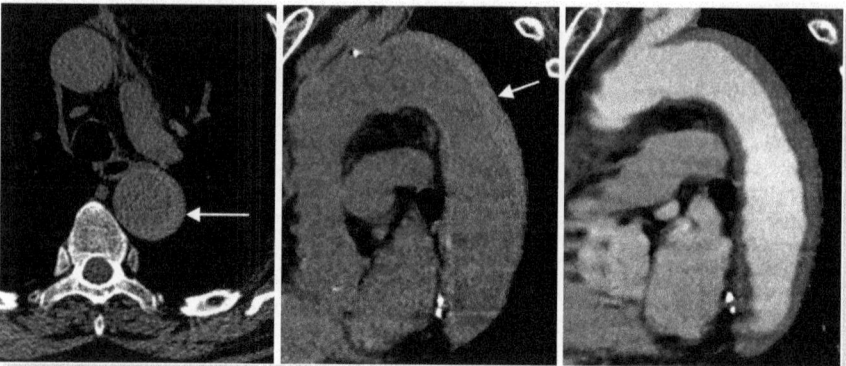

Figure 7: Intramural haematoma best identified on a plain scan as a hyperdence crescent (arrow)

- **T**-Thrombosis of false lumen. Long-term patency and partial thrombosis of the false lumen being associated with a higher risk of long-term complications.

The rationale of the system is in trying to capture the prognostic elements and thereby focus on the evidence for endovascular treatment of the descending thoracic dissection in both type B and type A dissections with distal involvement.

Intramural haematoma: This is an allied entity to dissection. It is characterised by similar presentation and represents thrombus within the wall of the aorta (Fig. 7). Evolution can be progression to frank dissection, or behaviour like complicated dissections or in the minority resolution (Figs 8A to E).

Treatment of Type B Dissection

The treatment strategy of type B dissection has evolved over the last decade. There has been consensus about medical management of all uncomplicated dissection being superior to any other intervention. The subset of patients who present with complicated dissection especially rupture or branch vessel ischaemia leading to malperfusion would be treated at the time of presentation if anatomically suitable and feasible for Thoracic Endovascular Aortic Repair (TEVAR). However, long-term follow-up of "uncomplicated dissection" has demonstrated disease progression which has raised the need to explore a strategy of early TEVAR to prevent late complication. A greater consensus has to evolve over identifying the subgroup of patients who would benefit from early treatment and also to define the optimum period for this treatment to be performed.

Uncomplicated type B dissection patients should be monitored closely in an intensive care setting with rigorous control of blood pressure. A target systolic blood pressure of 100–120 mmHg is ideal and achieved with intravenous beta blocking agents.[14] The main principle is to try and reduce the shear stress on the aortic wall.

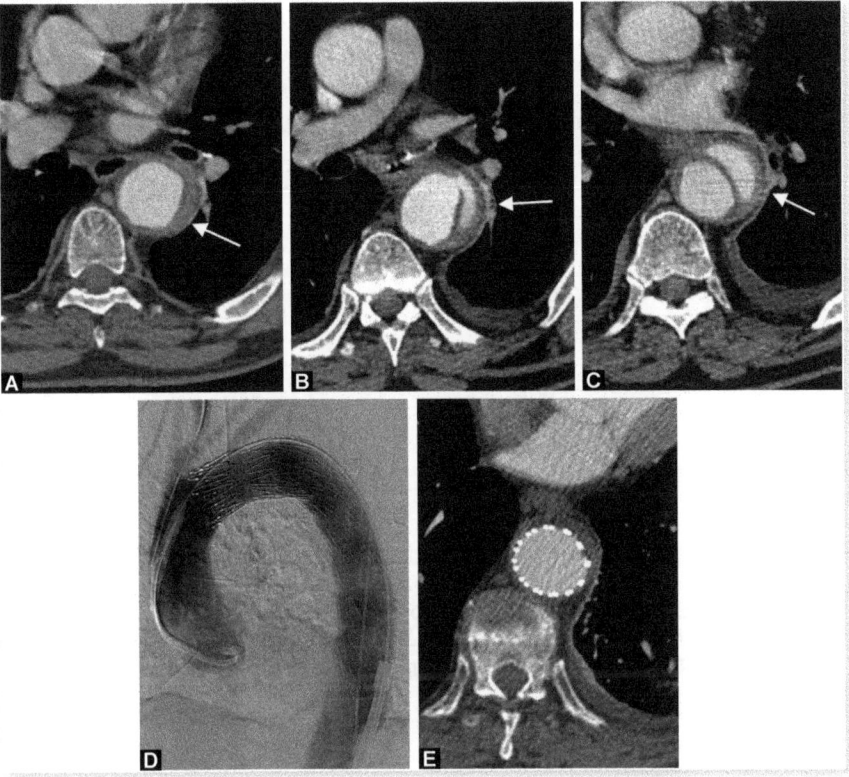

Figures 8A to E: (A) Intramural haematoma; (B and C) Progressing to a frank dissection; (D) In 48 hours (arrow), the primary entry tear is treated with a stent graft; (E) and aortic remodelling after 1 year post treatment

Complicated type B dissections which include aortic rupture, end organ ischemia, continuing pain despite full medical therapy and early false lumen expansion are an indication for treatment. TEVAR replaced open surgical repair with lower in-hospital mortality rates with a grade 1A recommendation.[15-17] The decision to perform a TEVAR to treat a type B dissection is preceded by a detailed assessment of the CT scan. The key features to be assessed include access vessels which ideally should be at least 7 mm in diameter to allow insertion of the commonly available stent grafts. Assessment of aortic branches, especially the left subclavian artery and left common carotid artery to define the landing zone is critical. Though, there has been a lot of discussion regarding covering of the left subclavian artery with or without a carotid subclavian bypass, the evidence for or against this is lacking. The key principle in treatment is to close the primary entry tear (Fig. 9). During the procedure of TEVAR, two of the key aspects are to define the true lumen and identify the primary entry tear. The use of ultrasound, trans-oesophageal echocardiography and intravascular ultrasound are important adjuncts as described above. The general oversize recommended of the stent graft is around 10%. The sizing is done to the proximal true lumen size and the size of the distal true lumen is not relevant as the membranes

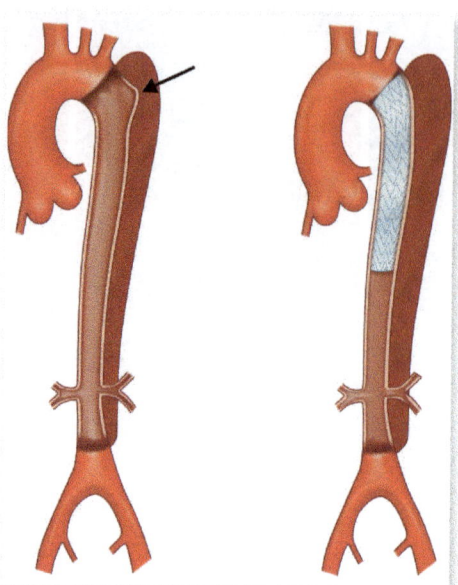

Figure 9: Type B dissection demonstrated by the presence of an primary entry intimal tear (arrow) distal to the origin of the left subclavian artery. The dissection extends into the visceral segment. The line diagram on the right demonstrate the closure of the primary entry tear with a stent graft

move back in acute dissections. The usual length of the stent is around 10 cm. Catheter manipulation in the arch should be avoided to minimize the risk of extending the dissection into the arch. For similar reasons, barbs in the stent graft are not recommended. A longer stent might be required if other tears are noticed. Balloon moulding is generally avoided to reduce risk of extending the dissection either proximally or distally. It is important to image the visceral and iliac vessels. Additional stenting or fenestration might be required to restore branch vessel perfusion.[18,19]

One of the concerns of stenting into a small true lumen distally would be the stent size mismatch. This could potentially lead to a distal stent graft induced new entry tear (dSINE) (Fig. 10).[20] If this happens, the false lumen could remain patent leading to late complications like aneurysmal dilatation. The problem of dSINE is more in chronic type B dissection than acute type B dissection as membranes in the acute phase tend to move back.[21] Various mechanisms of development of dSINE have been described. These involve changes in haemodynamics in relation to the rigid end of the stent graft against a fragile intimal flap especially if the distal stent graft is oversized in relation to the true lumen.[22] dSINE can be managed medically by lowering the blood pressure and/or extending the stent graft. The use of bare stents (PETTICOAT technique) has also been described with considerable success.[23]

The risk of treating dissection in the acute phase include peri-intervention stroke and retrograde type A dissection which is a dreaded complication with a high mortality rate. It was noted that retrograde dissections occur either at

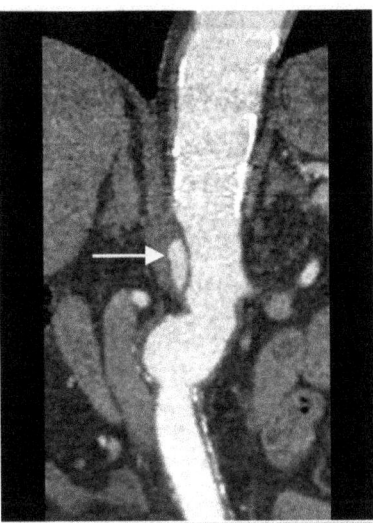

Figure 10: Distal stent graft induced new entry tear (dSINE)

the time of the procedure, immediately post-procedure or delayed which might be seen even after 3 months. It is thought that the dissection could be caused by stent factors, wire manipulation or progression of disease. The incidence of the complication varies from 3 to 4%, however the mortality from this could be as high at 40-50%[24]. The INSTEAD trial[25] which was a randomized trail comparing best medical treatment with TEVAR and best medical treatment alone indicated that TEVAR did not yield any benefits in comparison to best medical management at the end of 2 years and obviously was associated with a higher risk of complications associated with early TEVAR. However, the study did comment on the better false lumen thrombosis and aortic wall remodelling in the TEVAR group. The 5-year follow-up of these patients were reported in the INSTEAD XL[26] trial which reported an increased aorta specific survival at the end of 5 years. Though the numbers are small, long-term outcome data seem to suggest that endovascular scaffolding for initially uncomplicated type B dissection might offer a benefit in preventing late complications and reducing aorta-related deaths. Consensus is evolving on the fact that initially uncomplicated type B dissections does not preclude disease progression and there is a need to identify clinical and imaging groups that might benefit from early TEVAR. The timing of the early TEVAR in probably the subacute phase is still debated. Further studies are needed to define the optimal patient and optimal time for consideration of TEVAR in uncomplicated type B dissections.

Chronic type B dissection might cause ongoing aortic dilatation. The aortic lumen is extensively remodelled with increased fibrotic thickening of the dissection flap and a small true lumen causing treatment challenges. The role of TEVAR in chronic type B dissection is not well defined. Dissections confined to the thoracic aorta did better with false lumen thrombosis than dissections involving the abdominal aorta following treatment (Fig. 11). Fenestrated and branched grafts are required to treat thoraco-abdominal chronic dissections

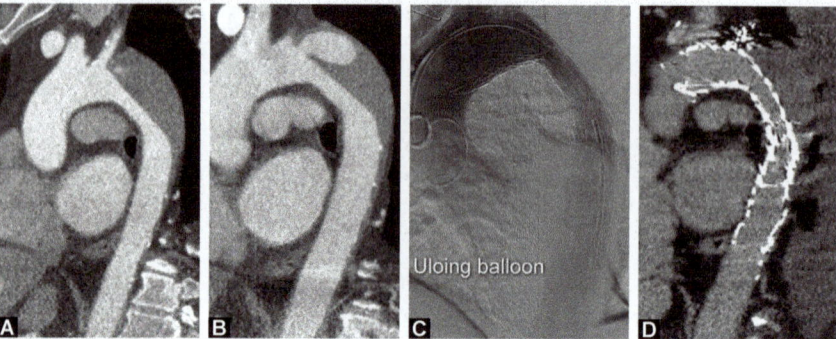

Figure 11: (A and B) Chronic dissection with a thick septum demonstrates aneurysm formation with a persistent primary entry tear in two scans a year apart. (C and D) This was stent grafted and CT demonstrates the unyeilding nature of the chronic septum which constricts the mid portion of the stent in a follow-up CT, (D) performed 6 months post-procedure. There is however, false lumen thrombosis

and the narrow true lumen space with an unyielding membrane complicates planning and deployment of these grafts. Data on long-term outcomes from these procedures are scarce.

Treatment of Type B Dissection: A Summary

- Consensus to treat complicated type B dissections
- Evolving data on long-term complications of medically treated uncomplicated type B dissection—uncomplicated dissection seems to be a misnomer and will require a new strategy to image and treat.
- Evolving technologies will decrease complications related to treating type 2 dissections early with TEVAR.

CONCLUSION

Multi-detector CT has revolutionised our understanding of the imaging of type B dissection. Clinical presentation of the complicated or uncomplicated dissection with the appropriate understanding of the dissection anatomy helps plan treatment. There is growing consensus towards a more aggressive approach in the treatment of type B dissections to improve long-term outcomes.

REFERENCES

1. Hagan PG, Nienaber CA, Isselbacher EM, et al. The International Registry of Acute Aortic Dissection (IRAD): new insights into an old disease. JAMA. 2000; 283:897-903.
2. Howard DP, Banerjee A, Fairhead JF, Perkins J, Silver LE, Rothwell PM, for the Oxford Vascular Study. Population-based study of incidence and outcome of acute aortic dissection and premorbid risk factor control: 10-year results from the Oxford Vascular Study. Circulation 2013;127:2031-37.

3. Roger V. Epidemiology of myocardial infarction. Med Clin North Am. 2007;91(4): 537-IX.
4. Hansen MS, Nogareda GJ, Hutchison SJ: Frequency of and inappropriate treatment of misdiagnosis of acute aortic dissection. Am J Cardiol. 2007;15;99(6):852-6. 10.1016/j.amjcard.2006.10.055.
5. Shiga T, Wajima Z, Apfel CC, Inoue T, Ohe Y. Diagnostic accuracy of transesophageal echocardiography, helical computed tomography, and magnetic resonance imaging for suspected thoracic aortic dissection: systematic review and meta-analysis. Arch Intern Med 2006;166:1350-56.
6. Rogers et al. Sensitivity of the aortic dissection detection risk Score, a novel guideline-based tool for identification of acute aortic dissection at initial presentation results from the international registry of acute aortic dissection. Circulation. 2011;123:2213-8.
7. Suzuki T, Distante A, Zizza A, et al. Diagnosis of acute aortic dissection by D-Dimer: the international registry of acute aortic dissection substudy on biomarker (IRAD-Bio) experience. Circulation 2009;119:2702-7.
8. Suzuki T, Katoh H, Tsuchio Y, et al. Diagnostic implications of elevated levels of smooth-muscle myosin heavy-chain protein in acute aortic dissection. Ann Intern Med. 2000;133:537-41.
9. LePage MA, Quint LE, Sonnad SS, Deeb GM, Williams DM. Aortic dissection: CT features that distinguish true lumen from false lumen. AJR Am J Roentgenol. 2001;177(1):207-211.
10. Chiu KW, Lakshminarayan R, Ettles DF. Acute aortic syndrome: CT findings. Clin Radiol. 2013;68:741-8.
11. Daily PO, Trueblood HW, Stinson EB, et al. Management of acute aortic dissection. Am Thorac Surg. 1970;10:237-247.
12. Suzuki T, Mehta RH, Ince H, Nagai R, Sakomura Y, Weber F, et al. Clinical profiles and outcomes of acute type B aortic dissection in the current era: lessons from the International Registry of Aortic Dissection (IRAD). Circulation 2003;108 (Suppl. 1):II312e7.
13. Dake MD, Thompson M, van Sambeek M, Vermassen F, Morales JP, for the DEFINE Investigators. DISSECT: a new mnemonic-based approach to the categorization of aortic dissection.
14. 2014 ESC Guidelines on the diagnosis and treatment of aortic diseases. European Heart Journal. 2014;35,2873-926 doi:10.1093/euheart/ehu281.
15. Sakalihasan N, Nienaber CA, Hustinx R, et al. Tissue Inflamation (by PET imaging) and Serologic Activity in the Evolution of Chronic Aortic Dissection. Eur Heart J Cardiovasc Imaging.
16. Estrera AL, Miller CC, Huynh TT, et al. Preoperative and operative predictors of delayed neurologic deficit following repair of thoracoabdominal aortic aneurysm. J Thorac Cardiovasc Surg 2003;126:1288-94.
17. Safi HJ, Estrera AL, Miller CC, et al. Evolution of risk for neurologic deficit after descending and thoracoabdominal aortic repair. Ann Thorac Surg. 2005; 80: 2173-79.
18. Lombardi JV, Cambria RP, Nienaber CA, et al. Prospective multicenter clinical trial (STABLE) on the endovascular treatment of complicated type B aortic dissection using a composite device design J Vasc Surg. 2012;55:629-40.

19. Canaud L, Patterson BO, Peach G, Hinchliffe R, Loftus I, Thompson MM. Systematic review of outcomes of combined proximal stent grafting with distal bare stenting for management of aortic dissection. J Thorac Cardiovasc Surg. 2013;145:1431-8.
20. Dong Z, Fu W, Wang Y, et al. Stent graft-induced new entry after endovascular repair for stanford type B aortic dissection. J Vasc Surg. 2010; 52:1450-7.
21. Yang CP, Hsu CP, Chen WY, et al. Aortic remodeling after endovascular repair with stainless steel-based stent graft in acute and chronic type B aortic dissection. J Vasc Surg. 2012;55:1600-10.
22. Janosi RA, Tsagakis K, Bettin M et al. Thoracic aortic aneurysm expansion due to late distal stent graft-induced new entry. Catheter Cardiovasc Interv.2015;85:E43-53.
23. Alsac JM, Girault A, El Batti S, et al. Experience of the zenith dissection endovascular system in the emergency setting of malperfusion in acute type B dissections. J Vasc Surg. 2014;59:645-50.
24. Eggebrecht H, Thompson M, Rousseau H, et al. Retrograde ascending aortic dissection during or after thoracic aortic stent graft placement: insight from the European Registry on Endovascular Aortic Repair Complications. Circulation. 2009;120(1 suppl):S276-S81.
25. Nienaber C, Rousseau H, Eggebrecht H, et al. Randomized comparison of strategies for type B aortic dissection: the INvestigation of STEnt grafts in Aortic Dissection (INSTEAD) trial. Circulation. 2009;120:2519-28.
26. Nienaber CA, Kische S, Rousseau H, et al. Endovascular repair of type B aortic dissection: long-term results of the randomized investigation of stent grafts in aortic dissection trial. Circ Cardiovasc Interv. 2013;6(4):407-16.

CHAPTER

6

Managing Superficial Femoral Artery Lesions: Metal, Drugs or More

Aniket Pradhan, Robert Fitridge

INTRODUCTION

The treatment of the superficial femoral artery (SFA) remains one of the most debated topics amongst vascular surgeons in everyday clinical practice. Excellent outcomes have been demonstrated in the endovascular treatment of the coronary, iliac and renal arteries. However, the SFA continues to be an 'Achilles heel' in endovascular therapy, exhibiting relatively poor primary patency rates (77-86% at one year) with contemporary techniques.[1]

Many reasons have been implicated for suboptimal outcomes in SFA intervention, including the anatomical position of the artery, which undergoes constant conformational changes (including extension/contraction, torsion, compression and flexion) (Fig. 1) and also the disease pattern which includes a high incidence of chronic total occlusions (CTO), calcified plaques and diffuse long segment disease. In most patients, SFA disease is associated with a concurrent inflow or outflow problem, which influences the effectiveness of the treatment.

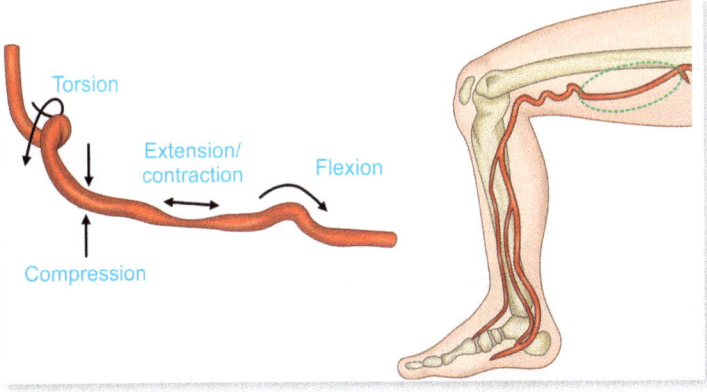

Figure 1: Mechanical stresses on the SFA

The patency of open surgical reconstruction of the femoral artery is excellent; however, bypass surgery is associated with significant morbidity, whereas patency of the endovascular procedures continues to be suboptimal but patient-related outcomes are very satisfactory, with a 30-day freedom from composite death, target limb amputation and early re-intervention of over 95% and same day or day 1 discharge of most patients.[2]

In this chapter we discuss the technical problems pertaining to SFA interventions and visit the literature on various modalities available for treating SFA disease.

SELECTING PATIENTS FOR OPEN SURGICAL OR ENDOVASCULAR TREATMENT OF THE SUPERFICIAL FEMORAL ARTERY

After confirmation of the presence of peripheral arterial disease (PAD) by physical examination and Doppler ankle-brachial indices (ABIs), further radiologic testing, such as arterial duplex scanning is usually performed. When intervention is planned, computed tomography angiography (CTA), magnetic resonance angiography (MRA), or catheter angiogram, may be performed to further localise and potentially treat the culprit lesion. Angiography is generally performed with the aim of proceeding with therapeutic intervention.

Treatment options for PAD are multifaceted and typically include a combination of medical therapy and surgery, either endovascular surgery, open surgery, or a hybrid combination of both techniques. However, to achieve optimal benefit when selecting patients for therapy, it is important to know which patients will require treatment for limb salvage and in addition, which patients are at higher risk for medical or postoperative complications. Not all patients with critical limb ischaemia (CLI) could or should undergo revascularisation. Those with extensive necrosis or infection or who are non-ambulatory may be best served with primary amputation. In almost every significant study treating PAD, patients with diabetes and kidney failure have inferior results with open or endovascular therapy. In addition, wound complications are reported to occur in as many as 40% of patients with an open lower extremity surgical procedure, in patients with renal impairment.

On initial diagnosis of PAD, patients may have no symptoms, exercise-induced claudication, lifestyle limiting claudication, rest pain, or tissue loss. (Table 1).

ANATOMICAL CLASSIFICATION OF ARTERIAL LESIONS

A classification system based on the anatomic distribution, number and nature of lesions (stenosis or occlusion) of the SFA and popliteal arteries were developed as part of the Trans-Atlantic Inter-Society Consensus Classification (TASC) II document. With the improvement of endovascular technologies and techniques, consensus recommendations have been developed around the TASC II classification.[3] TASC I and II recommend an endovascular-first approach for type A and B lesions (Fig. 2), and recommend surgery for most

Table 1: Severity classifications of lower limb ischaemia[3]

Fontaine classification		Rutherford classification	
Stage	Symptoms and signs	Stage	Symptoms and signs
1	None	0	None
2a	Intermittent claudication without pain on resting but with claudication at a distance of >200 m	1	Mild claudication
2b	Intermittent claudication without pain on resting but with claudication at a distance of <200 m	2	Moderate claudication
		3	Severe claudication
3	Nocturnal and/or resting pain	4	Rest pain
4	Necrosis and/or gangrene in the limb	5	Ischaemic ulceration not exceeding ulcer of the digits of the foot
		6	Severe Ischaemic ulcers or frank gangrene

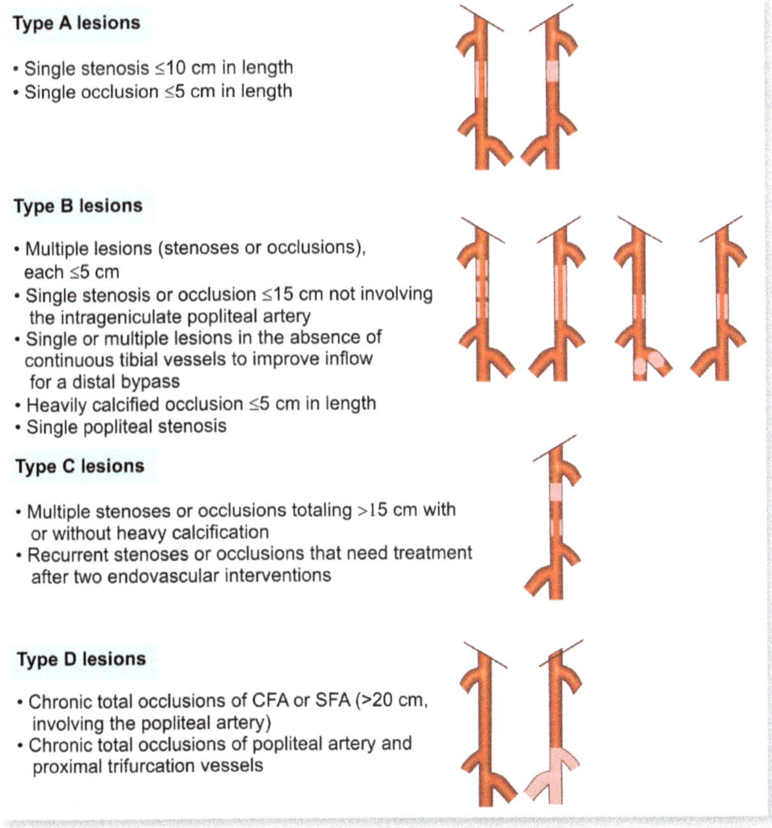

Type A lesions

- Single stenosis ≤10 cm in length
- Single occlusion ≤5 cm in length

Type B lesions

- Multiple lesions (stenoses or occlusions), each ≤5 cm
- Single stenosis or occlusion ≤15 cm not involving the intrageniculate popliteal artery
- Single or multiple lesions in the absence of continuous tibial vessels to improve inflow for a distal bypass
- Heavily calcified occlusion ≤5 cm in length
- Single popliteal stenosis

Type C lesions

- Multiple stenoses or occlusions totaling >15 cm with or without heavy calcification
- Recurrent stenoses or occlusions that need treatment after two endovascular interventions

Type D lesions

- Chronic total occlusions of CFA or SFA (>20 cm, involving the popliteal artery)
- Chronic total occlusions of popliteal artery and proximal trifurcation vessels

Figure 2: Trans-Atlantic Inter-Society Consensus II (TASC II) Classification of Femoro-popliteal Lesions. CFA, Common femoral artery; SFA, superficial femoral artery.[3]

type D lesions. Patients with type C lesions who are not good candidates for surgery may also benefit from an endovascular-first approach. Since 2000, the recommendations have evolved to reflect the technological advances in endovascular procedures such that type D lesions only include CTO of SFA > 20 cm, or occlusions involving the popliteal artery (Fig. 2).

BYPASS VS ENDOVASCULAR OPTIONS

TASC II recommends revascularisation for patients with CLI. The ACCF/AHA task force practice guidelines concluded that in CLI patients with complex lesions and having a life expectancy more than 2 years, bypass surgery was a reasonable initial treatment. For those who do not have an autogenous venous conduit available (or have limited life expectancy), endovascular treatment was a reasonable initial choice.

The Bypass versus Angioplasty in Severe Ischemia of the Leg (BASIL) trial was a multicentre randomized controlled trial that assigned 452 patients to a surgery-first or angioplasty-first approach.[4] The primary endpoint was amputation-free survival. The BASIL trial did not demonstrate a difference in overall survival or amputation-free survival. However, in those patients surviving over 2 years, bypass surgery was associated with improved overall survival and amputation-free survival. The BASIL trial also revealed that patients who received angioplasty followed by bypass surgery fared worse than patients who received surgery alone in both amputation-free survival and overall survival.[5] These findings contradict the widely held assumption that angioplasty can safely be performed as a temporizing measure before bypass and this has subsequently been the subject of significant debate.

Despite mixed results for angioplasty in the BASIL trial, there has not been an appreciable reversion to open surgical bypass as a first-line therapy for infrainguinal occlusive disease. The minimally invasive nature of PTA combined with improvements in technology and operator experience have only served to reinforce a widespread trend towards an aggressive endovascular-first approach for straight-forward as well as complex infrainguinal lesions.

ENDOVASCULAR TREATMENT

Definitions of Successful Intervention

The complexity of infrainguinal endovascular therapy has resulted in the creation of multiple definitions of success (Box 1). The measures of success

---

Box 1: Factors determining the type of intervention

1. The severity of presenting symptoms
2. The anatomical location and extent of disease
3. Presence or absence of venous conduit
4. The fitness and likely life expectancy of the patient

reported most commonly in the literature include clinical response with regard to symptom resolution and limb salvage, technical success, primary patency, assisted primary patency, secondary patency, and need for, or freedom from, target lesion revascularization (TLR). Depending on the study design and the intent of the investigators, significant variability exists in the use of these outcomes.

Clinical Response

The literature is characterised by significant heterogeneity in the reporting of clinical status for patients with infrainguinal PAD treated with endovascular therapy. The clinical variables that are evaluated most commonly and exhibit the greatest clinical relevance are resolution of symptoms, limb salvage, and patient survival.

Technical Success

The majority of studies have used angiographic criteria to define the technical success of infrainguinal endovascular therapy. Technical success is most often defined as the presence of antegrade flow through the treated lesion at the termination of the procedure.[6,7] Certain studies have added further refinements and other requirements, such as the presence of less than 25% to 30% residual stenosis, lack of flow-limiting dissection seen on angiography at the termination of the procedure, flow to the pedal arch, and vascular laboratory studies demonstrating a duplex-derived peak systolic velocity ratio (PSVR) of 1.5 or less at the treatment site or an ABI improvement of 0.15 or greater.[8,9] Conversely, technical failure has been defined as failure to revascularise the target lesion.[10]

Primary Patency

Primary patency has been interpreted in various ways in different studies. For arterial grafts, the definition of patency is clear, but in many cases of endovascular therapy, the artery was patent before treatment, so most investigators have included recurrent stenosis, as well as thrombosis, in the definition of patency after endovascular therapy. For the determination of primary patency, the degree of allowable restenosis varies between 30% and 50%, depending on the studies.

Assisted Primary Patency

The definition of assisted primary patency is simply primary patency (as defined earlier) with the assistance of a subsequent interventional procedure to maintain patency or treat a significant recurrent stenosis and is reported with Kaplan-Meier life-table analysis.

Secondary Patency

The definition of secondary patency differs from that of assisted primary patency in that it refers to patency that has been restored after occlusion of the treated arterial segment and is also reported with Kaplan-Meier life-table analysis.

Determinants of Outcome

The primary determinants of outcome for patients undergoing SFA endovascular therapy include lesion characteristics, pattern of vascular disease, patient demographics and comorbid diseases, clinical situation, and intraprocedural factors (Table 2).

TREATMENT OUTCOMES

Standard PTA

Standard percutaneous transluminal angioplasty (PTA) also known as plain old balloon angioplasty (POBA) is usually performed with noncompliant balloons which assume their intended diameter even at high pressures.

Table 2: Anatomical and patient factors influencing the outcome of endovascular treatment[11]

Favourable Status for Endovascular Therapy	Unfavourable Status for Endovascular Therapy
Lesion Characteristics	**Lesion Characteristics**
• Proximal lesion location • Stenosis • Short lesion length • Focal stenoses	• Distal lesion location • Occlusion • long lesion length • Multiple same segment stenoses
Pattern of Vascular Disease	**Pattern of Vascular Disease**
• Single-level disease • Normal 3-vessel runoff	• Multilevel disease • Poor (<3-vessel) runoff
Patient Demographics	**Patient Demographics**
• Male gender • Low comorbid disease burden	• Female gender • High comorbid disease burden (e.g. diabetes, ESRD)
Clinical Indications	**Clinical Indications**
• Claudication • Primary stenosis	• Critical limb ischaemia • Recurrent stenosis
Intraprocedural Factors	**Intraprocedural Factors**
• No residual stenosis or dissection • Robust haemodynamic response	• Presence of residual stenosis >30% or flow limiting dissection • Minimal haemodynamic response

In general, PTA of lesions less than 5 cm in length has a patency of 59% to 93% at 1 year.[12-14] Muradin et al.[15] undertook a meta-analysis to evaluate long term patency of SFA interventions from 19 studies between 1993 and 2000 and found that there was significant impact of occlusive (compared to stenotic) lesions and the presentation of CLI on long term outcomes; 3-year patency rates were 61% for stenosis in claudicants, 48% for occlusions in claudicants, 43% for stenoses in patients with CLI, and 30% for occlusions in patients with CLI.

Unsuccessful PTA often occurs secondary to heavily calcified eccentric stenoses, extensive dissection, acute thrombosis, vessel perforation, atheroemboli, or significant residual stenosis. Acute closure due to dissection, thrombosis, or both can occur in 4–7% of cases.

Long-segment Superficial Femoral Artery Lesions Angioplasty

Patients with CLI are often found to have long-segment occlusions of the SFA (TASC-D lesions). A study summarized the patency results after SFA intervention from the control arms (PTA-alone) of three device trials.[16] The primary patency of the 116 patients with a mean lesion length of 8.7 ± 3.1 cm (4–15 cm in length) was 28% at 12 months. They further summarised the randomized, controlled studies in the literature and found a combined 12-month primary patency rate of 37% in 191 patients treated with PTA for SFA lesions of a mean length of 8.9 cm. Standalone PTA for long SFA lesions has a high incidence of restenosis and in general carries a primary patency estimate rate of approximately 33% at 1 year.

Subintimal Angioplasty

Bolia et al. advocate intentional subintimal angioplasty (SIA) for long-segment lesions. They reported an initial technical success of 80% in 200 patients (mean lesion length 11.5 cm, range 2–37 cm).[17] Life table analysis excluding initial technical failures revealed primary patency rates of 71% and 58% at 1 and 3 years, respectively. There were 2 major (1%) and 13 minor (6.5%) complications, with a 30-day mortality rate of 1.5%. Unfortunately, most interventionalists have been unable to reproduce these excellent results.

Angioplasty Versus Stenting

With the application of endovascular therapy to lesions of increasing complexity, stent placement has become integral to the endovascular management of SFA disease. Both balloon-expandable and self-expanding stents have been used in the SFA. Balloon-expandable stents can be deformed from trauma or external compression, making self-expanding stents the preferred device type. Stents can be placed at the time of successful angioplasty (direct or primary stenting) or to salvage failed angioplasty (secondary stenting) at the time of intervention.

Three published trials provide randomization data between PTA and PTA with stenting using contemporary nitinol stents. The Femoral Artery

Table 3: Results of three randomized superficial femoral artery nitinol stent trials			
Study Name			
Variable	Schillinger	FAST	RESILIENT
Type	SC, R, Pros	MC, R, Pros	MC, R, Pros
Stent	Guidant Absolute	Bard Luminexx	Edwards LifeStent
Ischaemia	Claudication	Claudication	Claudication
Number of patients	104	244	206
PTA	53	121	72
Stent	51	123	134
Mean lesion length			
PTA	127 mm	46 mm	<150 mm
Stent	132 mm	44 mm	<150 mm
Procedural success			
PTA	68%	79%	72%
Stent	93%	95%	86%
Restenosis rate (12/24 months)			
PTA	63%/74%	39%/NA	62%/NA
Stent	37%/49%	32%/NA	20%/NA
Conclusion	PS > SS	PS = SS	PS > SS

Abbreviations: MC, multi-centre; NA, not applicable; Pros, prospective; PS, primary stenting; PTA, percutaneous transluminal angioplasty; R, randomized; SC, single centre; SS, secondary stenting

Stenting Trial (FAST Trial),[18] Schillinger SFA stent trial,[19] and the Resilient Trial[20] were conducted using prospective, randomized protocols (Table 3). The FAST trial did not show a benefit of stenting at a 12-month follow-up. This study used the Bard Luminex stent that has been shown in the femoral stenting in obstructions trial to have a high fracture rate. The Schillinger and Resilient trials showed benefit to primary stenting at 12 and 24 months using the Dynalink/Absolute and Edwards Lifestent NT, respectively. Both of these stents have been less prone to fracture. In general, a sustained benefit of primary stenting has been shown in longer rather than shorter lesions and in patients with claudication rather than CLI. Quality of life and improved functional capacity have also been favourably affected by primary stenting.

Long-segment SFA lesions have also proven challenging to treat with stents because dynamic forces in the SFA can lead to undesirable complications such as stent fracture. In the DURABILITY I trial,[21] 151 patients were prospectively recruited to receive a single, long non-overlapping stent in the SFA for lesions with a mean length of 9.6 cm. At 1 year, patients experienced a 79% freedom from target lesion revascularization and an 8% stent fracture rate. The 79% freedom from target lesion revascularization is comparable to results found in similar short-segment SFA stenting trials (Fig. 3).

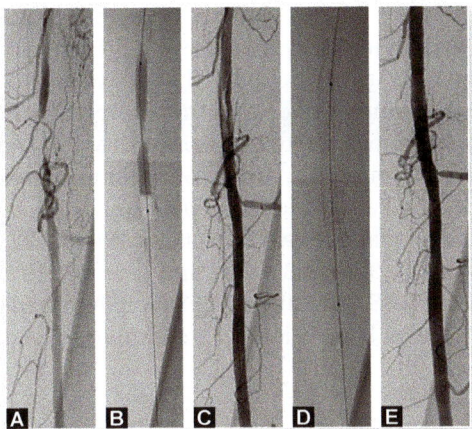

Figure 3: 77/M presenting with left hallux gangrene on a background of previous intermittent claudication. Ultrasound duplex detected a short length SFA lesion. (A) Subsequently an angiogram was performed under local anaesthetic which confirmed the ultrasound report; (B) A POBA was performed after crossing the lesion; (C) But there was a dissection noted; (D) Which was then stented with a BMS; (E) With a good result on completion angiogram

Drug-eluting Technology

Drug-eluting stents (DES) and drug-coated angioplasty balloons (DCB) are designed with the purpose of limiting the reactionary, proliferative process of neo-intimal hyperplasia. Researchers have hypothesised that these technologies would improve the patency rates observed in the SFA. A number of device specific trials have been conducted to test this hypothesis.

Drug-eluting Stents

The sirolimus-coated cordis SMART (Nitinol Self-Expandable) stent for the treatment of SFA disease (SIROCCO) I trial randomized 36 patients with SFA disease to treatment with either sirolimus-eluting or bare-metal stents. Although the sirolimus-eluting cohort demonstrated improved 1-year patency, the study failed to achieve the primary endpoint, which was improved mean in-stent restenosis at 2 years (22% in the sirolimus group versus 31% in the control group, P = NS). This trial also brought to light the issue of stent fracture, which occurred in six stents in SIROCCO I.[22]

The SIROCCO II trial was a randomized study that evaluated the use of slow-eluting sirolimus stents (N = 29) compared with bare-metal stents (N = 28) in patients presenting with chronic limb ischemia due to SFA occlusions or stenosis but failed to demonstrate a difference in the primary endpoint of improved mean in-stent restenosis.[23]

The Zilver PTX paclitaxel-eluting stent (Cook Medical, Bloomington, Indiana), was the focus of the largest trial of DES implantation in the SFA to date. Investigators randomized 236 patients to receive primary DES, and 238 to PTA[24] (Fig. 4). Of the PTA group, 120 patients had residual stenosis after angioplasty and were randomized to receive a provisional bare-metal stent (BMS) or DES. The primary endpoints in the trial were event-free survival (a combined endpoint defined as freedom from amputation, need for surgical revascularization, or worsening of two Rutherford classes) and primary patency at 12 months. The authors went on to follow the study cohort for 5 years.[25]

The primary DES had a superior primary patency in comparison to BMS placement. (83% vs 69%) at one year as well as (66% vs 43%) at five years The TLR with primary DES (90% vs 82%) at one year and (83% vs 68%) at five years was better than BMS. In addition, DES recipients had greater sustained improvement in "clinical benefit index," a combined outcome measure that

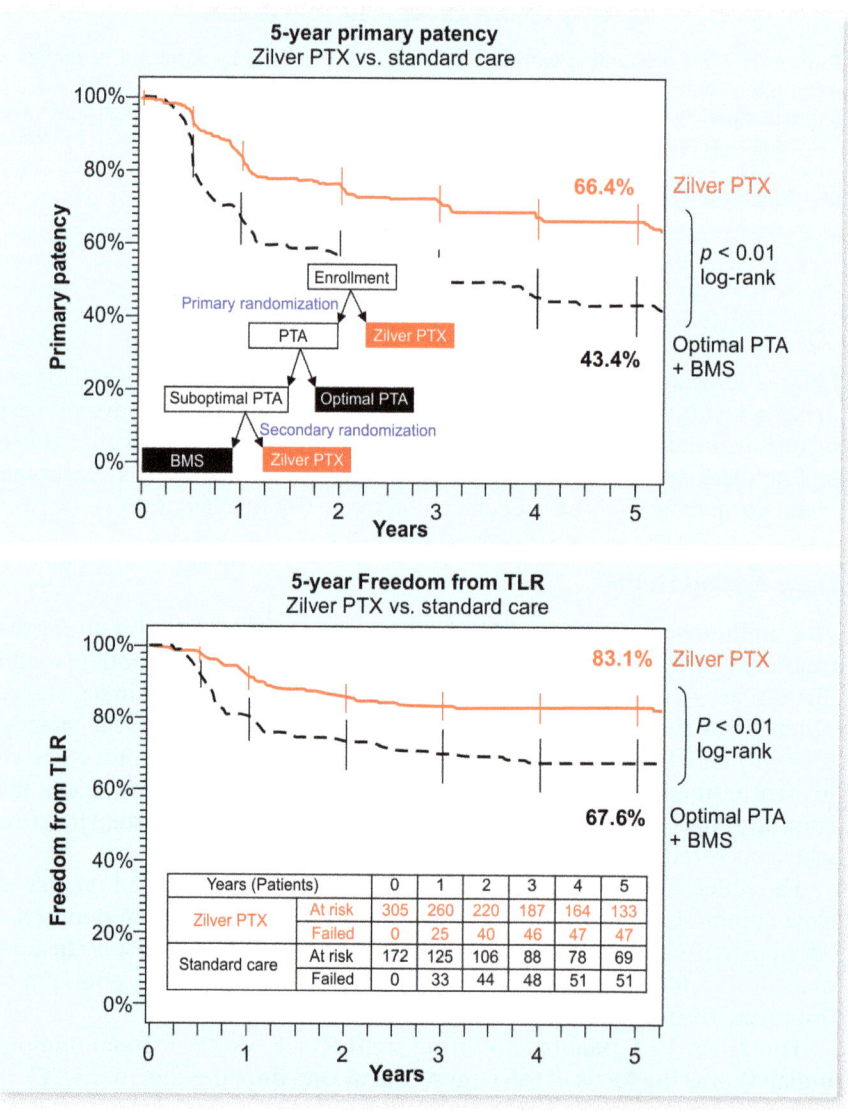

Figure 4: Zilver PTX DES five-year follow-up data[24]

included freedom from worsening claudication, ulceration, or tissue loss after the initial treatment at both one and five-year follow-up.

Covered Stents

Covered stents represent an alternative approach to endovascular treatment of SFA lesions. This approach is analogous to a surgical bypass, in that the entire region of disease is excluded with a graft. The Viabahn covered stent graft (Gore & Associates) consists of a nitinol stent frame lined internally with ePTFE (Expanded polytetrafluoroethylene). The device has evolved over time, with the addition of a heparin bioactive surface and, more recently, a contoured proximal edge. Results with the Viabahn stent graft have been studied in comparison to traditional surgical bypass, and to nitinol self-expanding stents in long SFA lesions (Fig. 5).

An early study randomised patients with SFA disease and symptomatic claudication to Viabahn stent grafting or open surgical bypass with ePTFE graft. Patency rates were similar between the two groups out to 4-year follow-up.[26]

The VIPER registry studied the use of newer-generation Viabahn stent grafts with a contoured edge in long SFA lesions (mean length, 19 cm). At 1 year, primary patency was 74%, and assisted patency was 87%. A secondary analysis of device oversizing found that primary patency increased to 87% if the device was minimally oversized (<20%).[27] Overall patency rates were similar for lesions longer than 200 mm, suggesting that Viabahn graft patency may not be as dependent on lesion length as standard stents.

The VIASTAR trial is a European-based randomized study of Viabahn versus bare-nitinol stent placement. Preliminary 12-month results from this study suggest restenosis rates of 27% with Viabahn stent grafting compared to 59% for bare-nitinol stents.[28]

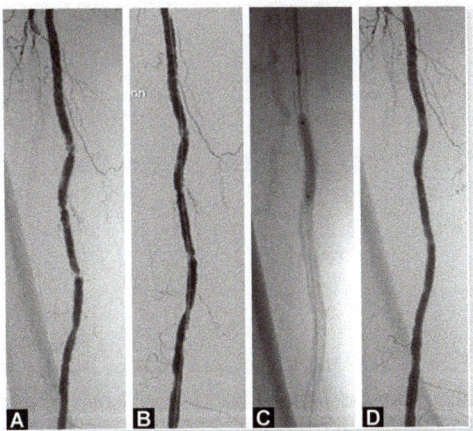

Figure 5: Viabahn 80-year-old lady with multiple co-morbidities presented with a critically ischaemic right foot. (A) An angiogram showed multiple high grade stenoses with highly calcified SFA throughout its entire length; (B) POBA showed no improvement in the luminal diameter; (C) The SFA was then lined with a Viabahn stent; (D) and an angioplasty was performed. The result showed good flow through the SFA with minimal recoil

Recently the use of Viabahn for in-stent re-stenosis is being investigated. The RELINE trial randomized 83 patients with BMS restenosis to treatment with POBA versus treatment with Viabahn endografts.[29] The 12-month patency data were highly favourable with primary patency of 74.8% in the Viabahn group compared to 28% patency in the angioplasty patients ($P<.001$). But this is being challenged by the results of the FAIR trial, which showed superior patency with DCB when used in in-stent re-stenosis.[30]

In the setting of acute thrombosis of a covered stent usually leads to higher morbidity as the collateral circulation is cut off due a covered nature of the stent. Also cost is a major consideration for this device.

Drug-coated Balloons

Drug-coated balloons (DCB) were developed to obtain the advantages of drug-eluting technology without actually leaving a foreign body in the form of a stent in the artery. Although stents are useful in preventing the elastic recoil of arteries after angioplasty, stents may actually increase neo-intimal hyperplasia by causing repetitive trauma and an increased inflammatory reaction. Stents also make the artery rigid and the different forces exerted during movement (see Fig. 1) become more prominent on the stent-free area, causing either new lesions or acute thrombosis. (Fig. 6). DCBs are designed to curb neo-intimal hyperplasia by delivering large doses of anti-cell proliferation agents directly to the site of vessel injury.

DCBs essentially function via the passive transfer of paclitaxel into the vessel wall by means of a carrier that helps the transportation of paclitaxel from the surface of the balloon to the vessel wall. Then, the paclitaxel particles that

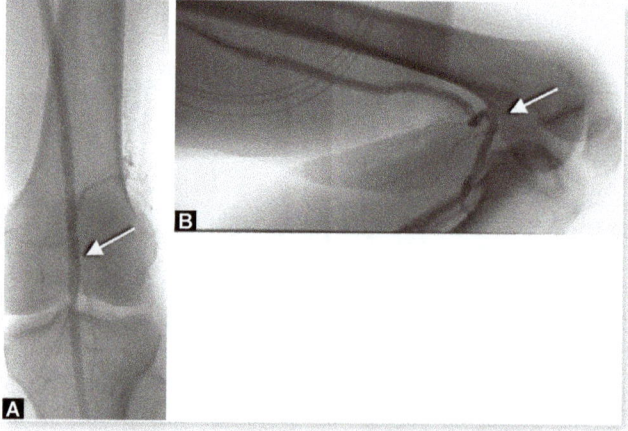

Figure 6: A 68/M with previous SFA stents put in for critically ischaemic limb. Presented for the second time with acute thrombosis of the stents after doing some gardening. (A) A transfemoral suction thrombectomy was performed with good result; Completion angiogram shows a patent and straight segment of artery (white arrow) after the stented section; (B) On repeating the angiogram with the leg folded beyond 90° the rigid segment of the SFA pushes the non-stented segment into a twist possibly causing the recurrent thrombosis.

adhere to the vessel wall are responsible for the drug-tissue concentrations over time. The crystallinity of the coating plays a very important role in paclitaxel-coated balloons and the uniformity of drug coating. The higher the crystallinity, the greater the drug uptake for DCBs. Small- to medium-sized paclitaxel crystals adhere to the injured vessel surface and continuously release paclitaxel over time into the underlying tissue.

There is considerable data on product-based studies. The THUNDER trial[31] was a randomized, controlled, multi-centre study comparing Paccocath paclitaxel-coated and conventional uncoated balloon catheters with respect to efficacy and tolerance in inhibiting restenosis. The TLR and LLL (late luminal loss) rates were 4% and 0.4 mm respectively as compared to the plain balloon group at 37% and 1.7 mm. The 5-year follow-up data showed that the TLR rates remained significantly lower in the DCB at 21% as compared to uncoated balloon at 56%.

The LEVANT II trial[32] was conducted across multiple centres using the Lutonix paclitaxel DCB (Bard Peripheral Vascular Inc.) in Europe and USA. 476 patients were randomised and treated. The study showed significantly improved primary patency and non-significantly decreased TLR with DCB versus plain balloon at 12 months. Primary patency in the DCB arm was 65.2% and in the control arm was 52.6%.

The IN.PACT SFA randomized trial[33] evaluated the safety and effectiveness of the DCB (IN.PACT Admiral, Medtronic, Santa Rosa, California) compared with standard PTA for the treatment of patients with symptomatic SFA disease. Primary patency in the DCB group was 82.2% at one year versus 52.4% in the plain balloon group. At two years the difference was stable and statistically significant (78.9% vs. 50.1%) (Fig. 7).

The drug-eluting technology definitely has an advantage over the POBA or the BMS in terms of early and mid-term (up to 2 years) TLR and primary patency (Table 4). The economic implications of widespread adoption of this approach needs to be considered.

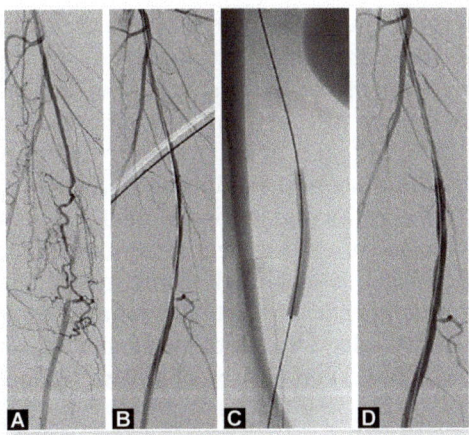

Figure 7: A 75/M presented with lifestyle limiting claudication. (A) Angiogram showed 12 cm long SFA occlusion; (B) The lesion was crossed and predilated; (C) A DCB was then used to dilate the SFA with completion angiogram showing good flow through (D) the occluded segment

Table 4: Summary of results for different therapies for SFA treatment

Therapy	Number of lesions	Lesion length (mm)	Primary patency		Freedom from TLR	
			12 months	24 months	12 months	24 months
PTA (POBA arm)						
Schlinger	53	127	37%	26%		47.2%
Zilver PTX	235	63	32.8%		67.6%	
LEVANT 2	543	63	56%		83.2%	
In.PACT	111	88	66.8%	50.1%	79.3%	71%
BMS						
FAST	244	46	88%			
Schlinger	51	132	63%	51%		63%
DES						
Zilver PTX	236	66	83.1%		90.5%	
DCB						
LEVANT II	543	63	83.7%		83.2%	
In.PACT SFA	220	89	89.8%	78.9%	97.5%	92%

Pit-falls in the Drug-eluting Technology Trials

The question whether DCBs are going to shift the SFA treatment paradigm away from stenting remains to be answered. Perhaps the most important difference between the DCB trials and DES trials is that the DCB trials perform screening via standard PTA. In both LEVANT 2 and IN. PACT SFA II, if the lesion did not respond well to the initial predilatation with balloon angioplasty to provide the investigator a reasonable assurance that the lesion would not require stenting, then that patient was not randomized to the control or treatment arm. Because these patients failed the initial screening angioplasty, they were considered a "screen fail" and were not placed in the study or the final results.

Although the definition of calcification is variable, the Zilver PTX trial appears to have included significantly more calcified lesions than the DCB trials. Calcification may be a significant issue that impacts the overall effectiveness of DCBs in real-world lesions. Fanelli et al. noted this limitation of DCBs in the conclusion of a recent peer-reviewed publication.[34]

The last significant gap is to directly compare the effectiveness of the two drug-eluting modalities in a variety of lesion types. In order to better understand the relative effectiveness of DCBs and DES in the superficial femoral artery (SFA), a direct comparison of the two technologies is needed.

Hybrid Procedures

Hybrid procedures that take into account the advantages of both surgery and endovascular therapy are frequently performed. The most common scenarios would be a common femoral endarterectomy and angioplasty and stenting of the SFA occlusion. Some have used tibial angioplasty to improve the runoff. It will be interesting to see the results of BASIL-2 trial which will be including hybrid procedures during randomisation and what effect they have on patency.

Health Economic Implications of SFA Treatment Modalities

The literature on health economic analysis of SFA therapy is sparse. A cost-effectiveness analysis based on a discrete event simulation model from a health service prospective in England included eight endovascular therapies (DES, DCB, BMS, brachytherapy, stent-grafts, cryoplasty) versus standard of care and concluded that DCBs may be a cost effective alternative to POBA with bail out stent.[35]

Katsanos et al.[36] undertook a systematic literature search to pool target lesion revascularisations. A model-based per patient cost impact and quasi-cost-effectiveness projection over 24 months based on pooled TLRs was calculated in the setting of the UK's National Health Service (NHS). The analysis showed that DCB and DES are associated with substantially lower TLR rates of around 18% and 19% over 24 months, compared with around 27% with a primary BMS strategy and around 36% with routine care without drug eluting technology. These improved clinical outcomes were found to be associated with limited increases in overall cost for the NHS budget.

Arguably, DES and DCB are not only protecting patients from recurrent symptomatic disease that may mandate reinterventions, but are also saving them from the inherent risk of potential complications, anxiety and inconvenience of having to undergo a repeat procedure.

Antiplatelet Therapy

Inclusion of clopidogrel is of paramount importance to prevent early thrombosis after a DCB or DES treatment for SFA disease. The duration of aspirin in most studies is life-long with addition of clopidogrel as a loading dose of 300 mg before a DCB or DES procedure.[24,32] Different durations of dual antiplatelet (DAP) therapy has been used post procedure in the reported trials. The Zilver PTX trial[24] used clopidogrel for two months post stenting, whereas the LEVANT trial[32] used then for a one month post stenting and for 3 months if a bail out BMS was used. The value of a longer period of DAP therapy is uncertain.

OTHER THERAPIES

Atherectomy Devices

Atherectomy—rotational, directional, or ablational (laser)—catheters are designed to remove plaque.

The SilverHawk Plaque Excision System (SilverHawk, Redwood City, California) is an excisional atherectomy device that uses a high-speed cutting blade, which excises a strip of plaque that is subsequently stored in a nosecone. Zeller et al[37] in a study of 131 lesions in 84 patients presenting with Rutherford category 2–5 ischemia treated using the SilverHawk device, showed that technical success was achieved in 86% of cases undergoing atherectomy alone and in 100% of cases using additional adjunctive modalities. Distal embolization is a concern with atherectomy, leading some to advocate the concomitant use of embolic protection devices.[38] Comparative trials have not been performed to confirm a real advantage over PTA.

Rotablator (Heart Technologies, Redmond, Washington) is an example of rotational atherectomy devices. A diamond-studded metal tip (Rotablator) spins rapidly, shaving atheroma from the vessel wall as it passes over a guide wire. The new channel is only as large as the catheter itself, requiring ancillary PTA. Of initially successful procedures, 30–40% fail within the first 6 months, limiting the enthusiasm for debulking.

The excimer laser (ClirPath, Colorado Springs, Colorado) uses a 308-nm ultraviolet wavelength and functions by ablating tissue on contact, without causing a rise in temperature in the surrounding tissue. In the Laser Angioplasty for Critical Limb Ischemia (LACI) trial, 423 lesions were treated in 145 patients who were poor candidates for surgical revascularization with 6-month limb salvage rate of 93%.[39]

The evidence to date, mostly single-centre observational studies, does not support the routine use of atherectomy or any debulking strategy, such as laser, for SFA lesions.

Biomimetic Stents

Conventional straight stents placed in the SFA are less compliant than the normal vessel and do not accommodate the shortening of the vessel when in flexion. This results in vessel redundancy being transferred to areas of the artery adjacent to the stented segment. The biomechanical incompatibility between a conventional straight stent and the artery can result in kinking and occlusion (see Fig. 6).

Understanding the biomechanics of the SFA and the effects of swirling flow have led to the development of a new generation of biomimetic stents.

Supera Stent

The Supera stent (Idev Technologies, Webster, TX) is a self-expanding nitinol stent with six pairs of interwoven nitinol wires in a closed-cell configuration (see Fig. 6). The Supera stent has biomimetic properties that confer higher radial strength, while enabling the stent to flex, bend, and otherwise move with the vessel so as to distribute the stress more evenly. In a recently published registry of 107 patients with complex SFA disease, freedom from restenosis by duplex ultrasonography was 85% at 12 months and 76% at 24 months.[30]

Among the 91 patients with follow-up X-rays, there were no stent fractures. These data suggest that newer nitinol stent designs may be associated with

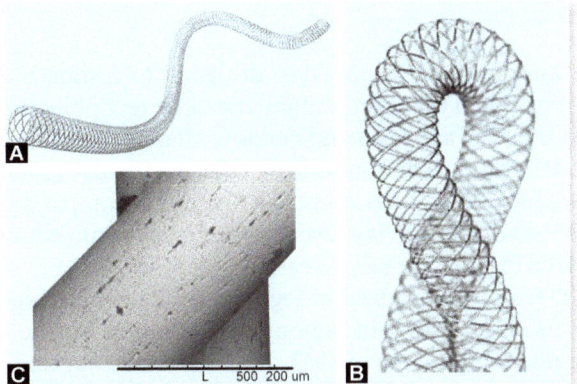

Figure 8: (A) The Supera interwoven nitinol stent is able to conform to the forces during movement in the superficial femoral and popliteal arteries; (B) A magnified image of the stent structure illustrating the degree of conformability; (C) Electron microscopy demonstrating a single nitinol wire (objective magnification 500×; scale bar = 200 μm).[31]

significantly lower rates of stent fracture, with associated lower rates of restenosis and stent failure. Optimal deployment of the Supera stent is critically dependent on accurate assessment of vessel diameter and vessel preparation. If the vessel is smaller in calibre than the selected stent size, or not adequately prepared with predilation to the same diameter as the outer dimension of the stent, the Supera may elongate during deployment. Such elongation may be associated with loss of both radial strength, precision in placement and stent failure (Fig. 8).[31]

BioMimics 3D Stent

The BioMimics 3D stent (Veryan Medical Ltd) is a *bio*mimetic stent that, by design, imparts curvature, generates swirling flow, and leads to a vasoprotective environment. The self-expanding stent is laser cut from a nitinol tube and has 3D helical centreline geometry set into the nitinol shape memory. The gentle transition of the BioMimics 3D stent, from the gradually reducing radial force of the end three crowns of the stent and the native artery, is specifically designed to reduce micro trauma, abnormal localised flow patterns, and kinking that could otherwise lead to restenosis, new atherosclerosis, and occlusion.

The MIMICS study is a prospective, 2:1, randomized, controlled trial conducted at eight German investigational centres with an independent imaging core lab comparing the safety and efficacy of the BioMimics 3D stent with a standard nitinol stent. The proportion of patients treated with the helical stent who maintained patency at 12 and 24 months was 80% and 72%, respectively, compared with 71% and 55% for the control group. The difference was significant through 24 months ($P = 0.05$). Freedom from clinically driven target lesion revascularization for the helical compared with straight stent was 91% versus 92% at 12 months and 91% versus 76% at 24 months.[40]

What to Expect?

Meaningful randomised trials need to designed to compare the emerging technologies with each other rather than the older technologies. The current focus of trials is device approval and needs to change to device superiority.

The REAL PTX study will randomize patients with SFA disease to either a DCB or DES. This trial will represent the first direct comparison of DCBs to DES in the SFA and will provide a very useful insight into when to choose a DCB versus DES for treating SFA disease.

The RAPID (randomised trial of leg flow paclitaxel eluting balloon and stenting versus standard plain balloon and stenting for the treatment of intermediate and long lesions of SFA) should increase our understanding of the role of DCBs in long SFA lesions.

BASIL-3 is a multi-centre randomised controlled trial of clinical and cost-effectiveness of drug-coated balloons, drug-eluting stents and plain balloon angioplasty with bail-out bare metal stent revascularisation strategies for severe limb ischaemia due to femoro-popliteal disease. Patients will be randomised, to have either a Plain Balloon Angioplasty with a Bare Metal Stent (if needed) or Drug Coated Balloon with a Bare Metal Stent (if needed) or a Drug Eluting Stent.[41]

CONCLUSION

- Anatomic location, varying stresses and highly calcific disease pattern in the SFA by far are the most important factors affecting long-term results of therapy.
- There is an on-going swing towards `endovascular first` therapy in the treatment of the SFA disease.
- Current role of primary surgery remains unclear in most practices.
- Adequate antiplatelet therapy post intervention is essential for long-term patency.
- The current role of POBA should be restricted to treating short length lesions due to the rates of re-intervention.
- DCBs should become the first-line strategy for treatment of SFA. For complex lesions DCB followed by BMS or primary use of DES should be considered (Fig. 9).
- Health economic evaluation of drug eluting technology shows definite advantage in the long run. This `spent now to save later` approach might pose a problem in the Indian medical scenario where patients fund most of the treatment on their own.
- Biomimetic technology may provide an interesting solution to the SFA conundrum.
- With newer technologies (atherectomy, cryoLASER, biomimetic stents) cost is a major deterring factor.
- Lack of randomised trials comparing new technologies with consistent end-points needs to be addressed to make an informed decision about the choice of therapy; drug, metal or more in the treatment of SFA disease.

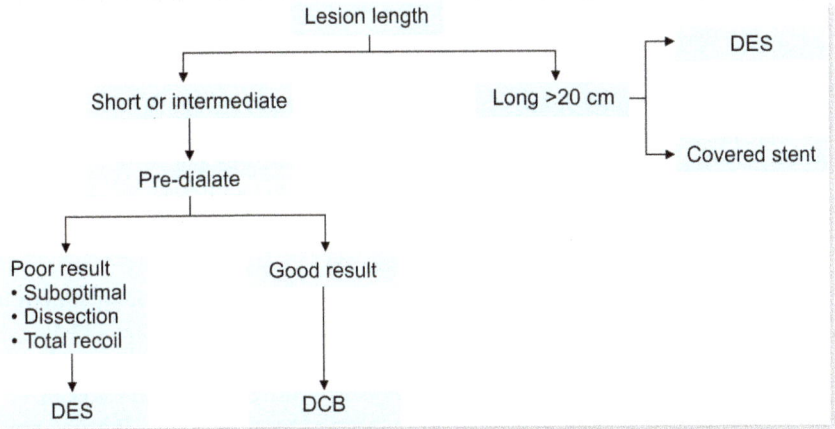

Figure 9: Suggested algorithm to manage the drug-eluting technology

REFERENCES

1. Laird JR, Katzen BT, Scheinert D, et al., RESILIENT Investigators. Nitinol stent implantation versus balloon angioplasty for lesions in the superficial femoral artery and proximal popliteal artery: twelve-month results from the RESILIENT randomized trial. Circ Cardiovasc Interv 2010;3:267-76.
2. Goodney PP, Beck AW, Nagle J, et al. RM. National trends in lower extremity bypass surgery, endovascular interventions, and major amputations. J Vasc Surg 2009;50:54-60.
3. Norgren L, Hiatt WR, Dormandy JA, Nehler MR, Harris KA, Fowkes FG. Inter-Society Consensus for the Management of Peripheral Arterial Disease (TASC II). J Vasc Surg. 2007;45 Suppl S:S5-67
4. Bradbury AW, et al. Bypass versus Angioplasty in Severe Ischaemia of the Leg (BASIL) trial: An intention-to-treat analysis of amputation-free and overall survival in patients randomized to a bypass surgery-first or a balloon angioplasty-first revascularization strategy. J Vasc Surg. 2010; 51:5S-17S.
5. Bradbury AW, et al. Bypass versus Angioplasty in Severe Ischaemia of the Leg (BASIL) trial: Analysis of amputation free and overall survival by treatment received. J Vasc Surg. 2010;51:18S-31S.
6. Laxdal E, et al: Subintimal angioplasty as a treatment of femoropopliteal artery occlusions. Eur J Vasc Endovasc Surg. 2003;25:578-82.
7. Hynes N, et al. Subintimal angioplasty as a primary modality in the management of critical limb ischemia: comparison to bypass grafting for aortoiliac and femoropopliteal occlusive disease. J Endovasc Ther. 2004;11:460-71.
8. Desgranges P, et al: Subintimal angioplasty: feasible and durable. Eur J Vasc Endovasc Surg. 2004;28:138-41.
9. Myers KA: Reporting standards and statistics for evaluating intervention. Cardiovasc Surg. 1995;3:455-61.
10. Florenes T, et al: Subintimal angioplasty in the treatment of patients with intermittent claudication: long term results. Eur J Vasc Endovasc Surg. 2004;28: 645-50.

11. Rutherford's Vascular Surgery, 2-Volume Set, 8th Edition Jack L. Cronenwett, MD and K. Wayne Johnston, MD, FRCSC ISBN: 978-1-4557-5304-8.
12. Jeans WD, Amstrong S, Cole SE, et al. Fate of patients undergoing transluminal angioplasty for lower-limb ischemia. Radiology. 1990;177: 559-64.
13. Blair JM, Gewertz BL, Moosa H, et al. Percutaneous transluminal angioplasty versus surgery for limb-threatening ischemia. J Vasc Surg. 1989;9:698.
14. Jamsen T, Manninen H, Tulla H, et al. The final outcome of primary infrainguinal percutaneous transluminal angioplasty in 100 consecutive patients with chronic critical limb ischemia. J Vasc Interv Radiol. 2002;13:455-63.
15. Muradin GS, et al. Balloon dilation and stent implantation for treatment of femoropopliteal arterial disease: meta-analysis. Radiology. 2001;221:137-45.
16. Johnston KW, Rae M, Hogg-Johnston SA, et al. Five-year results of a prospective study of percutaneous transluminal angioplasty. Ann Surg. 1987;206:403-13.
17. Bolia A, Bell PRF. Femoropopliteal and crural artery recanalization using subintimal angioplasty. Semin Vasc Surg. 1995;8:253-64.
18. Krankenberg H, Schluter M, Steinkamp HJ, et al. Nitinol stent implantation versus percutaneous transluminal angioplasty in superficial femoral artery lesions up to 10 cm in length: The Femoral Artery Stenting Trial (FAST). Circulation. 2007; 116:285-92.
19. Schillinger M, Sabeti S, Dick P, et al. Sustained benefit at 2 years of primary femoropopliteal stenting compared with balloon angioplasty with optional stenting. Circulation. 2007;115:2745-9.
20. Katzen B. Resilient trial. Presented at the International Symposium on Endovascular Therapy meeting Jan 22, Miami: Florida; 2008.
21. Bosiers M, et al. Nitinol stent implantation in long superficial femoral artery lesions: 12-month results of the DURABILITY I study. J Endovasc Ther. 2009;16:261-9.
22. Duda SH, et al. Sirolimus-eluting stents for the treatment of obstructive superficial femoral artery disease: six-month results. Circulation. 2002;106:1505-09.
23. Duda SH, et al. Sirolimus-eluting versus bare nitinol stent for obstructive superficial femoral artery disease: the SIROCCO II trial. J Vasc Interv Radiol. 2005;16: 331-8.
24. Dake MD, et al. Paclitaxel-eluting stents show superiority to balloon angioplasty and bare metal stents in femoropopliteal disease: twelve-month Zilver PTX randomized study results. Circ Cardiovasc Interv. 2011;4:495-504.
25. Dake M. The Zilver PTX randomized trial of treating femoropopliteal artery disease: 5-year results. Presented at: Vascular Interventional Advances (VIVA); November 4-7, 2014; Las Vegas, NV.
26. McQuade K, Gable D, Pearl G, Theune B, Black S. Four-year randomized prospective comparison of percutaneous ePTFE/nitinol self-expanding stent graft versus prosthetic femoral-popliteal bypass in the treatment of superficial femoral artery occlusive disease. J Vasc Surg. 2010;52:584-90; discussion 590-1.
27. Saxon RR. Heparin bonded stent-grafts in the SFA: VIPER one-year results. Paper presented at: International Symposium on Endovascular Therapy; January 18, 2012; Miami, FL.
28. Lammer J. Randomized trials of bare metal stents vs. covered stents in the SFA. Paper presented at: International Symposium on Endovascular Therapy; January 18, 2012; Miami, FL.

29. Bosiers M. RELINE study: Randomized comparison of endoluminal grafting with Viabahn vs. PTA for femoral artery in-stent restenosis—6 months results. Paper presented at: Leipzig Interventional Course; January 28-31, 2014; Leipzig, Germany.
30. Krankenberg H, Tübler T, Ingwersen M, et al. Drug-coated balloon versus standard balloon for superficial femoral artery in-stent restenosis: the randomized femoral artery in-stent restenosis (FAIR) trial. Circulation. 2015;132:2230-6.
31. Tepe G, Schnorr B, Albrecht T, et al. Angioplasty of femoral-popliteal arteries with drug-coated balloons: 5-year follow-up of the THUNDER trial. JACC Cardiovasc Interv. 2015;8(Pt A):102-8.
32. Rosenfield K, Jaff MR, White CJ, et al. Trial of a paclitaxel-coated balloon for femoropopliteal artery disease. N Engl J Med. 2015;373:145-53.
33. Tepe G, Laird J, Schneider P, et al. Drug-coated balloon versus standard percutaneous transluminal angioplasty for the treatment of superficial femoral and popliteal peripheral artery disease: 12-month results from the IN.PACT SFA randomized trial. Circulation. 2015;131:495-502.
34. Fanelli F, Cannavale A, Gazzetti M, et al. Calcium burden assessment and impact on drug-eluting balloons in peripheral arterial disease. Cardiovasc Intervent Radiol. 2014;37:898-907.
35. Kearns BC, Michaels JA, Stevenson MD, et al. Cost-effectiveness analysis of enhancements to angioplasty for infrainguinal arterial disease. Br J Surg. 2013;100:1180-8.
36. Katsanos K, Geisler BP, Garner AM, et al. Economic analysis of endovascular drug-eluting treatments for femoropopliteal artery disease in the UK. BMJ Open 2016;6: e011245.
37. Zeller T, et al: Long-term results after directional atherectomy of femoro-popliteal lesions. J Am Coll Cardiol. 2006;48:1573-8.
38. Lam RC, Shah S, Faries PL, et al. Incidence and clinical significance of distal embolization during percutaneous interventions involving the superficial femoral artery. J Vasc Surg. 2007;46:1155-59.
39. Laird JR, et al. Limb salvage following laser-assisted angioplasty for critical limb ischemia: results of the LACI multicenter trial. J Endovasc Ther 2006;13:1-11.
40. Zeller T, Gaines P et al: Helical Centerline Stent Improves Patency: Two-Year Results From the Randomized Mimics Trial. Circulation: Cardiovascular Interventions. 2016; 9: e002930.
41. http://www.birmingham.ac.uk/research/activity/mds/trials/bctu/trials/portfolio-v/Basil-3/index.aspx

CHAPTER

7

Subintimal Angioplasty

Neghal Kandiyil, Amman Bolia

CLINICAL RELEVANCE

Patients with peripheral arterial disease (PAD) secondary to chronic occlusions of their infrainguinal vessels can present with claudication (IC) or critical limb ischaemia (CLI). CLI and IC ischaemia are clinical diagnoses; CLI is based on the presence of ischaemic rest pain or tissue loss, whilst IC is defined as an exertional symptom affecting muscles of the lower limb secondary to PAD. Many of these patients will require revascularisation to avoid amputation, which can be performed by open surgical or endovascular revascularisation. Surgical revascularisation in the form of a bypass utilises an autologous vein as a conduit and achieves good long-term limb salvage rates.[1] However, surgical bypass is expensive, with increased risk in a patient population that often has significant cardiorespiratory and renal comorbidities. These factors may also compromise wound healing in an ischaemic limb. Subintimal angioplasty (SIA) was first introduced in 1987 as a minimally invasive percutaneous technique for the treatment of femoropopliteal occlusive disease in patients with intermittent claudication (IC).[2] The early positive results encouraged the procedure to be extended to the popliteal artery and the trifurcation vessels, where it has proved to be invaluable as an alternative treatment to surgical bypass in the treatment of critical limb ischaemia.

There has been a significant amount of clinical data showing that SIA of femoropopliteal occlusive disease for claudication is effective and durable.[2-20] In chronic CLI, it has become the first-line treatment in many patients with this condition.[4, 5,19-29]

The low cost and ease of technique of SIA has allowed treatment of a significant population of patients with occlusive disease PVD. The treatment has application in long superficial femoral artery (SFA), popliteal, and tibial occlusions and has the ability to reconstitute bifurcations and trifurcations that would otherwise not be possible with surgery. Also, reconstitution of long tibial occlusions including the foot arch can be performed, which would otherwise not be possible with surgery. In the treatment of CLI, subintimal angioplasty has made a significant impact with limb salvage rates between 70% and 94%.[27,29] In patients with claudication, primary-assisted patency rates of upto 64% at 5 years have been reported,[18] similar to those achieved by surgical bypass.[30]

INDICATIONS

Critical limb ischaemia due to occlusive arterial disease is the main indication. In our uni, SIA is also performed for short distance claudication due to occlusive disease, after conservative measures have failed, i.e. program of exercise and advice regarding lifestyle change.

Here are examples of where subintimal angioplasty is best performed (Figs 1 to 10):

1. Chronic femoropopliteal and tibial occlusions that have become hard and calcified, thus making it impossible for the guidewire to be negotiated through an "intraluminal" approach. A subintimal dissection plane is relatively easy to create in these situations.
2. Long occlusions of the femoropopliteal and tibial arteries, where it would be difficult to maintain an intraluminal position of the guidewire.
3. Previously failed intraluminal attempts at angioplasty may be suitable for a subintimal approach.
4. In proximal SFA occlusions in which there may be a very small stump or a flush occlusion; an intraluminal approach in these situations is difficult, if not impossible.
5. The presence of a large collateral vessel proximal to an occlusion that lacks a stump, which is necessary to engage the guidewire for transluminal angioplasty. This situation can be dealt with by creating a subintimal dissection above the collateral, thus avoiding persistent wire entry into the collateral.
6. One clear example of the benefit of SIA over surgery is that a popliteal occlusion which extends into the trifurcation vessels can be treated with subintimal angioplasty. Most of the time recanalisation of all three run off vessels can be achieved.
7. Subintimal Angioplasty can bail you out of trouble. If an arterial perforation occurs during attempted intraluminal crossing of an occlusion; a subintimal dissection above the perforation can avoid the site of the perforation by negotiating the plane of dissection away from the site of the perforation.
8. It has been shown that SIA can recanalise native SFA occlusions in patients who have undergone femoropopliteal bypass grafting that have subsequently occluded.[31,32] Similarly, tibial occlusions can be recanalised after failure of a femoro-distal bypass graft.[32]
9. In patients who are not fit for a CFA/SFA endarterectomy. Recanalisation of both these vessels may be achieved by the subintimal approach, thus reconstituting the bifurcation.

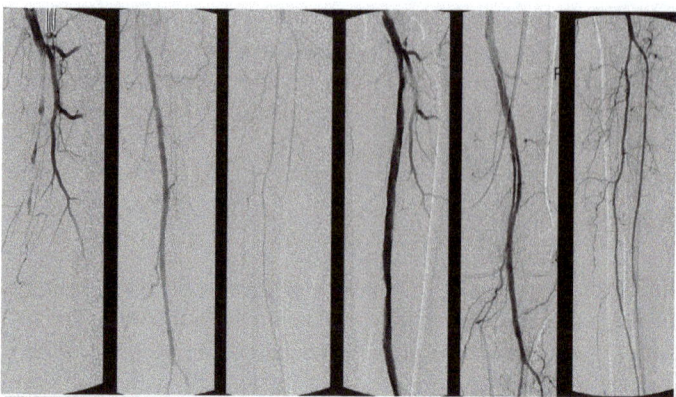

Figure 1: There is a near full-length occlusion of the SFA, reconstituting at the adductor canal level. This was successfully recanalised. Notice the dissection flap just above the knee joint level, which is where re-entry was achieved

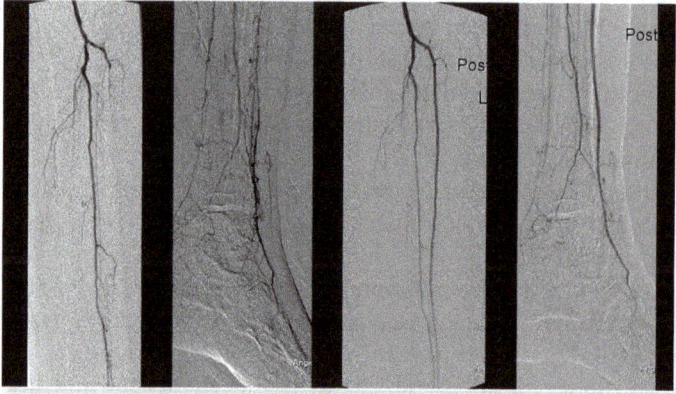

Figure 2: A long occlusion of the anterior tibial artery has been recanalised

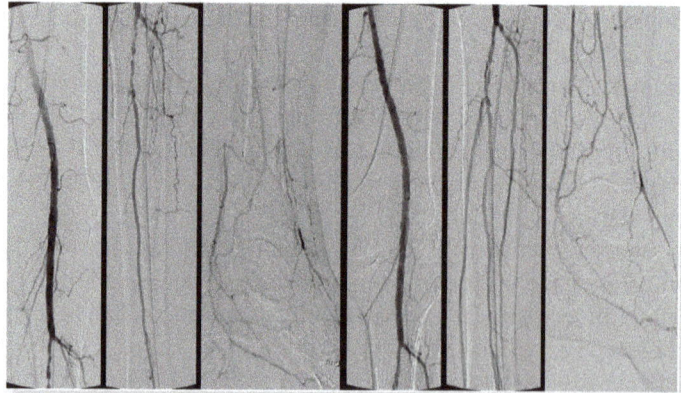

Figure 3: There is some disease in the tibioperoneal trunk, a long occlusion of the Anterior tibial and a full-length occlusion of the posterior tibial artery. All the lesions were successfully treated

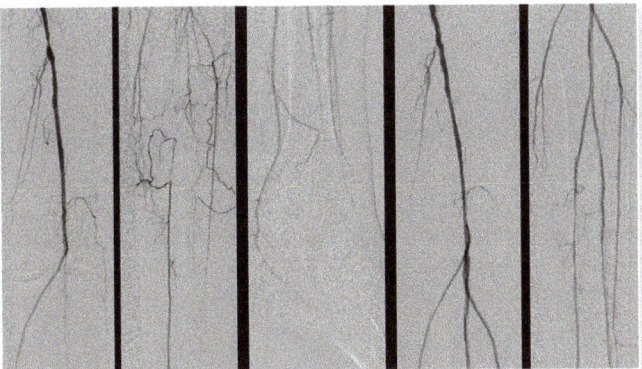

Figure 4: There is a popliteal occlusion extending from mid-popliteal level into all three run-off vessels. The trifurcation has been reconstituted

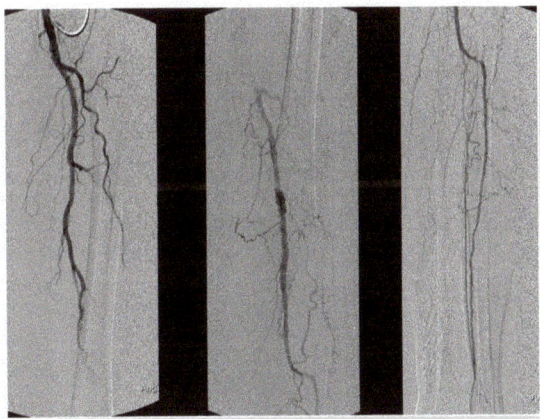

Figure 5: There is a flush occlusion of the SFA, upto the adductor canal level

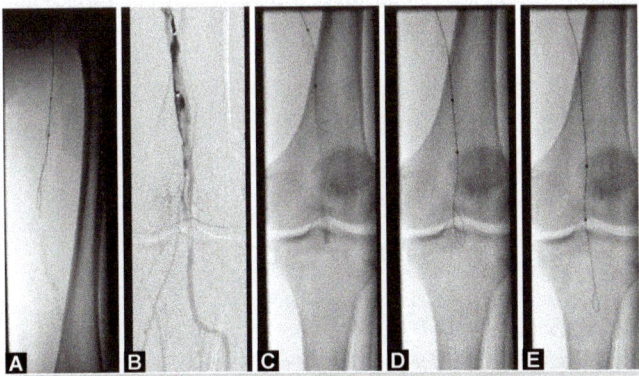

Figures 6: (A) A loop is seen in the middle of the SFA occlusion seen in Figure 5, (B) Contrast injection in the subintimal space shows some communication to the true lumen just beyond the knee joint level, (C) There is a pocket of remnant contrast in the subintimal channel seen just beyond the knee joint level, (D) Wire loop is seen within the 'pocket', (E) Following entry into the true lumen, the loop diameter can be seen, narrower than when in the subintimal space. At this point, the loop will be felt to move completely freely

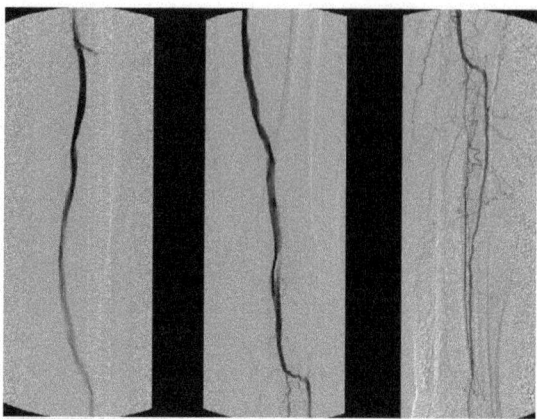

Figure 7: Final result of the recanalised SFA occlusion seen in Figure 5. Dissection flap can be seen above the point of re-entry

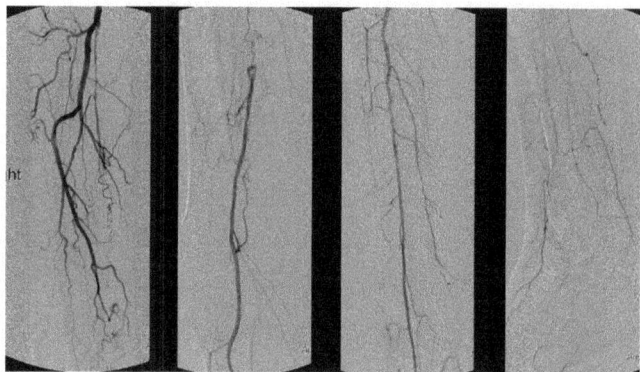

Figure 8: There is a long SFA occlusion and one vessel run-off, being the peroneal artery. All 3 run-off vessels are available at the ankle level

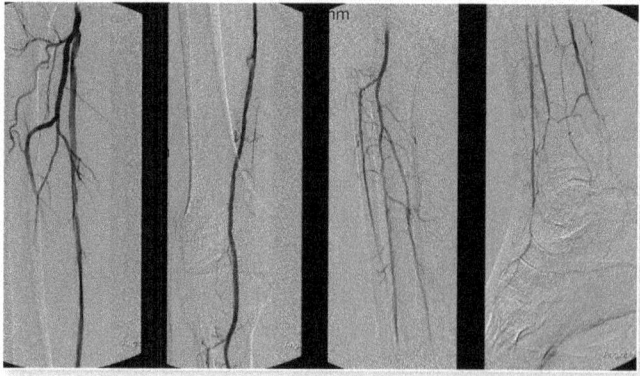

Figure 9: As well as the SFA, the anterior and posterior tibial arteries shown in Figure 8 have been recanalised to achieve the best haemodynamics, and faster flow, which aids patency on the recanalised SFA

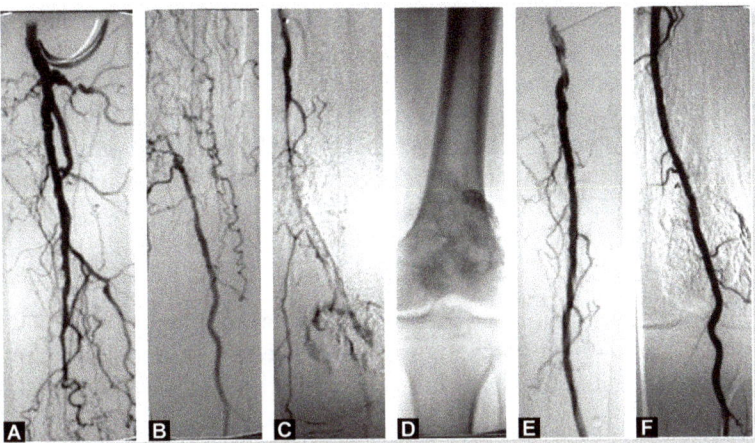

Figure 10: (A and B) show a 5 cm distal SFA occlusion; (C and D) Show that a large perforation occurred, (E and F) The subintimal approach enabled an alternative dissection (away from the perforation site) and a successful outcome was achieved

CONTRAINDICATIONS

1. Fresh occlusions (less than 3 months old); subintimal and intraluminal angioplasties are unlikely to be successful. This is due to the softness of the thrombus, which fails to be displaced when the lumen is being reestablished with a balloon. Any such attempt of angioplasty significantly increases the risk for distal embolism.
   It is important to elicit a careful history from the patient, so that any evidence of sudden worsening of symptoms should alert one to the possibility of a fresh thrombus. In these situations, a duplex scan may confirm the presence of a fresh thrombus with the demonstration of echolucency of the occluding material. CT-angiogram in certain instances may give you clues to acute emboli; contrast surrounding a filling defect, 'rimming effect' is a specific finding for acute emboli. Subacute thrombus is more difficult to characterize on CT and also well developed collaterals may give you a false impression of a chronic thrombus, as most of these acute/subacute lesions have an underlying stenosis.
   A very good indicator of acute/subacute thrombus is a positive "guidewire test," an easy passage of the guidewire through the occluding material, will indicate the presence of a soft thrombus and therefore unfavorable occlusion for recanalisation. Also, under fluoroscopy, contrast injected above the occlusion can show this rimming effect or a typical cut off appearance of contrast.
2. In patients who have a popliteal aneurysm, there is significant immediate or delayed risk of vessel perforation, if an occlusion with a popliteal aneurysm is crossed with a subintimal technique.
3. Heavy calcification or fine cylindrical arterial calcification, as seen in renal failure or long-term diabetic patients, can be problematic in subintimal angioplasty. Whilst it is usually not difficult to initiate a dissection, it is very

difficult to re-enter the true lumen distally due to this form of calcification. This is where re-entry devices such as the OUTBACK™ Re-entry catheter (Cordis) or Pioneer Plus catheter (Medtronic) are useful.

When re-entry has been achieved in these calcified vessels, the chances of re-coil are fairly high and may result in an unfavorable outcome. This will require prolonged inflation or if flow limiting, reinforcement with stents.

EQUIPMENT

Angiography equipment with high quality digital subtraction and road map facilities using a 40 cm image intensifier are desirable. Good zooming and magnification facilities the procedure, particularly when working in the small vessels of the foot.

The technique is requires minimum amount of materials and is very cost effective.

The equipment needed:
1. A standard Teflon-coated, 0.035-inch, 180-cm-long guidewire is used for entry into the artery through the needle.
2. Once entry has been achieved and a catheter introduced, the wire is substituted for a hydrophilic wire (Terumo) in either standard or stiff format, depending on the nature of the lesion. Once again, these wires are 0.035-inch in diameter, 180-cm long with a curved tip and a 3-cm floppy end.
3. The most widely used catheter, particularly for flush occlusions where there is no available stump or only a small stump, is the 4-Fr short angled catheter ('Bolia Mini-cath', Terumo Medical Corporation, Tokyo, Japan) which comes in a 20-cm length with a 30 or 60° curved tip. Similar-shaped catheters, for example Bernstein (Boston Scientific, Natick Massachusetts, USA), vertebral, or Vanchi 2 catheter (Cook) may also be used. However, the advantage of the Bolia Mini-cath is two-fold; firstly, being 4-Fr and short in length, it facilitates entry into the common femoral artery when there is only a short length of wire engaged within the vessel. Secondly, the Bolia Mini-cath is easier to handle and manipulate than the longer catheters, particularly important when entering the origin of the SFA or initiating a dissection at this level through an ipsilateral antegrade common femoral artery puncture.
4. Two most commonly used balloons are a 5 mm × 4 cm with a length of 80 cm for the femoropopliteal segment, and a 3 mm × 2 cm with a length of 135 cm for infra-popliteal disease. Both these balloon catheters are used in a 5-Fr format; necessary to overcome resistance offered by long length occlusions in the infra-inguinal and infra-popliteal segments. A simple inflation device consisting of a 10-ml high-pressure syringe with a flow switch is used for quick inflations and deflations.
5. If small vessels in the foot are encountered, re-entry may be achieved with a 0.018 hydrophilic wire using a Glidewire Advantage (Terumo), which comes in a 180- or 300-cm length. Another stiffer wire V-18™ or V-14™ wire (Boston scientific) that may be useful in narrow caliber calcified tibial and foot vessels.

6. Closure device; a closure device is most useful in patients who have had tibial angioplasty of a long Tibial occlusion, as prolonged manual compression of the groin will reduce the flow into the tibial vessel and may cause re-occlusion. The authors currently prefer Exoseal (Cordis) or an Angioseal (St Jude Medical) vascular closure device, unless contraindicated.

Medication

Most patients who undergo these procedures are pretreated with aspirin, 75–150 mg/day. Heparin, 3000 to 5000 international units (IU), is used during the procedure. In tibial occlusions; a vasodilator Tolazoline (a non-selective competitive α-adrenergic receptor antagonist) can also be given intra-arterially in a dose of 5 mg before crossing a lesion and usually 5 mg at the conclusion of the procedure to prevent vasospasm. When vasospasm does occur, Glyceryl trinitrate (GTN) is used in 100 µg increments upto a total dose of 500 µg. The authors also recommend a GTN patch that is applied to the foot for the treated leg to deliver 5 mg of GTN over a 24-hour period, after the treatment of the infra-popliteal vessels. This sustains vasodilation, especially in the capillary vessels and improves the flow in the immediate post-procedure period.

TECHNIQUE

Anatomy and Approach of SIA

Access into the Artery

SIA has its main application in the femoropopliteal and tibial arteries. As there is a need for increased force to get past the occlusion, an ipsilateral antegrade puncture is important; unless there is a specific reason to the contrary. Relative contraindications for antegrade puncture include a high common femoral artery bifurcation, scarring from previous surgery, infection at puncture site or severe obesity where an antegrade puncture may be difficult. In these instances, a crossover from the contralateral CFA or a popliteal approach is more appropriate.

The puncture is usually directed at the mid to lower part of the common femoral artery. This can be performed with either ultrasound or with palpation. With palpation, one can work out the length of common femoral artery that is available for puncture (the part of the artery that is overlying the superior pubic ramus, against which it will have to be compressed at the conclusion of the procedure). As a general guide, the mid-portion of the common femoral artery is approximately at the level of the mid-portion of the femoral head. For flush occlusions or when there is only a small stump of the SFA, a high common femoral puncture is recommended. The site of puncture is determined by the level of the upper brim of the superior pubic ramus at which pulsations of the artery can be felt. The artery superior to this level will be the external iliac artery and must not be punctured or the chance of retroperitoneal bleeding will be increased. The high puncture will therefore have to be directed about 1 cm or so below the palpable brim of the superior pubic ramus. A puncture at this level will mean that there is at least 1.5 to 2 cm of the common femoral artery (CFA) before it bifurcates, thus allowing the Bolia Mini-cath to be positioned for manipulation into the SFA origin occlusion. It cannot be emphasized enough the importance of a correctly sited puncture; the authors opt to check the position of the puncture relative to the femoral bifurcation and superior pubic ramus by injecting contrast through the puncture needle prior to the introduction of a guidewire.

Depending on the operator's experience, an ultrasound can alternately be used to precisely puncture 1.5 to 2 cm from the bifurcation. Ultrasound has specific advantages over the palpation technique; it allows you to avoid areas where calcified plaque can make advancement of the wire troublesome. Also, ultrasound can prevent posterior wall puncture and avoid small branch vessel perforation, therefore reducing the complication rate of pseudoaneurysms.[33]

Cannulating the SFA

After a correct high puncture, a standard Teflon-coated guidewire is advanced, where it usually enters the profunda artery. An angled 4-Fr short catheter (Bolia Mini-cath) is advanced over guidewire. Do not place an introducer sheath at this time as it will make it difficult to access the SFA. A diagnostic angiogram is carried out through this catheter position to outline the full length of the occlusion and all the vessels down to the foot. It is important to obtain a detailed diagnostic study, so that should a complication occur, such as embolism, one has an exact idea of which vessels were patent pre-intervention and which vessels have occluded post-intervention. Heparin, 3000 IU, is injected intra-arterially as soon as the decision for angioplasty of the artery is made, a further 2000 IU of heparin can be given if procedural time is prolonged.

With an appropriate oblique projection (right anterior oblique for a right SFA occlusion) and small puffs of contrast material, the catheter tip is slowly withdrawn from the profunda artery into the common femoral artery. The tip of the catheter is directed away from the profunda to the occluded SFA origin. Then, with the use of a road map facility, a curved hydrophilic guidewire is advanced into the origin of the SFA when a small stump is available. If no stump is available, one will usually have an idea of where the origin of the SFA should be, at the level where the profunda artery dips downward away from the line of the common femoral artery as seen on the appropriate oblique projection. An angled hydrophilic guidewire is then run along the junction of the common femoral and profunda arteries. Usually, the wire will be seen to engage at the origin of the SFA. Once engagement is achieved, the wire is advanced into the occlusion, and if necessary, the Mini-cath is positioned at the entry point of the SFA to provide support, so that the wire can enter the occlusion rather than being pushed away from it.

Crossing the Occlusion

After the wire has entered the occlusion, the Mini-cath is advanced into the occlusion and the wire is then manipulated into a loop. The loop is advanced

5 to 10 cm further, and when this position is achieved, the purpose of the Mini-cath is over, and it is replaced by a balloon catheter which is usually 5 or 6 mm in diameter x 4 cm in length on an 80 cm shaft. The loop is then advanced further, with the balloon catheter following immediately behind it. When the loop stops advancing, the balloon catheter is advanced towards the leading edge of the loop for support, which will allow the loop to be advanced further. The length of the loop is shortened every so often, and when the end of the occlusion is reached, the length of the loop must be 5 cm or less. A little twisting and forward action allows re-entry to be achieved in the distal part of the artery, and in most cases this takes place without effort (Fig. 6). If the loop fails to re-enter the artery, it is usually due to diffuse disease beyond the end of the occlusion. In such situations the dissection can be extended further until the disease free part of the artery is reached, where the loop has its most favourable situation for re-entry. There is a natural tendency for the loop to re-enter at the junction between the diseased and non-diseased segment of the artery (the line of "demarcation"). It is important to mentally mark the level beyond which one does not want a subintimal channel to extend, at the time of the baseline angiogram. For Femoropopliteal occlusion, extension of the subintimal tract into the below knee popliteal artery puts the runoff vessel patency at risk and unless they are also occluded it should be avoided. Also, by crossing the below knee popliteal artery, you can compromise the surgical option of a finite element method (FEM)—below knee popliteal bypass. The authors recommend withdrawing the guidewire and re-attempting to re-enter the true lumen proximally should this occur. Failure to re-enter using standard techniques may result in a re-entry device being employed. (See below).

Recanalisation of the Artery

Once the entire length of the occlusion has been crossed the balloon is inflated from the distal part to the proximal part of the occlusion. High-pressure (10 to 12 atm) but short inflations are carried out throughout the length of the occlusion. The balloon is usually inflated twice, once from distal to proximal and then from proximal to distal part of the occlusion. The balloon catheter is then positioned beyond the occlusion before the guidewire is taken out. Injection of contrast material through the catheter will confirm rapid flow in the distal vessels beyond the recanalised segment, which is a measure of a successful outcome. The catheter is gradually withdrawn to a level proximal to the recanalised segment, and during withdrawal, small puffs of contrast material are used to ensure that the channel is open and flowing. A final angiogram of the newly recanalised segment is carried out. Although the recanalised segment almost invariably appears smooth and disease free, the measure of a successful outcome is usually determined by the speed of flow rather than cosmetic appearances. A completion angiogram of the distal vessels ensures that if any emboli have been released, they will be detected and dealt with appropriately. At the conclusion of the procedure a further dose of tolazoline (5 mg) can be given to facilitate peripheral vasodilation and reduce peripheral resistance. It helps to enhance flow through the recanalised segment. Aspirin, if not contraindicated, is prescribed for patients who have undergone successful recanalisation, the usual dose being 150 mg daily for 3 months tailored to 75 mg/day thereafter indefinitely. Some authors opt for dual anti-platelet therapy with the addition of Clopidogrel (75 mg/day) or Ticlopidine (500 mg/day) for 1 month post-procedure. This regime may be of benefit, particularly in those patients with known aspirin resistance.

Subintimal Angioplasty of the Tibial Vessels

Tibial occlusions can be treated by subintimal angioplasty using a similar technique (Figs 2 to 4). Generally, short occlusions are usually easily crossed intraluminally, but subintimal angioplasty can be used for longer occlusions (>3 cm) or if difficult to cross intraluminally. In tibial occlusive disease, it is important to use a 0.035-inch guidewire and balloon catheter with a 5-Fr shaft. The larger guidewire and catheters are needed when a long tibial occlusion must be crossed, such as an occlusion 30 cm long. The 0.035 system overcomes the resistance of the long occlusion, and this system has enough strength in the system to a allow progression of the catheter-wire combination throughout the length of the occlusion. The system can be further strengthened with the use of a stiff hydrophilic guidewire if necessary. The most popular balloon catheter for this procedure is one with a 3 mm diameter, 2 cm long balloon on a 135 cm long 5-Fr shaft. However, if the vessels in the foot are of narrow caliber, you can exchange for a 0.018 or 0.014 system (V-18TM or V-14™ wire-Boston scientific or Terumo GLIDEWIRE ADVANTAGE® Guidewire) before re-entry into these pedal vessels.

Once again, the aim is to form a loop in the hydrophilic guidewire that allows one to cross the entire length of the lesion with minimal risk of perforation. In addition, from experience, this loop is desirable for achieving dissection throughout the length of the tibial artery and also for achieving re-entry back into the true lumen distally. Because the intima becomes thinner as the distal arterial tree is approached, it is usually not difficult to re-enter the true lumen in the distal tibial artery. However, it is important to keep the length of the loop short, so that the softer part (floppy tip) of the guidewire forms the leading edge of the loop and therefore reduces the chance of perforation in these small delicate vessels. Once the lesion is crossed, the catheter or balloon is advanced into this area, the wire is removed and a small volume of contrast is injected to see if the catheter tips is within the dissection (contrast accumulates with no flow) or the catheter/balloon tips is in the true lumen (rapid flow away in normal vessel) there is rapid flow in vessel. Once true lumen is confirmed, a more secure guidewire is placed (Teflon standard wire 0.035) and balloon dilation is performed.

In cases where there is a long femoropopliteal occlusion with concomitant trifurcation occlusive disease, a single vessel runoff it is of vital importance for true-lumen re-entry to occur (Fig. 4). This does not necessarily occur using the standard aforementioned technique as the guidewire will have a natural tendency to take the path of least resistant which does not always equate to the least diseased crural vessel. Therefore, you can direct the wire into the main crural vessel by using an angled catheter, the authors use the vertebral catheter (Terumo, Radifocus® Angiographic Catheter). This technique rarely fails, but if this occurs a retrograde puncture in the distal crural vessels can be performed. The crural vessel occlusion can be crossed using an 0.018 wire with the above technique. Another solution to the problem has been addressed with Subintimal Arterial Flossing with Antegrade-Retrograde Intervention (SAFARI by Spinosa et al.)[34] This technique has not been used by the authors and therefore is not described in this chapter.

Re-entry Devices

Depending of level of experience, subintimal revascularisation of chronically occluded femoropopliteal or crural vessels has an associated with a failure rate between 10-15%.[35,36] The main limitation is the failure to re-enter the distal true lumen after crossing the occlusion subintimally. You should always have in mind the area where you should stop the subintimal dissection; otherwise you risk the patency of the crural vessels and risk ruining a potential surgical option. Also, Inadvertent lengthening of the subintimal dissection may itself cause complications including loss of patent branches and collaterals distal to the treated occlusion.

Re-entry devices are a valuable tool to re-enter the true lumen. The two most commonly used re-entry devices are the Outback LTD Re-Entry Catheter (Cordis Corp, NJ, USA) and the Pioneer catheter (Medtronic Inc, Minnesota, USA) recently updated to the Pioneer Plus Catheter Plus 120. The Outback catheter is a 120 cm single-lumen, over-the-wire (0.014-inch), 6-Fr compatible system that uses simple orthogonally orientated radio-opaque nose-cone markers allowing fluoroscopically targeted true lumen re-entry with a 22G nitinol cannula. The Pioneer Plus catheter is a 6-Fr compatible dual-lumen, over-the-wire (0.014') device that utilizes intra-vascular ultrasound to direct the housed re-entry needle into the true lumen.

The Outback device is the most commonly used device, and there is good evidence of its success, by a systematic review of all Outback device literature. The pooled Outback catheter success rate was 90% (95% CI of 85-94)[19] with only a complication rate of approximately 4% (95% CI 1.6 to 8.3%), which included one death from late bleeding and ensuing myocardial infarction, minor bleeding, flow limiting dissection and perforation. Interestingly, more than 40% of limbs had a residual stenosis >30% at the end of the procedure, with the majority of these needing stenting. This most likely reflects the heavy burden of calcified disease evident within this patient sub-population.

The main limitation of the device is its cost, with Outback LTD and Pioneer catheter costing approximately $1750 and $3000, respectively. The Pioneer system requires the added cost of a separate ultrasound console and expertise in using intravascular ultrasound. Although, even with these prices, the cost of a surgical bypass with the number of days stay in hospital usually justifies the use of this device.

POST-PROCEDURAL AND FOLLOW-UP CARE

Patients who have had SIA do not need any special attention when compared to conventional angioplasty. Most patients are taking aspirin at the start of the procedure, but if they are not taking it. They should receive 150 mg/day for at least 3 months. During angioplasty, patients receive 3000 to 5000 IU of heparin, but do not receive any further anticoagulants after the procedure. If the procedure has involved the tibial vessels, it is preferable that patients be given a patch containing 5 mg of GTN that is released gradually over a period of 24 hours. The patch is normally applied to the treated foot.

If a high puncture has been made, we would almost always use an Angioseal (St Jude Medical, Minneapolis, MN). It is advisable to inform the nursing staff on the ward that a high puncture has been made and a keen eye should be kept on the patient's blood pressure and pulse. It the blood pressure fall or the pulse rise (or both), retroperitoneal bleeding may be a possibility and the medical staff must be informed promptly. In straightforward situations in which a high puncture has not been made, patients may start mobilisation after 4-6 hours of bed rest.

Patients are followed-up in an outpatient clinic for clinical assessment by a vascular surgeon. The history will usually reveal any improvement in claudication or critical limb ischaemia. A history and clinical examination are performed as a matter of routine 3 weeks and 3 months following the procedure, after which patients are discharged if all is well. Secondary patency rate can be improved with Duplex surveillance; any re-stenoses may be treatable with drug eluting balloons. Duplex scanning is recommended at 1, 3, 6, and 12 months after the procedure and then at yearly intervals.

Controversies, Complications and Outcomes of Subintimal Angioplasty

In the past, subintimal angioplasty was a controversial technique. This was mainly because of conventional teaching used to state all angioplasties must be performed intraluminally and if a dissection did occur, the procedure had to be terminated. This has proved incorrect, as subintimal angioplasty has been practiced for nearly 30 years, and when performed correctly has produced excellent results.

The preferred approach by the authors for subintimal angioplasty is an ipsilateral common femoral artery puncture to treat flush occlusions and all occlusions below this level. However, some advocate a crossover or a popliteal approach. The crossover approach is still necessary when either the ipsilateral groin is unavailable (scarring or infection) or the patient is grossly obese, and the antegrade approach would be difficult. It is worth noting that the crossover approach has disadvantages. Firstly, you will lose the feel of the guidewire and therefore one's ability to perform delicate manipulations is reduced. Secondly, you will lose the force required to get through very long and calcified occlusions. Thirdly, if an embolic complication occurs, it becomes difficult to perform percutaneous embolectomy. Also, a contralateral puncture puts unaffected leg at risk from the emboli and arterial damage.

The popliteal approach can be used if a contralateral access is difficult or an antegrade SFA occlusion has failed. It can be used to treat either flush occlusions, or occlusions with a large proximal collateral and no entry point. However, there are some significant disadvantages. Firstly, tibial vessel disease cannot be treated at the same time as the SFA lesion without having to make an additional puncture. This is particularly important in patients with critical limb ischaemia, who often have tandem lesions in the femoropopliteal and tibial arteries. Additionally, any embolic complication in which the embolus is located in the midportion of the popliteal artery or below would be impossible to aspirate percutaneously without having to make an additional puncture.

The use of an introducer sheath is the usually practice for percutaneous interventions. However, the majority of flush SFA occlusions can be treated successfully without the need to use an introducer sheath. The sheath can get in the way, if the flush SFA occlusion is near the puncture site and the proximal SFA cannot be treated adequately. Also, the sheath occupies space in the common femoral artery and can makes manipulations difficult.

There is continuing debate regarding the use of selective stenting, routine stenting with or without drug eluting stent, following subintimal recanalisation of femoropopliteal occlusions. Although the literature is inconclusive, we can extrapolate studies where the use of balloon-mounted stainless steel stents following successful intraluminal angioplasty that failed to demonstrate any benefit over angioplasty alone.[37,38] One study even found a detriment effect of increased occlusion rate with systematic stenting.[39] Conversely, recent studies including the Resilient trial report that for moderate length lesions in the femoropopliteal segment routine stenting is associated with improved patency than angioplasty alone.[40,41] These results may reflect improvement in stent design compared to the previous studies. However, it is important not to extrapolate intraluminal angioplasty studies to subintimal angioplasty. The key difference is that the new channel created between the intimal and medial vessel layers by SIA is devoid of endothelium and isolated from the intraluminal prothrombotic atheroma. This may in itself improve long-term patency rates without the need for stents as re-stenosis is frequently secondary to neo-intimal hyperplasia or atherosclerotic progression.

To date there are no randomized controlled trials comparing routine long stenting with subintimal angioplasty alone or selective stenting. However, there are comparative studies such as in Hong et al., where long stenting was an independent predictor of restenosis (hazard ratio [HR]: 2.0) compared to spot stenting after adjustment of confounding factors. Long stenting, especially involving the P2 or P3 segment of the popliteal artery, was independently associated with 7.5-fold increases in restenosis risk (p <0.001).[42] Another study by Treiman et al.[43] showed good short-term patency rates, but poor medium-term results (3 years and beyond) in 29 patients who underwent SIA and routine stenting for CLI secondary to femoropopliteal. In the authors view after reviewing the literature; only spot stenting should be employed where there is suboptimal haemodynamic flow. Stenting in these areas improves the angiographic appearance, and haemodynamic flow of a suboptimal SIA.

COMPLICATIONS

There are four main complications of subintimal angioplasty; vessel perforation, peripheral embolism, retroperitoneal bleeding after a high puncture, and elastic recoil. Most of these can be resolved percutaneously without a major adverse event.[44] The overall incidence of patients requiring surgery for a complication was ≤1%.

Perforation

Due to the more extensive nature of the procedure, perforation of an occluded segment during subintimal angioplasty appears marginally more common than with transluminal angioplasty (RR, 2.06; 95% CI, 1.19-3.56; $P = 0.01$).[44] Perforation can usually be successfully resolved by forming an alternative dissection tract proximal to the site of the perforation and on the contralateral side of the vessel and then performing the procedure in the standard way (Fig. 10).[45] This treats the perforation in two ways: First, it diverts the flow of blood along the path of least resistance away from the perforation and more distally into the leg. Second, the atheroma is shifted to the damaged side of the vessel, where it compresses the site of perforation.

If the perforation is large as assessed by substantial leakage of contrast material into the tissues, particularly in a hypertensive patient, it may be difficult to find an alternative dissection tract. In such situations, an embolisation coil is placed immediately above the site of the perforation to re-create the occlusion and stop the flow of blood into the perforation. The majority of these patients are then recalled for a repeat attempt, usually in a few weeks. Experience indicates that most of these patients achieve a successful outcome, and the presence of the embolisation coil does not hinder the procedure or affect the outcome.[46]

If perforation may occur during balloon dilation, initially a balloon Tamponade above or at the site of the perforation is used to create a seal. The balloon is inflated at low pressure (2 to 4 atmospheres) over a 2 to 3 minute period and repeated up to 4 times if necessary. In most cases, this may seal the perforation adequately, however if this method fails, a covered stent is deployed.

Embolism

The incidence of embolic complication occurs in about 5% of patients. The majority of these small emboli can be removed by percutaneous embolectomy with a large (8-Fr) non-tapered catheter (Angiomed) or (3-F CAT3, Indigo catheter) in the tibial vessels with a specialised 50-ml Luer lock suction syringe. If the embolus is large and fails to attach itself to the embolectomy catheter despite adequate suction, an alternative way of dealing with it is to "push and park." as described by Higginson.[47] This is only possible if there is more than one run-off vessel. The embolus can be pushed with either the already available non-tapered embolectomy catheter or a balloon catheter to advance it into one of the runoff vessels. Because the embolus is likely to advance down a straight line, it usually ends up in the peroneal artery, thus relieving one of the other vessels and allowing flow to continue down to the foot. Surgical embolectomy is rarely required after subintimal angioplasty, when using these techniques.

Retroperitoneal Haematoma

A flush occlusion of the SFA sometimes requires a high antegrade puncture of the common femoral artery. In these situations, the puncture should be high enough to allow manipulations, so that one can enter the SFA occlusion but not so high that the risk of retroperitoneal haematoma is increased. In our unit, nursing staff caring for the patient should be warned, so they can increase the frequency of patient observations. Also, a group and save is obtained, to expedite the need for urgent blood transfusions. We are increasingly using closure devices for high punctures, but we have to be wary that if the puncture is too high the angle that the artery dips in the pelvis can cause the closure device to fail. Closure devices have also proved useful for patients taking multiple antiplatelet agents, heparin and those that need to mobilize early.

Elastic Recoil

Elastic recoil is a physiological property in arteries, that allows these vessels to conform and become more resilient to movement in the legs.[48] Injured vessels, such as what occurs in angioplasty may undergo elastic recoil or negative remodeling, which results in loss of luminal dimensions without a further increase in neointimal area. The elastic recoil phenomenon is unpredictable. The segment of elastic recoil fails to remain open despite multiple balloon dilations, the distal limb will not receive any blood flow either from the recanalised segment or from the collaterals. In other words, the flow in the artery beyond the occluded segment becomes static and an emergency situation has been created. The focus of recoil can be ascertained by puffing small amounts of contrast along the artery length and confirming which segment caused the most stasis. The majority of these situations have been treated successfully by placement of a long self-expanding stent at the site of the occlusion, where the recoil is maximal. The incidence of this complication, where stenting is employed is 1% or less.

OUTCOMES

SIA has a sharp learning curve; our first 200 procedures demonstrated a technical success rate of 80%;[4] this increased to 90% in the subsequent 200 cases. Yilmaz et al. reported an initial technical success rate of 83% for the first 30 patients, 92% in the next 37, and 100% in the last 29.[7] This learning curve may explain the poorer results of SIA from centres with little experience with this technique. London et al. provided the first major report of the technique of subintimal angioplasty in 200 consecutive femoropopliteal artery occlusions with a mean length of 11 cm.[4] The technical success rate was 80%. The primary patency rate of technically successful procedures at 12 and 36 months was 71% and 58%, respectively, with the symptomatic patency rate being 73% and 61%, respectively. The majority of reports on the results of subintimal angioplasty quote a primary success rate of between 80% and 90%,[2,4,6,7,9,10,16,18,28,49] with the latter rate being more likely as experience increases.

Some of the best results thus far have been reported by Sultan et al., five year results[49] and Florenes et al.[18] Excellent patency rates in excess of 60% at 60 months follow-up have been demonstrated. The likely high success rate has been attributed to conscientious surveillance where restenoses could be diagnosed and treated early.

Subintimal angioplasty has made its greatest impact in critical limb ischaemia because it has a very effective role to play in the recanalisation of multiple long tibial artery occlusions, which is the predominant disease in patients with critical limb ischaemia.[22,24,26-28] Studies have reported limb salvage rates of 94% at 36 months in patients who had critical limb ischaemia and tibial vessel disease.[27] This is important in cases of CLI for which SIA may allow minor limb amputation of wounds or ulcers to heal, and provide time for improved collateralisation of the diseased arterial segment, thereby eliminating symptom recurrence if the recanalised segment should re-occlude.

KEY POINTS

- Subintimal angioplasty is effective and durable technique for claudication and critical limb ischaemia.
- Subintimal angioplasty has an early learning curve, which can be learnt from tertiary centres that deal with large volume of cases.
- Subintimal angioplasty has an extended role in situations in which intraluminal angioplasties have or would fail, it has several bail out roles described above.
- Limb salvage rates of around 90% at 1 year can be expected with subintimal angioplasty.
- Primary success rates of 80-90% are achievable, and complications requiring surgery are low.
- Stents should not be used routinely, as it prohibits repeat subintimal angioplasties; however, spot stenting is very useful to combat focal flow limiting dissections or elastic recoil.
- Keep in mind, there is a surgical option, and you should not compromise this option by overzealous subintimal angioplasty.

REFERENCES

1. Bradbury AW, Adam DJ, Bell J, Forbes JF, Fowkes FG, Gillespie I, et al. Bypass versus Angioplasty in Severe Ischaemia of the Leg (BASIL) trial: An intention-to-treat analysis of amputation-free and overall survival in patients randomized to a bypass surgery-first or a balloon angioplasty-first revascularization strategy. J Vasc Surg. 2010;51(5 Suppl):5S-17S.
2. Bolia A, Brennan J, Bell PR. Recanalisation of femoro-popliteal occlusions: improving success rate by subintimal recanalisation. Clin Radiol. 1989;40(3):325.

3. Kocher M, Cerna M, Utikal P, Kozak J, Sisola I, Thomas RP, et al. Subintimal angioplasty in femoropopliteal region-Mid-term results. Eur J Radiol. 2010;73(3):672-6.
4. London NJ, Srinivasan R, Naylor AR, Hartshorne T, Ratliff DA, Bell PR, et al. Subintimal angioplasty of femoropopliteal artery occlusions: the long-term results. Eur J Vasc Surg. 1994;8(2):148-55.
5. Bolia A, Bell P. Femoropopliteal and crural artery recanalization using subintimal angioplasty. Semin Vasc Surg. 1995;8 (3):253-64.
6. Reekers JA, Kromhout JG, Jacobs MJ. Percutaneous intentional extraluminal recanalisation of the femoropopliteal artery. Eur J Vasc Surg. 1994;8(6):723-8.
7. Yilmaz S, Sindel T, Yegin A, Luleci E. Subintimal angioplasty of long superficial femoral artery occlusions. J Vasc Interv Radiol. 2003;14(8):997-1010.
8. Yilmaz S, Sindel T, Ceken K, Alimoglu E, Luleci E. Subintimal recanalization of long superficial femoral artery occlusions through the retrograde popliteal approach. Cardiovasc Intervent Radiol. 2001;24(3):154-60.
9. Laxdal E, Jenssen GL, Pedersen G, Aune S. Subintimal angioplasty as a treatment of femoropopliteal artery occlusions. Eur J Vasc Endovasc Surg. 2003;25(6):578-82.
10. McCarthy RJ, Neary W, Roobottom C, Tottle A, Ashley S. Short-term results of femoropopliteal subintimal angioplasty. Br J Surg. 2000;87(10):1361-5.
11. Siablis D, Diamantopoulos A, Katsanos K, Spiliopoulos S, Kagadis GC, Papadoulas S, et al. Subintimal angioplasty of long chronic total femoropopliteal occlusions: long-term outcomes, predictors of angiographic restenosis, and role of stenting. Cardiovasc Intervent Radiol. 2012;35(3):483-90.
12. Bausback Y, Botsios S, Flux J, Werner M, Schuster J, Aithal J, et al. Outback catheter for femoropopliteal occlusions: immediate and long-term results. J Endovasc Ther. 2011;18(1):13-21.
13. Sidhu R, Pigott J, Pigott M, Comerota A. Subintimal angioplasty for advanced lower extremity ischemia due to TASC II C and D lesions of the superficial femoral artery. Vasc Endovascular Surg. 2010;44(8):633-7.
14. Scott EC, Biuckians A, Light RE, Burgess J, Meier GH 3rd, Panneton JM. Subintimal angioplasty: Our experience in the treatment of 506 infrainguinal arterial occlusions. J Vasc Surg. 2008;48(4):878-84.
15. Scott EC, Biuckians A, Light RE, Scibelli CD, Milner TP, Meier GH 3rd, et al. Subintimal angioplasty for the treatment of claudication and critical limb ischemia: 3-year results. J Vasc Surg. 2007;46(5):959-64.
16. Trocciola SM, Chaer R, Dayal R, Lin SC, Kumar N, Rhee J, et al. Comparison of results in endovascular interventions for infrainguinal lesions: claudication versus critical limb ischemia. Am Surg. 2005;71(6):474-9; discussion 9-80.
17. Desgranges P, Boufi M, Lapeyre M, Tarquini G, van Laere O, Losy F, et al. Subintimal angioplasty: feasible and durable. Eur J Vasc Endovasc Surg. 2004;28(2):138-41.
18. Florenes T, Bay D, Sandbaek G, Saetre T, Jorgensen JJ, Slagsvold CE, et al. Subintimal angioplasty in the treatment of patients with intermittent claudication: long term results. Eur J Vasc Endovasc Surg. 2004;28(6):645-50.
19. Kitrou P, Parthipun A, Diamantopoulos A, Paraskevopoulos I, Karunanithy N, Katsanos K. Targeted True Lumen Re-Entry with the Outback Catheter: Accuracy, Success, and Complications in 100 Peripheral Chronic Total Occlusions and Systematic Review of the Literature. J Endovasc Ther. 2015;22(4):538-45.

20. Tisi PV, Mirnezami A, Baker S, Tawn J, Parvin SD, Darke SG. Role of subintimal angioplasty in the treatment of chronic lower limb ischaemia. Eur J Vasc Endovasc Surg. 2002;24(5):417-22.
21. Akesson M, Riva L, Ivancev K, Uher P, Lundell A, Malina M. Subintimal angioplasty of infrainguinal arterial occlusions for critical limb ischemia: long-term patency and clinical efficacy. J Endovasc Ther. 2007;14(4):444-51.
22. Lazaris AM, Tsiamis AC, Fishwick G, Bolia A, Bell PR. Clinical outcome of primary infrainguinal subintimal angioplasty in diabetic patients with critical lower limb ischemia. J Endovasc Ther. 2004;11(4):447-53.
23. Lipsitz EC, Ohki T, Veith FJ, Suggs WD, Wain RA, Cynamon J, et al. Does subintimal angioplasty have a role in the treatment of severe lower extremity ischemia? J Vasc Surg. 2003;37(2):386-91.
24. Molloy KJ, Nasim A, London NJ, Naylor AR, Bell PR, Fishwick G, et al. Percutaneous transluminal angioplasty in the treatment of critical limb ischemia. J Endovasc Ther. 2003;10(2):298-303.
25. Nydahl S, Hartshorne T, Bell PR, Bolia A, London NJ. Subintimal angioplasty of infrapopliteal occlusions in critically ischaemic limbs. Eur J Vasc Endovasc Surg. 1997;14(3):212-6.
26. Vraux H, Hammer F, Verhelst R, Goffette P, Vandeleene B. Subintimal angioplasty of tibial vessel occlusions in the treatment of critical limb ischaemia: mid-term results. Eur J Vasc Endovasc Surg. 2000;20(5):441-6.
27. Ingle H, Nasim A, Bolia A, Fishwick G, Naylor R, Bell PR, et al. Subintimal angioplasty of isolated infragenicular vessels in lower limb ischemia: long-term results. J Endovasc Ther. 2002;9(4):411-6.
28. Varty K, Nydahl S, Nasim A, Bolia A, Bell PR, London JM. Results of surgery and angioplasty for the treatment of chronic severe lower limb ischaemia. Eur J Vasc Endovasc Surg. 1998;16(2):159-63.
29. Hynes N, Mahendran B, Manning B, Andrews E, Courtney D, Sultan S. The influence of subintimal angioplasty on level of amputation and limb salvage rates in lower limb critical ischaemia: a 15-year experience. Eur J Vasc Endovasc Surg. 2005;30(3):291-9.
30. Allen BT, Reilly JM, Rubin BG, Thompson RW, Anderson CB, Flye MW, et al. Femoropopliteal bypass for claudication: vein vs. PTFE. Ann Vasc Surg. 1996;10(2):178-85.
31. Walker SR, Papavassiliou VG, Bolia A, London N. Subintimal angioplasty of native vessels in the management of occluded vascular grafts. Eur J Vasc Endovasc Surg. 2001;22(1):41-3.
32. Nasim A, Sayers RD, Bell PR, Bolia A. Recanalisation of the native artery following failure of a bypass graft. Eur J Vasc Endovasc Surg. 1995;10(1):125-7.
33. Gabriel M, Pawlaczyk K, Waliszewski K, Krasinski Z, Majewski W. Location of femoral artery puncture site and the risk of postcatheterization pseudoaneurysm formation. Int J Cardiol. 2007;120(2):167-71.
34. Spinosa DJ, Harthun NL, Bissonette EA, Cage D, Leung DA, Angle JF, et al. Subintimal arterial flossing with antegrade-retrograde intervention (SAFARI) for subintimal recanalization to treat chronic critical limb ischemia. J Vasc Interv Radiol. 2005;16(1):37-44.

35. Jacobs DL, Motaganahalli RL, Cox DE, Wittgen CM, Peterson GJ. True lumen re-entry devices facilitate subintimal angioplasty and stenting of total chronic occlusions: Initial report. J Vasc Surg. 2006;43(6):1291-6.
36. Morgenstern BR, Getrajdman GI, Laffey KJ, Bixon R, Martin EC. Total occlusions of the femoropopliteal artery: high technical success rate of conventional balloon angioplasty. Radiology. 1989;172(3 Pt 2):937-40.
37. Grimm J, Muller-Hulsbeck S, Jahnke T, Hilbert C, Brossmann J, Heller M. Randomized study to compare PTA alone versus PTA with Palmaz stent placement for femoropopliteal lesions. J Vasc Interv Radiol. 2001;12(8):935-42.
38. Becquemin JP, Favre JP, Marzelle J, Nemoz C, Corsin C, Leizorovicz A. Systematic versus selective stent placement after superficial femoral artery balloon angioplasty: a multicenter prospective randomized study. J Vasc Surg. 2003;37(3):487-94.
39. Vroegindeweij D, Vos LD, Tielbeek AV, Buth J, vd Bosch HC. Balloon angioplasty combined with primary stenting versus balloon angioplasty alone in femoropopliteal obstructions: A comparative randomized study. Cardiovasc Intervent Radiol. 1997;20(6):420-5.
40. Chalmers N. Letter by Chalmers regarding article "Nitinol stent implantation versus balloon angioplasty for lesions in the superficial femoral artery and proximal popliteal artery: twelve-month results from the RESILIENT randomized trial". Circ Cardiovasc Interv. 2010;3(5):e22;
41. Schillinger M, Sabeti S, Dick P, Amighi J, Mlekusch W, Schlager O, et al. Sustained benefit at 2 years of primary femoropopliteal stenting compared with balloon angioplasty with optional stenting. Circulation. 2007;115(21):2745-9.
42. Hong SJ, Ko YG, Shin DH, Kim JS, Kim BK, Choi D, et al. Outcomes of spot stenting versus long stenting after intentional subintimal approach for long chronic total occlusions of the femoropopliteal artery. JACC Cardiovasc Interv. 2015;8(3):472-80.
43. Treiman GS, Treiman R, Whiting J. Results of percutaneous subintimal angioplasty using routine stenting. J Vasc Surg. 2006;43(3):513-9.
44. Hayes PD, Chokkalingam A, Jones R, Bell PR, Fishwick G, Bolia A, et al. Arterial perforation during infrainguinal lower limb angioplasty does not worsen outcome: results from 1409 patients. J Endovasc Ther. 2002;9(4):422-7.
45. Nasim A, Sayers RD, Dunlop P, Bell PR, Bolia A. Intentional extraluminal recanalisation of the femoropopliteal segment following perforation during percutaneous transluminal angioplasty. Eur J Vasc Endovasc Surg. 1996;12(2):246-9.
46. Bolia A. Subintimial angioplasty, the way forward. Acta Chir Belg. 2004;104(5):547-54.
47. Higginson A, Alaeddin F, Fishwick G, Bolia A. "Push and park": an alternative strategy for management of embolic complication during balloon angioplasty. Eur J Vasc Endovasc Surg. 2001;21(3):279-82.
48. Vykoukal MGDaD. Changing Paradigms in the Management of Peripheral Vascular Disease: The Need for Integration of Knowledge, Imaging, and Therapeutics. Springer.1-30.
49. Sultan S, Hynes N. Five-year Irish trial of CLI patients with TASC II type C/D lesions undergoing subintimal angioplasty or bypass surgery based on plaque echolucency. J Endovasc Ther. 2009;16(3):270-83.

SUGGESTED READING

1. Bolia A, Bell PRF. Femoropopliteal and crural artery recanalisation using subintimal angioplasty. Semin Vasc Surg. 1995;3:253-64.
2. Bolia A. Percutaneous intentional extraluminal (subintimal) recanalisation of crural arteries. Eur J Radiol. 1998;28:199-204.
3. Reekers JA, Bolia A. Percutaneous intentional extraluminal (subintimal) recanalisation: how to do it yourself? Eur J Radiol. 1998;28:192-8.

CHAPTER 8

Current Concepts in Managing Tibial Vessel Disease

Kapil Mathur, Satheesh Ramamurthy, T Vidyasagaran

SURGERY VS ENDOVASCULAR DEBATE

The rapid adoption of the endovascular-first strategy can be attributed not only to continuously evolving technology and improved vascular imaging but also to the expanding skill level of endovascular specialists and the dissemination of these skills. However, the difficulty in recommending the endovascular-first strategy for complex lesions is demonstrated by the inability of the TASC (Inter-Society Consensus for the Management of Peripheral Arterial Disease) Steering Committee to arrive at a consensus after their multispeciality convention at Örebro, Sweden in 2009. A criticism of the TASC II classification was that it did not include an infrapopliteal classification and hence a subsequently published update provided a separate classification of infrapopliteal disease severity (Fig. 1).[1]

The difficulty in providing recommendations is not surprising given the paucity of prospective data to determine the appropriate and beneficial role of endovascular interventions. This is in part because endovascular options are almost universally preferred for less complex lesions and surgical bypasses for more complex lesions with consequently worse clinical outcomes. Though the BASIL[2-4] trial included patients with infrainguinal rather than isolated infrapopliteal involvement, it is still the most relevant as one-third of the bypass group and 62% of the endovascular group patients had infrapopliteal disease. First published in 2005,[2] its final results with separate intention to treat and by treatment received analyses were published in 2010.[3,4]

TASC II document[5] pertaining to the treatment of femoropopliteal lesions states that endovascular therapy is the treatment of choice for TASC A lesions and surgery is the treatment of choice for TASC D lesions but when it comes to TASC B and C lesions, the recommendations adopt a preference of endovascular over surgery for B lesions and surgery over endovascular therapy for C lesions. It also recommends taking into consideration the patient's co-morbidities, fully informed patient preference and the operator's own long-term results with each modality. In addition to this, the BASIL trial's results

TASC A lesions

Single focal stenosis, ≤5 cm in length, in the target tibial artery with occlusion or stenosis of similar or worse severity in the other tibial arteries

TASC B lesions

Multiple stenoses, each ≤5 cm in length, or total length ≤10 cm or single occlusion ≤3 cm in length, in the target tibial artery with occlusion or stenosis of similar or worse severity in the other tibial arteries

TASC C lesions

Multiple stenoses in the target tibial artery and/ or single occlusion with total lesion length >10 cm with occlusion or stenosis of similar or worse severity in the other tibial arteries

TASC D lesions

Multiple occlusions involving the target tibial artery with total lesion length >10 cm or dense lesion calcification or nonvisualisation of collaterals. The other tibial arteries occluded or dense calcification

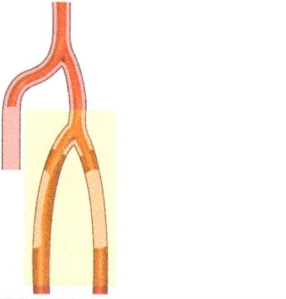

Figure 1: TASC classification of infrapopliteal lesions. The unshaded area represents the target lesion; area inside the shaded rectangle represents typical background disease. (Reprinted from The TASC Steering Committee)[1]

suggested that though bypass surgery with autogenous vein offered the long-term amputation free survival the subset of patients who are not expected to live for more than 2 years should be first offered balloon angioplasty.[3,4] These findings were endorsed in the updated American College of Cardiology

Foundation/American Heart Association guidelines for the management of patients with peripheral arterial disease.[6]

The PREVENT III study was the largest prospective randomised study of vein bypasses for advanced lower extremity ischaemia and its surgical results serve as a benchmark for current practice. They reported a primary, primary assisted and secondary graft patency of 61%, 77% and 80%, respectively at 1 year and patient survival and limb salvage rates of 84% and 88%, respectively.[7]

There is no randomised controlled data comparing only infrapopliteal angioplasty with surgical distal bypass Fernandez[8] et al., reported their outcomes after tibial balloon angioplasty of a 123 limbs with a primary patency, assisted primary patency and secondary patency of 33%, 50% and 56% at 1 year with a limb salvage rate of 75%. More recently, a large single-centre study from the UK[9] reported medium term outcomes after tibial angioplasty of 527 limb with a primary patency of 48.5% and 32.9% at 1 year and 3 years with a limb salvage of 92.7% at 3 years.

This data makes us better prepared at clinical decision making on treatment options, but regardless of the mode of revascularisation selected, the goal should be to restore straight-line blood flow to the foot, especially in the setting of tissue loss. Michael Conte[10] masterly summarised the key factors involved in selecting the revascularisation strategy by favouring bypasses in those patients with average surgical risk with a life expectancy of 2 or more years, major tissue loss with multilevel or TASC C/D pattern of diseases and availability of GSV (Great Saphenous Vein) or good quality alternate vein and endovascular means for those with high surgical risk, limited life expectancy, minor tissue loss with TASC A/B/C pattern of disease and inadequate venous conduit.

Though there appears to be a consensus for treatment of short infrapopliteal lesions, endovascular interventions for complex infrapopliteal disease is still controversial. Andrej Schmidt[11] et al. from Leipzig, Germany reported their results from balloon angioplasty of lesions >80 mm in infrapopliteal vessels (average lesion length of 184 mm) of 77 limbs with a 100% limb salvage at a mean follow-up of 15 months despite high rates of restenosis and occlusion on follow-up arteriography at 3 months, perhaps explained by a temporary perfusion enhancement enough to bring about ulcer healing. In the same study, despite a restenosis rate of 68.8% at 3 months there was clinical improvement in 76% with no major amputations, which makes us question whether restenosis is a clinically relevant end-point after tibial revascularisation.[12]

ENDOVASCULAR ADJUNCTS—DRUG-COATED BALLOONS

On the other hand, durable infrapopliteal vessel patency is a desired revascularisation goal and leads to faster and more sustained complete wound healing. Paclitaxel drug-eluting balloons (DEB) were introduced to achieve this goal. On the back of consistently good results supporting the safety and efficacy in randomised multi-centre trials of IN.PACT DEBs in femoropopliteal lesions[13] and also two single-centre studies (one was retrospective[14] and the other was randomised[15]) suggesting that the IN.PACT Amphirion DEB (IA-DEB) (Medtronic, Santa Rosa, California) reduces infrapopliteal vessel restenosis and re-intervention rates, the IN.PACT DEEP[16] randomized multi-centre trial was conducted to test the hypothesis of superior efficacy of IA-DEB versus PTA. The trial however failed to meet its primary efficacy end-point of IA-DEB superiority over PTA and also the 2.4-fold higher amputation rate in the study arm lead to safety concerns which convinced the manufacturer to withdraw the product from the market.

Despite the negative results of the study, the IN.PACT DEEP study remains a benchmark trial in CLI patients with the PTA arm showing an extraordinarily low 12-month binary restenosis rate of 35% and major amputation rate of 3.6%. As the results of the study applied only to the concerned device, the IN.PACT Amphirion DEB, the results of the BIOLUX P-II randomized trial, which is BIOTRONIK'S-First in Man study of the Passeo-18 LUX (Biotronik AG, Buelach, Switzerland) drug releasing PTA Balloon Catheter vs. the uncoated Passeo-18 PTA balloon catheter in subjects requiring revascularisation of infrapopliteal arteries, were eagerly awaited. The 12-month results published[17] show that though there were no safety concerns identified, the results were not superior to those of uncoated balloons. So, for the time being at least, what looked to be a sure winner, given the results in single-centre studies and in other territories, seems to need more convincing data to recommend its use.

Endovascular Adjuncts—Stents

The use of stents in below the knee arteries has not matched their use in other vascular territories. There is a lack of definitive data supporting a primary stent-based strategy in the infrapopliteal vascular bed due to the diffuse nature of atherosclerosis in these vessels;[1,2,6] however, the use of bare metal stents in a "bail-out" or "salvage" situation is supported, with acceptable short and medium-term results, especially in high risk patients for surgical bypasses.[18]

The evidence for the primary use of drug eluting stents is more convincing.
- The ACHILLES trial,[19] which randomized patients between PTA (percutaneous transluminal angioplasty) and DES (drug eluting stents) using the Cypher Select Sirolimus Eluting Stent (Cordis Corporation, Bridgewater, NJ, USA), found superior patency rates in the DES group at 1 year (75% vs 57.1%) though no differences in death, amputation rates or clinical status improvement and hence should be interpreted with caution.
- Infrapopliteal BMS (bare metal stents) were compared with DES in the DESTINY[20] trial using the Everolimus-eluting Xcience V (Abbot Vascular, Abbott Park, IL, USA) and Yukon-BTX[21,22] trial using the sirolimus-eluting YUKON stent (Translumina, Hechingen, Germany) with both showing improved patency at 1 year and the YUKON-BTX also reporting improved event-free survival at 3 years.
- The IDEAS[23] Randomized Controlled Trial compared paclitaxel-coated balloons (PCB) vs DES in long (>70 mm) infrapopliteal lesions in patients with Rutherford categories 3-6 and found significantly less restenosis but this did not result in any significant difference in target lesion revascularisation.

Endovascular Adjuncts—Atherectomy Devices and Others

Early elastic recoil and frequent dissections after PTA and incomplete stent expansion in severely calcified tibial arteries has led to the search for alternate strategies like plaque debulking using an atherectomy device. Atherectomy has been heralded as an effective debulking technique in calcified and advanced lesions (TASC C and D) and can be indicated in heavily calcified or PTA-resistant lesions.[24] The merits of an initial debulking strategy is that it allows for the native vessel and intrinsic vessel characteristics to be maintained such that if further intervention is required in the future for restenosis, all interventional options are still available. Atherectomy may also provide the ability to treat longer lesions without the need for a lengthy endoprosthesis and further can preserve side branches as compared to a balloon-stent approach.

Four different methods of atherectomy have been utilised for treatment of femoropopliteal or small-vessel infrapopliteal disease: plaque excision (directional) atherectomy, rotational atherectomy/aspiration, laser atheroablation, and orbital atherectomy. Directional atherectomy devices utilize carbide rotating cutter disks that resect and remove the atherosclerotic plaque. As with the use of all atherectomy devices, distal embolization is a risk. The SilverHawk™ (with one blade), the TurboHawk™ (with four contoured blades) and the HawkOne™ (single device to treat different morphologies) from Covidien-Medtronic (Minneapolis, Mn) are all FDA approved and come in size ranges from 1.5 to 7 mm. The Definitive LE (Determination of Effectiveness of SilverHawk/TurboHawk Peripheral Plaque Excision Systems for the Treatment of Infrainguinal Vessels/Lower Extremities) trial of 800 patients (96 tibial CLI cases) treated with stand-alone directional atherectomy recently reported a 12-month freedom from amputation of 95% and primary patency rate of 71% for their CLI cohort (N-201).[25]

Excimer laser atherectomy (Spectranetics Corp, Colorado Springs, Colo) has an advantage of not only debulking, but also being able to penetrate the proximal fibrous cap in chronic total occlusions, enhancing crossing capability. In the LACI trial, which was a multicenter study to evaluate the efficacy of excimer laser-assisted angioplasty in CLI patients with complex femoropopliteal and tibioperoneal occlusive disease, the authors describe a "step-by-step" technique of advancing the laser catheter without a guidewire for a distance of 1-2 cm in lesions resistant to guidewire navigation.[26]

However, a study which compared early and late outcomes of tibial intervention with angioplasty vs atherectomy-assisted interventions, found that the adjunctive use of atherectomy offered no improvement in primary outcomes over PTA alone and hence questioned its generalised use as an adjunct to PTA to treat all lesions, given the increased cost and operative time.[27] The study included 418 interventions out of which 79 were performed with atherectomy–33 using the Excimer laser atherectomy (Spectranetics Corp, Colorado Springs, Colo), 13 directional using the SilverHawk directional atherectomy (ev3 Endovascular Inc, Plymouth, Minn), and 33 orbital using the Diamondback 360 orbital atherectomy (Cardiovascular Systems Inc, St Paul, Minn).

Other devices, such as the Peripheral Cutting Balloon® (Boston Scientific Corporation, Natick, MA) which uses a non-compliant balloon with four atherotomes, the AngioSculpt® Scoring Balloon (Angioscore, Inc., Fremont, CA) which uses a semi-compliant balloon with a flexible nitinol scoring element and the CryoPlasty® PolarCath™ Peripheral Dilatation System (Boston Scientific Corporation, Natick, MA) which uses liquid nitrous oxide to cool the surface of the balloon to −10°C, have been shown to be effective in treating infrapopliteal disease.[28-30] However current literature reviews have failed to show superior efficacy when compared with conventional, less expensive therapies.[1]

The list of technological advances in tibial revascularisation is long and not limited to the major ones mentioned above. Advances in guidewire technology with respect to tip load, tip stiffness, hydrophilic/hydrophobic coating of the tip and body, guidewire flexibility, ability to shape, shaping memory, shaft support, torque transmission, trackability, and pushability along with low-profile and lengthy tibial balloons and support catheters have been critical in below the knee interventions.

BALLOON ANGIOPLASTY TECHNIQUES

Advances and dissemination of techniques and skills have been equally important to the rapid rise of below the knee angioplasty. The initial approach would be transluminal, using a drilling technique for crossing chronic total occlusions (CTO) but in case of difficulty there are several other approaches described. The subintimal angioplasty technique which is used successfully in the superficial femoral artery can be extended to the tibial arteries with some modification but must be preferably avoided in calcified arteries.[31] The advantages of this technique include its ability to cross long chronic occlusions, the option of recanalisation of more than one tibial vessel and extending its use to pedal vessels by recanalising the pedal arch.[32]

Extreme cases, seen especially in diabetics with calcified tibial arteries, can necessitate the use of techniques, such as subintimal arterial flossing with antegrade-retrograde intervention (SAFARI), the pedal-plantar loop technique and transcollateral angioplasty.[33] What these techniques have in common is that they give importance to the integrity of the plantar arch and allow for the concept of complete revascularisation of all three tibial arteries instead of just one. In situations where the conventional antegrade approach has failed to cross the lesion, patent leg vessels distal to the lesion can be visualised because of collateral circulation and access can be obtained by direct puncture with a 21 G needle. A guidewire is then passed through this and if it crosses the length of the tibial occlusion it can be retrieved proximally and used to balloon dilate the lesion (Fig. 2). Spinosa[34] et al. described the SAFARI technique where the distal guidewire has entered the subintimal space and is recovered through a catheter introduced antegradely into the subintimal space.

The pedal plantar loop technique, described by Manzi et al. in 2009,[35] is based on the recanalisation of both pedal and plantar arteries and their anatomical anastomosis in order to restore direct arterial in-flow from both

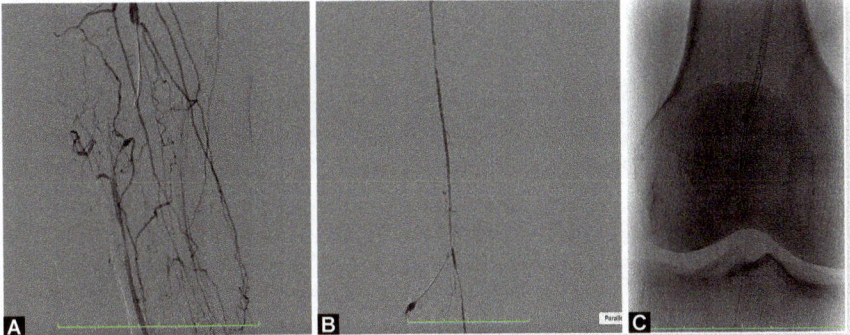

Figure 2: Retrograde pedal access in a patient with great toe gangrene. (A) Occlusion of the popliteal artery, tibioperoneal trunk, posterior tibial and peroneal arteries with a patent but severely diseased proximal anterior tibial artery (AT), antegrade recanalisation was unsuccessful; (B) Retrograde pedal access was obtained by puncturing the distal AT with a 21G needle; (C) The 0.018" guidewire was manipulated into an antegrade catheter and exteriorized

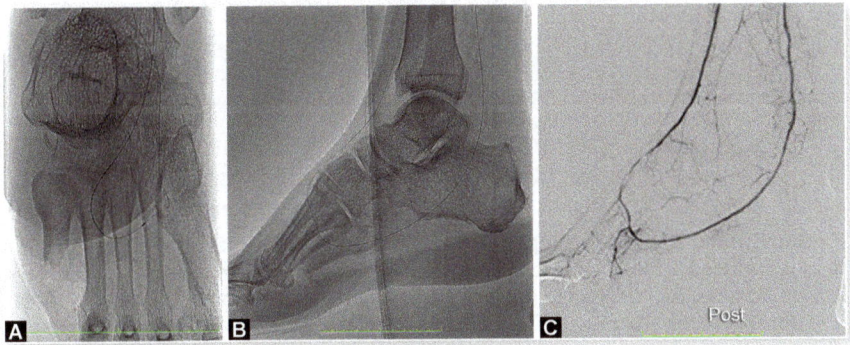

Figure 3: Pedal plantar loop technique in a patient with severe distal ischaemia and a non-healing 5th toe stump. (A) Anteroposterior view showing "figure of 8" pattern with guidewire traversing through the 1st interosseous space; (B) Lateral view of pedal plantar loop; (C) Completed plantar arch

anterior and posterior tibial vessels (Figs 3A and B). Several variations of this technique have been described, including one by Palena and Manzi[36] which describes recanalising occlusions through an antegrade pedal approach in the opposing circulatory pathway of the foot when a retrograde puncture is not possible. In trans-collateral angioplasty, the recanalization is per-formed through a highly developed collateral artery which provides access to the occluded target vessel (Fig. 4).[37]

There have been vast strides in below the knee interventions with exciting new technology available, but for the moment, balloon angioplasty remains the mainstay of endovascular interventions. Between open vascular bypasses and endovascular therapy, significant disagreement still exists as to which therapy works best in candidates for both types of intervention. Randomised controlled data should soon be available to us from the BEST-CLI trial[38] and the BASIL 2 trial[39] which will help us to make more informed

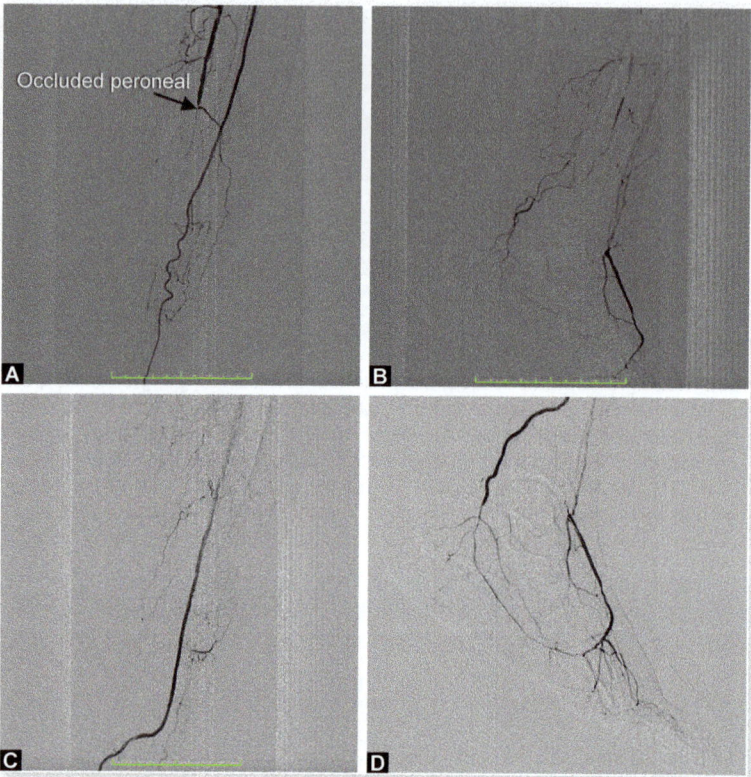

Figure 4: Trans-collateral angioplasty in a patient with heel ulceration. (A) The Posterior tibial is occluded at the origin and the peroneal and AT occlude at mid-leg with a collateral arising from the AT continuing inferiorly; (B) There is reformation of the lateral plantar and dorsalis pedis arteries; (C) To provide angiosome-directed direct revascularization of the heel ulceration, the lateral plantar artery is approached through the posterior communicating branch of the peroneal artery; (D) Good flow is seen in the lateral plantar and the pedal arch via the posterior communicating peroneal collateral

decisions on the best modality of treatment for a given patient. At present, the choice of therapy for a patient with a TASC C/D lesion with acceptable surgical risk and good quality venous conduit remains a highly individual one, considerably influenced by the physician's own skills, past results and interests.

EDITOR'S COMMENTS

The jury is still out on the ideal management of BTK lesions. In recent times, four RCTs have examined the efficacy of DEBs in BTK atherosclerotic disease, two of which have been briefly discussed above by the authors. In the **IDEAS** trial, 50 patients were randomized to infrapopliteal DEB angioplasty (25 arteries in 25 limbs) or primary DES placement (30 arteries in 27 limbs). The binary restenosis rate was significantly lower in DES (28% vs 57.9%; $P =$

0.0457). There were no significant differences in TLR (7.7% in DES vs 13.6% in DEB; $P = 0.65$). At 6 months, five patients died (two in DEB vs three in DES; $P = 1.00$) and three suffered a major amputation (one in DEB vs two in DES; $P = 1.00$). In the **IN.PACT DEEP** trial, 358 patients with CLI were randomized 2:1 to IN.PACT Amphirion DEB angioplasty or standard PTA at 13 European sites. After 12 months, the decision was made to recall the IN.PACT Amphirion DEB based on a trend toward a higher rate of major amputation in the DEB arm. The other two are the DEBELLUM and DEBATE BTK trials.

In the **DEBELLUM** trial consecutive patients with 122 lesions in the femoral-popliteal and/or infrapopliteal arteries were randomized to DEBs or standard PTA. The preliminary 1-year results on the BTK lesions confirmed a better outcome with DEBs over standard PTA in terms of LLL (0.66 ± 0.9 mm DEB vs 1.69 ± 1.5 mm PTA; $P < 0.05$), TLR (15.3% DEB vs 47.0% PTA; $P < 0.05$), and primary patency (84.6% DEB vs 41.1% PTA; $P < 0.05$). However, major adverse events (defined as major or minor amputation, thrombosis, or death) did not differ significantly between DEBs and standard PTA presumably because of the limited number of lesions and patients treated.

The **DEBATE-BTK** trial investigated the efficacy of a paclitaxel DEB for the reduction of restenosis in diabetic patients with CLI. Binary restenosis, assessed by angiography in >90% of patients, occurred in 20 of 74 (27%) lesions in the DEB group versus 55 of 74 (74%) lesions in the standard PTA group ($P < 0.001$), TLR in 12 (18%) versus 29 (43%) ($P = 0.002$), and target vessel occlusion in 12 (17%) versus 41 (55%) ($P < 0.001$). There was one major amputation, which occurred in the standard PTA group ($P = 0.9$).

ONGOING BTK TRIALS WORLDWIDE

Swedish RCT: SWEDEPAD trial is testing the hypothesis that DEB is superior to standard PTA in terms of important clinical outcomes, when applied on femoral-popliteal and/or infrapopliteal PAD. This trial has two separate parallel studies, SWEDEPAD 1 and SWEDEPAD 2, each defined by the severity of PAD. Patients with CLI are allocated to SWEDEPAD 1 and patients with IC are allocated to SWEDEPAD 2. The primary outcome measures are amputation rate (SWEDEPAD 1) and health-related quality of life (SWEDEPAD 2).

Italian RCT: The ACOART-BTK trial is a DEBs versus standard PTA trial in the treatment of infrapopliteal disease in patients with CLI.

Singapore: The SINGA-PACLI trial is another RCT, which is aiming to study the results of DEBs compared to standard PTA for the treatment of infrapopliteal disease in patients with CLI.

Concerns remain about angioplasty with DEBs having an adverse effect through downstream drug distribution into tissue distal to the lesion location, which may affect wound healing.

Despite RCTs having demonstrated technical superiority of DEBs over standard PTA, there are still certain issues to be addressed prior to their widespread use as a primary treatment for patients with BTK disease. One is the lack of a significant difference in major amputation or mortality rates between DEBs and standard PTA. Another issue is the cost implication.

REFERENCES

1. The TASC Steering Committee. An Update on Methods for Revascularization and expansion of the TASC Lesion Classification to Include Below-the-Knee Arteries: A Supplement to the Inter-Society Consensus for the Management of Peripheral Arterial Disease (TASC II). Journal of Endovascular Therapy. 2015;22(5): 663-77.
2. Adam DJ, Beard JD, Cleveland T, et al. Bypass versus angioplasty in severe ischaemia of the leg (BASIL): multicentre, randomised controlled trial. Lancet. 2005;366:1925-34.
3. Bradbury AW, Adam DJ, Bell J, et al. Bypass versus Angioplasty in Severe Ischaemia of the Leg (BASIL) trial: an intention-to-treat analysis of amputation-free and overall survival in patients randomized to a bypass surgery-first or a balloon angioplasty-first revascularization strategy. J Vasc Surg. 2010;51(5 suppl):5S-17S.
4. Bradbury AW, Adam DJ, Bell J, et al. Bypass versus Angioplasty in Severe Ischaemia of the Leg (BASIL) trial: analysis of amputation free and overall survival by treatment received. J Vasc Surg. 2010;51(5 suppl):18S-31S.
5. Norgren L, Hiatt WR, Dormandy JA, et al. Inter-Society Consensus for the Management of Peripheral Arterial Disease (TASC II). J Vasc Surg. 2007;45(suppl S):S5-S67.
6. Rooke TW, Hirsch AT, Misra S: 2011 ACCF/AHA Focused update of the guideline for the management of patients with peripheral arterial disease (updating the 2005 guideline). J Vasc Surg. 2011;54:e32-58.
7. Conte MS, Bandyk DF, Clowes AW, et al. Results of PREVENT III: a multicenter, randomized trial of edifoligide for the prevention of vein graft failure in lower extremity bypass surgery. J Vasc Surg. 2006;43:742-51.
8. Fernandez N, McEnaney R, Marone L, et al. Predictors of failure and success of tibial interventions for critical limb ischemia. J Vasc Surg. 2010;52:834-42.
9. K Mathur, MK Ayyappan, J Hodson, et al. Factors Affecting Medium-Term Outcomes After Crural Angioplasty in Critically Ischemic Legs. Vascular and Endovascular Surgery. 2015; 49(3-4):63-8.
10. Conte MS. Critical appraisal of surgical revascularization for critical limb ischemia. J Vasc Surg. 2013;57:8S-13S.
11. Schmidt A, Ulrich M, Winker B, et al. Angiographic patency and clinical outcome after balloon-angioplasty for extensive infrapopliteal arterial disease. Catheter Cardiovasc Interv. 2010;76:1047-54.
12. Rana MA and Gloviczki P. Endovascular Interventions for Infrapopliteal Arterial Disease: An Update. Semin Vasc Surg. 25:29-34.
13. Werk M, Albrecht T, Meyer DR, et al. Paclitaxel-coated balloons reduce restenosis after femoro-popliteal angioplasty: evidence from the randomized PACIFIER trial. Circ Cardiovasc Interv. 2012;5:831-40.
14. Schmidt A, Piorkowski M, Werner M, et al. First experience with drug-eluting balloons in infrapopliteal arteries: restenosis rate and clinical outcome. J Am Coll Cardiol. 2011;58:1105-9.
15. Liistro F, Porto I, Angioli P, et al. Drug-eluting balloon in peripheral intervention for below the knee angioplasty evaluation (DEBATE-BTK): a randomized trial in diabetic patients with critical limb ischemia. Circulation. 2013;128:615-21.

16. Zeller T, Baumgartner I, Schenert D, et al of the IN.PACT DEEP Trial Investigators. Drug-Eluting Balloon Versus Standard Balloon Angioplasty for Infrapopliteal Arterial Revascularization in Critical Limb Ischemia: 12-Month Results From the IN.PACT DEEP Randomized Trial. J Am Coll Cardiol. 2014;64:1568-76.
17. Zeller T, Beschomer U, Pilger E, Bosiers M, Deloose K, Peters P, et al. Paclitaxel-Coated Balloon in Infrapopliteal Arteries. 12-Month Results From the BIOLUX P-II Randomized Trial (BIOTRONIK'S-First in Man study of the Passeo-18 LUX drug releasing PTA Balloon Catheter vs. the uncoated Passeo-18 PTA balloon catheter in subjects requiring revascularization of infrapopliteal arteries). J Am Coll Cardiol Intv. 2015;8(12):1614-22.
18. Donas KP, Torsello G, Schwindt A, Schönefeld E, Boldt O and Pitoulias GA. Below knee bare nitinol stent placement in high-risk patients with critical limb ischemia is still durable after 24 months of follow-up. J Vasc Surg. 2010;52:356-61.
19. Scheinert D, Katsanos K, Zeller T, et al. A prospective randomized multicenter comparison of balloon angioplasty and infrapopliteal stenting with the sirolimus-eluting stent in patients with ischemic peripheral arterial disease: 1-year results from the ACHILLES trial. J Am Coll Cardiol. 2012;60:2290-5.
20. Bosiers M, Scheinert D, Peeters P, et al. Randomized comparison of everolimus-eluting versus bare-metal stents in patients with critical limb ischemia and infrapopliteal arterial occlusive disease. J Vasc Surg. 2012;55:390-8.
21. Rastan A, Tepe G, Krankenberg H, et al. Sirolimus-eluting stents vs. bare-metal stents for treatment of focal lesions in infrapopliteal arteries: a double-blind, multi-centre, randomized clinical trial. Eur Heart J. 2011;32:2274-81.
22. Rastan A, Brechtel K, Krankenberg H, et al. Sirolimus-eluting stents for treatment of infrapopliteal arteries reduce clinical event rate compared to bare-metal stents: long-term results from a randomized trial. J Am Coll Cardiol. 2012;60:587-91.
23. Siablis D, Kitrou PM, Spiliopoulos S, et al. Paclitaxel-coated balloon angioplasty versus drug-eluting stenting for the treatment of infrapopliteal long-segment arterial occlusive disease: the IDEAS randomized controlled trial. JACC Cardiovasc Interv. 2014;7:1048-56.
24. Tan TW, Semaan E, Nasr W, Eberhardt RT, Hamburg N, Doros G, et al. Endovascular revascularization of symptomatic infrapopliteal arteriosclerotic occlusive disease: comparison of atherectomy and angioplasty. Int J Angiol 2001;20:19-24.
25. McKinsey JF, Zeller T, Rocha-Singh KJ, Jaff MR, Garcia LA; DEFINITIVE LE Investigators. Lower extremity revascularization using directional atherectomy: 12-month prospective results of the DEFINITIVE LE study. JACC Cardiovasc Interv. 2014;7(8):923-33.
26. Laird JR, Zeller T, Gray BH, Scheinert D, Vranic M, Reiser C, et al. Limb Salvage Following Laser-Assisted Angioplasty for Critical Limb Ischemia: Results of the LACI Multicenter Trial. J Endovasc Ther. 2006;13:1-11.
27. Todd Jr KE, Ahanchi SS, Maurer CA, Kim JH, Chipman CR and Panneton JM. Atherectomy offers no benefits over balloon angioplasty in tibial interventions for critical limb ischemia. J Vasc Surg. 2013;58:941-8.
28. Cardon JM, Jan F, Vasseur MA, et al. Value of cutting balloon angioplasty for limb salvage in patients with obstruction of popliteal and distal arteries. Ann Vasc Surg. 2008;22:314-8.

29. Kiesz RS, Scheinert D, Peeters PJ, et al. Results from the International Registry of the AngioSculpt scoring balloon catheter for the treatment of infra-popliteal disease. J Am Coll Cardiol. 2008;51(10 suppl B):75.
30. Das T, McNamara T, Gray B, et al. Cryoplasty therapy for limb salvage in patients with critical limb ischemia. J Endovasc Ther. 2007;14:753-62.
31. Lyden SP. Techniques and outcomes for endovascular treatment in the tibial arteries. J Vasc Surg. 2009;50:1219-23.
32. Kawarada O, Yokoi Y, Sekii H, et al. Retrograde crossing through the pedal arch for totally occluded tibial artery. J Interv Cardiol. 2008;21:342-6.
33. Pernès J-M, Auguste M, Borie H, Kovarsky S, Bouchareb A, Despujole C, et al. Infrapopliteal arterial recanalization: A true advance for limb salvage in diabetics. Diagnostic and Interventional Imaging. 2015;96:423-34.
34. Spinosa DJ, Leung DA, Harthun NL, Cage DL, Fritz Angle J,Hagspiel KD, et al. Simultaneous antegrade and retrogradeaccess for subintimal recanalization of peripheral arterialocclusion. J Vasc Interv Radiol. 2003;14:1449-54.
35. Manzi M, Fusaro M, Ceccacci T, Erente G, Dalla Paola L and Brocco E, et al. Clinical results of below-the-knee intervention using pedal-plantar loop technique for the revascularization of foot arteries. J Cardiovasc Surg (Torino). 2009;50:331-7.
36. Palena LM and Manzi M. Antegrade pedal approach for recanalizing occlusions in the opposing circulatory pathway of the foot when a retrograde puncture is not possible. J Endovasc Ther. 2014;21(6):775-8.
37. Fusaro M, Agostini P, Biondi-Zoccai G. "Trans-collateral"angioplasty for a challenging chronic total occlusion of thetibial vessels: a novel approach to percutaneous revasculariza-tion in critical lower limb ischemia. Catheter Cardiovasc Interv. 2008;71(2):266-72.
38. Farber A, Rosenfield K, Menard M. The BEST-CLI trial: a multidisciplinary effort to assess which therapy is best for patients with critical limb ischemia. Tech Vasc Interv Radiol. 2014;17(3):221-4.
39. Popplewell MA, Davies H, Jarrett H, Bate G, Grant M, Patel S, et al; BASIL-2 Trial Investigators. Bypass versus angioplasty in severe ischaemia of the leg - 2 (BASIL-2) trial: study protocol for a randomised controlled trial. Trials. 2016;17:11.

CHAPTER

9

Failing Vascular Grafts

Cho Ee Ng, Vish Bhattacharya

INTRODUCTION

Infrainguinal bypass grafts have been carried out since the 1960s to relieve the symptoms of claudication or to relieve rest pain and promote wound healing. The long saphenous vein has been the conduit of choice but arm veins, cadaveric veins and umbilical veins have also been used. DeBakey first described the use of Dacron grafts and Sauvage and DeBakey introduced the internal and external velour into their grafts to promote graft healing. Despite half a century of research no ideal graft has yet been made which would allow the internal surface to completely endothelialise and consequently, maintain long-term patency.

Infrainguinal bypass grafts may fail within 30 days and this is typically due to technical failures such as 'missed' valves when using the long saphenous vein, stenosis at the proximal or distal origins, kinking at various points in the graft tunnel, or poor choice of a diseased conduit. Failure after 30 days is likely to be due to intimal hyperplasia which is mainly due to continued smoking. Beyond 2 years, blockage of graft is related atherosclerosis in the native vessel which can affect the inflow tract, proximal or distal anastomoses or distal run off vessels.[1]

The autogenous long saphenous vein bypass graft is the gold standard for bypass in the limbs. However, it is well known that almost 30-40% of lower extremity grafts develop significant stenosis within the first year after implantation.[2]

PATHOPHYSIOLOGY

Histological studies revealed vein harvesting and implantation in the arterial environment effects the entire length of the bypass graft.[2] Within 24 hours of arterial flow endothelial cells are focally absent or appear elevated by endothelial oedema and inflammatory cells.[1,3] Platelets, inflammatory cells and fibrin adhere to the denuded epithelium where they release growth factors such as basic fibroblastic growth factor, vascular endothelial growth factor and insulin like growth factor. The endothelial layer is restored by 10 days to 2 weeks but in long human bypass graft it takes far longer than in the short grafts used in animal experiments.[4] After one year or so, the vein grafts exhibit nitrous oxide mediated endothelium dependant relaxation.[2]

The media also undergoes changes following implantation, initially becoming oedematous with focal haemorrhage. Affected by the increase compressive stress the smooth muscle cells show some evidence of apoptosis. During this early phase, almost 70% of medial smooth muscle cells are lost. However, the remaining smooth muscle cells develop structural changes consistent with increased intracellular processes and enter the cell cycle as soon as 48 hours.[2]

The adventitia consisting of fibroblasts surrounded by loose connective tissue with vasa vasorum and vasa nervosum also undergo changes after implantation. The newly implanted vein graft is assumed to receive oxygenation by passive diffusion from the luminal arterial blood.[5] Which were fed a diet that sustains plasma cholesterol levels of approximately 225 mg/dl. Grafts were excised from five animals for analysis on each of postoperative days 3, 7, 14, 30, 60, and 90. Cholesterol content increased from 69 ± 24 µg/100 mg (mean $\pm$ standard deviation). The vasa vasorum which are initially thrombosed with fragmented collagen fibres have been shown to return to normal functioning adventitia within 7 days. This not only helps nourish the graft but also controls the passage of inflammatory cells to promote recovery. The fibroblasts however have been shown in some balloon injury models to migrate into the developing intima and add to intimal hyperplasia.[2,4]

After three weeks, the media and the adventitia is replaced with wide spread fibrous collagen and traces of elastin. The endothelium appears normal, there is new formation of a thickened intima rich with collagen surrounded by ground substance and a relatively thin media. There is full return of barrier function and return of vasoactive activity after three months in a vein graft.[6]

In cases where the vein graft inflammation fails to resolve there is fibrosis and consequently, vein graft stenosis and development of intimal hyperplasia.[2]

PREDICTORS OF GRAFT FAILURE

It has been shown that continued smoking postoperatively, but not a prior history of smoker is predictor of graft failure. Several studies have shown that female gender is also an adverse predictor of graft failure. The use of synthetic graft and a presence of critical ischaemia at the time of surgery are also predictors of graft failure. The presence of a postoperative complication whether procedure related or general and high-grade lesions based on TASC (TransAtlantic Inter-Society Consensus) classification at the time of surgery are additional important factors.[7]

DUPLEX US SCANNING AFTER VEIN GRAFTING

The rational for duplex ultrasonography (US) surveillance if is to detect graft stenosis and therefore improved patency rate.[8]

Duplex US surveillance has shown that the peak systolic flow of the velocity is the most sensitive indicator of graft stenosis and ratios of more than 2-2.5 are representative of significant stenosis, although some reports suggest that a higher value of 3-3.5 is more appropriate for intervention. Other values that can signify a graft stenosis are a peak systolic flow velocity of more than 200 cm/second at any point of the graft or mid graft peak systolic flow velocity of less than 45 cm per second.[9] When the peak systolic velocity reaches >2, there is reduction of 50% of the diameter and across section reduction of 70% and this is considered haemodynamically significant.

Surveillance for autologous or prosthetic grafts by duplex US has not been confirmed by any large randomised controlled studied, but various publications have reached different results. Studies by Ferris, Hobbs and Moffidi have shown that intraoperative early duplex US surveillance can detect technical failure in grafts at high risk for future stenosis.[9-12] Lundell et al. have shown, in a study of 165 grafts, that there was significant benefit at 3 years in assisted primary and secondary patency for autologous graft but no benefit in patency for the surveillance of prosthetic grafts.[13] Bergamini reported on another large randomised study of 615 bypasses and found significant improvement in secondary patency and limb salvage for grafts followed by US scan when compared with clinical surveillance alone.[9,14]

Duplex US remains the gold standard for surveillance of failing grafts although contrast enhanced magnetic resonance angiogram (MRA) have accurately measured volume of bypass grafts. MRAs have yet to be done routinely for surveillance despite proven to be useful for suspected graft abnormalities, as the usage is dependent on availability, local expertise and costs. One has to be aware of the small risk of renal disease and nephrogenic systemic fibrosis.[9] Moreover, MRAs have the tendency for over diagnosis due to turbulence being identified as stenosis although this may improve with the advancement of technology.[15]

In contrasting studies, some authors have found no benefit in Duplex US graft surveillance. Davies et al. in 2005 carried out a multicentric prospective randomised controlled trial of 594 patients with a patent vein graft at 30 days after surgery. The patients were randomised to either clinical or duplex follow up at 6 months, 9 months, 12 months and 18 months postoperatively. They found out that the amputation rates were 7% in each group and vascular mortality rates 3% versus 4% over 18 months. Greater number of patients in the clinical group had vein graft stenosis at 18 months but no difference was observed in primary patency, primary-assisted patency and secondary patency between the clinical group and the duplex US group (about 70-80% in each group).[16]

In the case of the prosthetic graft arteriography or an MR angiogram is usually better as a duplex may not be able to image the surface of the graft sufficiently especially where the graft has been externally supported.[17]

METHODS OF PREVENTING GRAFT FAILURE

Antiplatelet drugs have been used typically to prevent platelet aggregation that leads to hyperplastic intimal thickening. The CASPAR study (Clopidogrel and

AcetylSalicylic acid in bypass surgery for Peripheral ARterial disease) showed a benefit for dual-antiplatelet agent Aspirin and Clopidogrel in prosthetic grafts without an increase in bleeding risk. The Dutch Bypass Oral anticoagulants or Aspirin study (BOA) compared oral anticoagulant to Aspirin in a large randomised trial that included vein grafts and prosthetic grafts. The investigators found that oral anticoagulation was better for prevention of vein graft occlusion whereas aspirin at 80 mg a day reduced occlusion in prosthetic grafts.[18]

Currently, there are no pharmacological agents available which is able to prevent stenosis let alone reverse it. Vitamin K antagonist appear to have a role in maintaining patency of a vein graft, much like aspirin does for prosthetic graft, however evidence for this is not conclusive.

MANAGEMENT OF FAILING GRAFTS

When a stenosis is found on Duplex US scanning, the ideal treatment is angioplasty with or without stenting (Fig. 1).

The other alternative is open repair of the stenosed segment or revision of the proximal or distal anastomosis. In some cases, this may be associated with thrombus formation in which case the treatment would involve thrombolysis as well as angioplasty (Fig. 2) or thrombectomy and open revision of the defect.

McCullum and Schermerhorn reported a 10 years' study of grafts carried out between 2000 and 2010. Ninety one failing grafts were treated with surgical revision and 84 with endovascular treatment with a follow-up of 30 months. They noted that some lower extremity bypass graft stenoses were 'unfavourable' lesions which did not respond well to endovascular management. Their study showed that multiple lesions, lesions more than 2 cm, lesions in grafts which are less than 3 months old, and lesions less than 3 mm in diameter fared worse than those with 'favourable' lesions when treated with endovascular therapy. These 'unfavourable' lesions had better freedom from failure after surgery than endovascular treatment. 'Favourable' lesions fared better after endovascular treatment but not after surgical revision.[19]

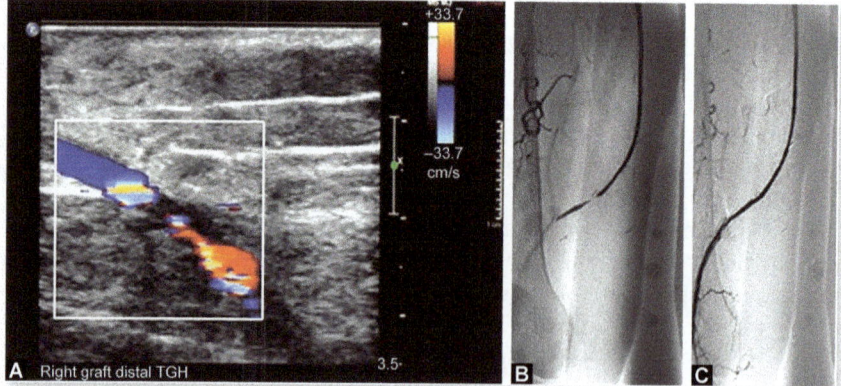

Figure 1: (A) Duplex US showing severe stenosis in a vein graft, (B) Pre-intervention angiogram showing level of stenosis and virtually no flow into popliteal artery, (C) Post-angioplasty angiogram showing good filling of popliteal artery

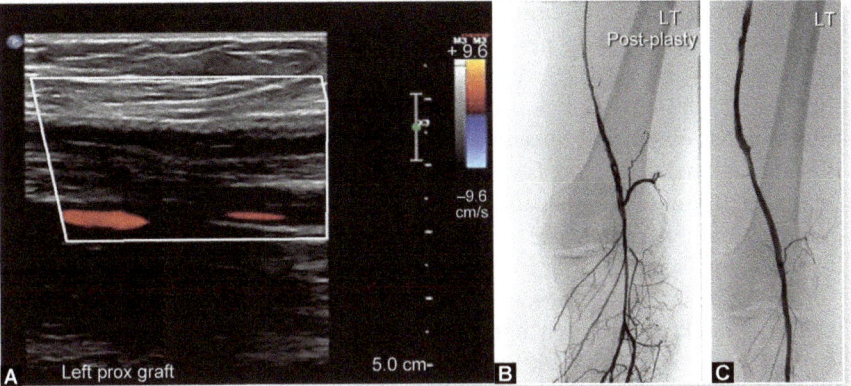

Figure 2: (A) Duplex US showing severe stenosis in a failing vein graft and evidence of fresh thrombus, (B) Pre-intervention angiogram showing poor flow in graft due to stenosis and thrombus, (C) Post-thrombolysis and angioplasty 24-hour angiogram showing good filling of vein graft and popliteal artery

Mathur and Vohra have reported on the long-term outcome of graft angioplasty of bypasses between 2003-2010. One hundred and seventy eight graft angioplasties were performed in 114 bypasses grafts in 103 limbs in 98 patients.[20]

Park et al. reviewed 258 vein grafts carried out between 2003 and 2011. The results of open surgery, endovascular and conservative treatment were reviewed for the failing vein grafts. They found that in a follow-up period of nearly 8 years, 64% grafts were patent with no stenosis seen, 16% of grafts were 'failing' and 15% of grafts had occluded completely. The 16% 'failing' grafts had a total 50 treatments as some needed reintervention. Graft occlusion was more common in the 8 conservatively managed grafts. Severe restenosis of more than 75% was more common following endovascular surgery than open surgical repair. Reintervention free graft patency was superior in the open group compared to the endovascular group (87% vs 42%).[21] Their conclusion was that open surgical revision of graft stenoses had better overall outcome.

MANAGEMENT OF COMPLETELY OCCLUDED GRAFTS

Vein graft occlusion is expected between 19-23% of cases between 2-5 years following infrainguinal bypass. Consequently, the American Heart Association Practice Guidelines in 2005, recommend regular evaluation for at least 2 years.[17]

Two historic landmark trials, the TOPAS (Thrombolysis or Peripheral Artery Surgery) and the STILE (Surgery vs Thrombectomy for Ischaemic Lower Extremity) trials compared thrombectomy and thrombolysis for occluded vein grafts. The TOPAS trial in 1996 showed that the length of the occlusion determined the success of lysis, with lesions of 30 cm or longer responding better to thrombolysis than thrombectomy. The STILE trial showed that open thrombectomy was best for chronic occlusion and thrombolysis was best for recently occluded grafts. At 12 months' amputation and mortality was the same in both groups. However adverse events were more in the thrombolysis group.

Bonhomme and colleagues carried out a study of 106 thrombolytic procedures between 1993 and 2008. They observed a high initial success rate with 76% success rate after catheter directed thrombolysis. Unfortunately, they noted a 58% reocclusion rate at 45 months follow-up. They noted that thrombosed *vein* grafts, grafts inserted beyond 2 weeks, poor run off and failure to identify causative stenosis were determinants of poor long-term outcome. They concluded that thrombolysis should be restricted to selected cases like grafts with recent occlusion, prosthetic or vein grafts of longer than one year duration and in patients with critical limb ischaemia.[22]

Comerota and colleagues, in a series of 124 patients, have shown that those with graft occlusion longer than 14 days have a significantly better outcome when treated surgically, with a new bypass being the best surgical option. However, in patients with acute limb ischaemia less than 14 days, successful thrombolysis of occluded lower extremity bypass grafts improves limb salvage. The authors noted that the patients with occluded prosthetic grafts suffer more major morbid events compared with occluded autogenous grafts.[23]

Another notable option is the use of self-expanding stents throughout the vein graft for vein grafts that have shrunken causing the occlusion rather than thrombosed. Again there is little evidence to establish its clinical usefulness. Mathur and colleagues in a small series of 18 patients have shown acceptable revascularization in the short-term although a long-term solution to the problem remains.[24]

CONCLUSION

Surveillance of vein grafts using Duplex remains the gold standard for follow-up despite some studies to the contrary. Whenever possible lesions causing stenosis should be treated with angioplasty if they are less than 5 cm. Surgical revision is ideal for longer stenosis. All patients with grafts at risk should be put on prophylactic dual antiplatelet treatment provided here are no contraindications. Once the graft is completely occluded, thrombolysis has better results if performed early.

Surgical options, including graft revision, is better if the occlusion has been present for more than 2 weeks. Presently, surgical intervention for management of these occlusion include graft thrombectomy or revision using simple vein patch, placement of a new graft or amputation. Thrombectomy alone, is associated with consistently poor long-term graft patency. Placement of a new vein graft to bypass the lesion remains the most favourable option for long-term limb salvage following a secondary procedure.

REFERENCES

1. Davies MG, Hagen PO. Reprinted Article "pathophysiology of vein graft failure: A review." European Journal of Vascular and Endovascular Surgery. 2011. p. S19-29.
2. Owens CD, Gasper WJ, Rahman AS, Conte MS. Vein graft failure. J Vasc Surg. NIH Public Access. 2015;61(1):203-16.

3. Berguer R, Higgins RF, Reddy DJ. Intimal hyperplasia. An experimental study. Arch Surg. 1980;115(3):332-5.
4. Owens CD, Ho KJ, Conte MS. Lower extremity vein graft failure: a translational approach. Vasc Med. 2008;13(1):63-74.
5. Boerboom LE, Olinger GN, Liu TZ, Rodriguez ER, Ferrans VJ, Kissebah AH. Histologic, morphometric, and biochemical evolution of vein bypass grafts in a nonhuman primate model. I. Sequential changes within the first three months. J Thorac Cardiovasc Surg. 1990;99(1):97-106.
6. Dilley RJ, McGeachie JK, Prendergast FJ. A review of the histologic changes in vein-to-artery grafts, with particular reference to intimal hyperplasia. Arch Surg. 1988;123(6):691-6.
7. Hallihan PD, Choileain NN, Myers E, Redmond HP, Fulton GF. Predictors of Time to Graft Failure Following Infrainguinal Arterial Reconstruction. Surg Sci. 2011;2:166-72.
8. Troutman DA, Madden NJ, Dougherty MJ, Calligaro KD, Calligaro KD, Syrek JR, et al. Duplex ultrasound diagnosis of failing stent grafts placed for occlusive disease. J Vasc Surg. Elsevier. 2014;60(6):1580-4.
9. Majdalany BS, Rybicki FJ, Dill KE, Bandyk DF, Francois CJ, Gerhard-Herman MD, et al. ACR Appropriateness Criteria®; follow-up of lower-extremity arterial bypass surgery. Reston (VA): Agency for Healthcare Research and Quality (AHRQ); 2013: 10.
10. Ferris BL, Mills JL, Hughes JD, Durrani T, Knox R, Moody P, et al. Is early postoperative duplex scan surveillance of leg bypass grafts clinically important? J Vasc Surg. Elsevier. 2003;37(3):495-500.
11. Hobbs SD, Pinkney T, Sykes TCF, Fox AD, Houghton AD, II) I-SC for the M of PAD (TASC, et al. Patency of infra-inguinal vein grafts—effect of intraoperative Doppler assessment and a graft surveillance program. J Vasc Surg. Elsevier. 2009;49(6):1452-8.
12. Mofidi R, Kelman J, Berry O, Bennett S, Murie JA, Dawson ARW, et al. Significance of the early postoperative duplex result in infrainguinal vein bypass surveillance. Eur J Vasc Endovasc Surg. Elsevier. 1998;34(3):327-32.
13. Lundell A, Lindblad B, Bergqvist D, Hansen F. Femoropopliteal-crural graft patency is improved by an intensive surveillance program: A prospective randomized study. J Vasc Surg. 1995;21(1):26-34.
14. Bergamini TM, George SM, Massey HT, Henke PK, Klamer TW, Lambert GE, et al. Intensive surveillance of femoropopliteal-tibial autogenous vein bypasses improves long-term graft patency and limb salvage. Ann Surg. Lippincott, Williams, and Wilkins. 1995;221(5):507-15; discussion 515-6.
15. Giannoukas AD, Androulakis AE, Labropoulos N, Wolfe JHN. The role of surveillance after infrainguinal bypass grafting. Eur J Vasc Endovasc Surg. 1996; 11(3):279-89.
16. Davies AH, Hawdon AJ, Sydes MR, Thompson SG, VGST Participants. Is duplex surveillance of value after leg vein bypass grafting? Principal results of the Vein Graft Surveillance Randomised Trial (VGST). Circulation. American Heart Association Journals. 2005;112(13):1985-91.
17. Hirsch AT, Haskal ZJ, Hertzer NR, Bakal CW, Creager MA, Halperin JL, et al. ACC/AHA 2005 Practice Guidelines for the Management of Patients With Peripheral Arterial Disease (Lower Extremity, Renal, Mesenteric, and Abdominal Aortic). Circulation. 2006;113(11):e463-5.

18. Samson RH. Future improvements in graft performance The Impact of Drug Therapy on Surgical Bypass. Endovasc Today. 2015;June Suppl:20-2.
19. McCallum JC, Bensley RP, Darling JD, Hamdan AD, Wyers MC, Hile C, et al. Open surgical revision provides a more durable repair than endovascular treatment for unfavorable vein graft lesions. J Vasc Surg. Elsevier; 2016;63(1):142-7.
20. Mathur K, Vohra RK, Hodson J, Kuyumdzhiev S, Duddy MJ, Hopkins JD. Infrainguinal Vein Graft Stenoses: Long-Term Outcomes of Graft Angioplasty. Eur J Vasc Endovasc Surg. 2016;52(2):189-97.
21. Park K-M, Park YJ, Yang S-S, Kim D-I, Kim Y-W. Treatment of failing vein grafts in patients who underwent lower extremity arterial bypass. J Korean Surg Soc. Korean Surgical Society; 2012;83(5):307-15.
22. Bonhomme S, Trotteur G, Van Damme H, Defraigne JO. Thrombolysis of occluded infra-inguinal bypass grafts: Is it worthwhile? Acta Chir Belg. 2010;110(4):445-50.
23. Comerota AJ, Weaver FA, Hosking JD, Froehlich J, Folander H, Sussman B, et al. Results of a prospective, randomized trial of surgery versus thrombolysis for occluded lower extremity bypass grafts. Am J Surg. Elsevier. 1996;172(2):105-12.
24. Mathur K, Ayyappan MK, Hodson J, Hopkins J, Duddy MJ, Tiwari A, et al. Stenting as a bail-out option after failed percutaneous transluminal angioplasty in infrainguinal vein bypass grafts. Vascular. SAGE Publications; 2015;1708538115602835.

CHAPTER

10

Recent Advances in Management of Ischaemic Stroke

Souvik Sen, Ravish Kothari, Neil Patel, Lauren D Giamberardino

INTRODUCTION

Stroke is the fifth leading cause of death, the leading cause of preventable disability, and a major source of healthcare costs in the United States.[1] In 2010, Americans were paying approximately $74 billion in stroke-related medical costs. Approximately 795,000 Americans suffer from a new or recurring stroke every year, an average of one stroke every 40 seconds. Stroke claims more than 137,000 lives per year. Stroke mortality remains higher in the Southeastern region defined as the "Stroke Belt", including the following eight states: Alabama, Arkansas, Georgia, Louisiana, Mississippi, North Carolina, South Carolina, and Tennessee.[2] As the United States population continues to grow, the prevalence of stroke is also predicted to increase. By 2030, it is estimated that nearly 4% of the United States population will have suffered a stroke. Individuals over the age of 65 have an increased risk of stroke and this population is expected to grow substantially over the next two decades, resulting in an increase prevalence of stroke as a whole.[3]

Stroke, cerebrovascular accident, or "brain-attack" is defined as a sudden onset of neurological deficits of a vascular origin lasting for greater than or equal to twenty four hours, and confirmed on brain scan (CT or MRI).[4] Stroke occurs when an area of the brain does not receive adequate blood flow due to a blocked or ruptured blood vessel, resulting in deprivation of oxygen and nutrients and a buildup of toxic metabolites. The decrease in blood supply can lead to severe and lasting damage to neural tissue. Blockages can be caused by a blood clot or rupture of a blood vessel and can result in the loss of function in the affected area of the brain. Damage to neural tissue may manifest in sensory, motor, and speech deficits. Signs and symptoms of a stroke include the onset of one-sided weakness or numbness and difficulty with vision, speaking, thinking, or coordination.[1] Sometimes these symptoms will improve within twenty four hours, often within minutes, with no evidence of stroke seen on a brain scan and is referred to as a "mini stroke" of transient ischaemic attack (TIA). A transient ischaemic attack is caused by a temporary clot. The individuals affected by mini strokes are at an even higher risk for a stroke subsequently.[1]

Strokes can be classified into two categories: ischaemic or lack of blood supply to the brain and haemorrhagic or bleeding in and around the brain. The ischaemic strokes are 87% more common and are similar in mechanism to a heart attack, in that ischaemic strokes are caused by the hardening of the blood vessels (atherosclerosis) or a blood clot (thrombus). A haemorrhagic stroke results from a ruptured blood vessel in the brain, increasing pressure and swelling. Strokes can be treatable if diagnosed early, although frequently they go untreated because of a missed diagnosis.[5]

The American Heart and Stroke Associations recommend using FAST (facial droop, arm/limb weakness, speech difficulty, time to dial 911) as a simple screening tool used to quickly recognize a stroke and improve outcomes. Abnormal facial droop is present when on side of the face does not move at all or unequally compared to the opposite side. When one arm drifts either slightly or considerable compared to the other, this is abnormal and can be an early sign of a stroke. An individual showing early signs of a stroke may also have slurred speech, use inappropriate words, or may be unable to speak at all. When these abnormalities are present, it is important to call 911 as soon as possible.[6]

STROKE PREVENTION

Guidelines for the Primary Prevention of Stroke

According to the American Heart and Stroke Associations, 80% of strokes are preventable. The current standards for prevention strategies for ischaemic stroke include blood thinners, cholesterol lowering medications, lifestyle changes, and treatment of risk factors such as high blood pressure.[5]

The 2014 American Heart Association/American Stroke Association Guidelines for the Primary Prevention of Stroke suggests that modifiable risk factors to include high blood pressure, high cholesterol, diabetes, physical inactivity, diet and nutrition, obesity, and cigarette smoking can be crucial in the primary prevention of stroke. High blood pressure is the most important modifiable stroke risk factor because the treatment of high blood pressure is one of the most effective strategies for preventing both ischaemic and haemorrhagic strokes. Patients who have high blood pressure should be treated with antihypertensive drugs with a target blood pressure of 140/90 mmHg. Patients with high cholesterol are estimated to have a high ten year risk for cardiovascular events and should seek treatment with a statin for primary prevention of stroke. Individuals affected by diabetes should seek a comprehensive program that includes thigh control of high blood pressure and glycaemic control to reduce microvascular complications and the risk of stroke. Capable adults should take part in moderate to vigorous aerobic physical activity for at least 40 minutes per day and three to four days a week. Additionally, epidemiological studies and randomised trials have determined that diets low in sodium, high in potassium, and rich in fruits and vegetables may help reduce the risk of stroke. Such diets included the Mediterranean and DASH style diets. Overweight (BMI = 25 to 29 kg/m^2) and obese (BMI >30 kg/m^2) individuals should aim for weight reduction in order to lower blood pressure and thus reducing the risk of stroke. Finally, cigarette smoking is known to increase the risk of ischaemic stroke and subarachnoid hemorrhages. Studies have shown a reduction in stroke risk due to smoking cessation and community-wide smoking bans. To assist active smokers in quitting, both drug therapy (nicotine replacement) and counselling are recommended.[9]

Guidelines for the Secondary Prevention of Stroke

Individuals who have suffered an ischaemic stroke or TIA are at high risk for a recurrent cardiovascular event. On average, these individuals are at a 3-4% risk for a recurrent ischaemic stroke within the first year. The estimated risk for individuals is dependent upon many additional factors including comorbidities and adherence to preventive therapies. Due to the increased risk of recurrent ischaemic events, the American Heart Association and American Stroke Association have prepared the Guidelines for the Prevention of Stroke in Patients with Stroke and Transient ischaemic Attack for prevention of future ischaemic events among survivors of stroke or TIA.[10]

Most imperative in the prevention of secondary stroke is the treatment of high blood pressure, defined as systolic blood pressure greater than or equal to 140 mmHg or a diastolic pressure greater than or equal to 90 mmHg. The prevalence of high blood pressure among patients with a recent ischaemic stroke is approximately 70%, therefore patients with documented blood pressures greater than or equal to 140 mmHg systolic or greater than or equal to 90 mmHg in the days following an initial stroke or TIA should be started on a blood pressure therapy regimen. For patients who have an initial stroke or TIA assumed to be of atherosclerotic origin and are documented to have a LDL-C level greater than or equal to 100 mg/dl, a statin therapy with lipid lowering effects is recommended in an effort to reduce the risk of recurrent events. All patients, after an initial stroke or TIA, should also be screened for diabetes by testing fasting plasma glucose, haemoglobin A1c, or an oral glucose tolerance test. However, haemoglobin A1c may be more accurate in the immediate time period following the event. Pre-existing American Diabetic Association guidelines for glycaemic control is recommended for patients with stroke or TIA who may also be pre-diabetic or diabetic. Nutritional assessments should also be conducted on these patients to test for signs of over nutrition or under nutrition and patients should be referred for individualized nutritional counselling as necessary. Patients with stroke or TIA should reduce their sodium intake to approximately 2.4 g per day or less than 1.5 g per day to further reduce blood pressure. More evidently, these patients should also follow diets like the Mediterranean and DASH diets that are low in sodium, high in potassium, and rich in fruits and vegetables to reduce their recurrent stroke risk. Capable adults should also make an effort to participate in moderate to vigorous aerobic physical activity at least three to four times a week. These sessions should last on average 40 minutes and should be sufficient enough to break a sweat or noticeably raise the heart rate (i.e. walking briskly, exercise bicycle). Healthcare providers should also strongly advise those patients who have had a stroke or TIA and have smoked in the last year to quit and avoid second hand tobacco smoke. In an effort to help patient quit smoking, providers can offer counselling, nicotine replacement products, and oral smoking cessation medications.[10]

STROKE TREATMENT

A current treatment of ischaemic stroke revolves around salvaging the penumbra or area that is functionally impaired, due to a lack of oxygen, but structurally sounds. When stroke patients reach the emergency department in a timely fashion, they are subjected to brain scans (CT or MRI) and can be treated with a clot busting medication called Tissue Plasminogen Activator (tPA), the gold standard treatment for ischaemic strokes. Tissue Plasminogen Activator works by dissolving the blood vessel blockage, restoring blood flow to the stroke affected part of the brain. If administered within a three our window from stroke symptom onset, tPA may significantly improve the chances of recovering from stroke. The National Institute of Neurological Disorders and Stroke (NINDS) study suggests that patients who received tPA in accordance with a strict protocol were at least 30% more likely to recover within three months of the stroke without any significant disability. In some medical centres with interventional capabilities, endovascular catheter based clot retrieval devices can be used (up to eight hours from stroke symptom onset) and further improvement of the stroke deficits may occur.[9] When arteries (i.e. common carotid artery) show signs of plaque buildup or blockages, additional medical procedures may be necessary such as: carotid endarterectomy, angioplasty, or stent placement. Carotid endarterectomy, or carotid artery surgery, is a procedure in which blood vessel blockage is surgically removed from the carotid artery. Physicians may also use balloon angioplasty and implantable steel screens called stents to dilate the blood vessel and increase blood flow.

Endovascular procedures may also be used to treat certain haemorrhagic strokes similar to the procedure used for treating ischaemic strokes. This less invasive procedure involves the use of a catheter introduced through a major artery in the leg or arm that is guided to the cause of the hemorrhage and then deposits a mechanical agent, such as a coil, to prevent rupture or further bleeding. For strokes caused by a bleed within the brain or by an abnormal tangle of blood vessels or arteriovenous malformation (AVM), surgical treatment may be a consideration to stop the bleeding. If the bleed is caused by a ruptured aneurysm, swelling of the vessel that causes a rupture, a metal clip can be placed surgically at the base of the aneurysm to secure it.[10]

RECENT ADVANCEMENT IN STROKE TREATMENT

New Randomised Clinical Trials of Endovascular Stroke Treatment

Intra-arterial Fibrinolysis and/or First-generation Mechanical Embolectomy Devices

SYNTHESIS

A prospective, randomized, open-label blinded-end point, two arm superiority trial, SYNTHESIS Expansion enrolled 362 patients with ischaemic stroke eligible for IV tPA within 4.5 hours of stroke symptom onset and were eligible for possible endovascular treatment within six hours. The only imaging required for enrollment was non-enhanced computed tomography (CT). Patients were randomized 1:1 to either standard dose IV tPA or endovascular therapy (intra-arterial (IA) tPA, mechanical clot disruption or retrieval, or a combination of these approaches). The median stroke symptom onset to treatment was 2.75 hours in the IV tPA arm and 3.75 hours in the endovascular treatment arm. Among those patients receiving endovascular treatment, 66% were treated with IA tPA and thrombus disruption with a guidewire only; in 34% of the participants a device was fully deployed and stent retrievers were used in 14%. Rates and efficacy of recanalization were not published. However, there was no difference in the primary end point of percentage with good outcome (modified Rankin Scale (mRS) 0–1), death at three months, or symptomatic intracerebral haemorrhage (sICH) at seven days.[11]

IMS III

The Interventional Management of Stroke III (IMS III) was a prospective, randomized, open-label blinded-end point, two arm superiority trial enrolling patients with major ischaemic stroke (NIHSS ≥10), receiving IV tPA within three hours and likely to or known to have a major cerebral artery (MCA) occlusion. Patients presenting with hypodensity in greater than one-third of the MCA territory on non-enhanced CT were excluded. Patients were randomized 1:2 to standard dose IV tPA or to IV tPA at 0.6 mg/kg followed my endovascular therapy with a device and/or IA tPA if occlusion persisted and intervention could begin within five hours and completed within seven hours of stroke symptom onset. In the endovascular treatment group, groin puncture was completed at an average of 208 ± 47 minutes post-stroke onset. In the endovascular treatment group, 77% received endovascular intervention, IA tPA alone was administered to 41%, 59% received device with or without IA tPA, and in only 1.5% a stent retriever was used. Recanalization occurred 325 ± 52 minutes post-stroke onset, resulting in Thrombolysis In Cerebral Infarction (TICI) grade of 2b/3 in 41% of participants. There was no significant difference in outcome between the IV tPA only group and the endovascular treatment group for the primary end point of the percentage of patients with a good outcome (mRS 0–2) or death at 90 days. In the endovascular treatment group, there was no difference in outcome between those treated ≤90 minutes versus >90 minutes from IV tPA to groin puncture. However, the participants with mRS 0–2 at 90 days increased with increasing recanalization.[11]

MR RESCUE

A prospective, randomized, open-label blinded-end point, two arm superiority trial, MR and Recanalization of Stroke Clots Using Embolectomy (MR RESCUE), enrolled 118 patients with larger artery occlusion and anterior circulation ischaemic stroke within eight hours of stroke symptom onset and ineligible for IV tPA or presenting with persistent vessel occlusion after IV tPA. Patients were divided into subgroups by pretreatment CT or MRI, those with a favourable penumbral pattern and those with an unfavourable penumbral pattern, using imaging criteria based on a previous study. Subsequently, patients were randomly assigned 1:1 to standard medical care or endovascular therapy (MERCI or Penumbra device with optional IA tPA). Average stroke symptom onset to groin puncture in the endovascular group was 6.35 ± 1.2 hours. 25% of the endovascular group resulted in a TICI 2b/3 recanalisation. Mean scores on mRS at 90 days did not differ between the endovascular group and the standard medical care group. Endovascular therapy was not superior to standard medical care in patients with a favourable penumbral pattern or in patients with an unfavourable penumbral pattern.[11]

Stent Retrievers

MR CLEAN

The Multicenter Randomized Clinical Trial of Endovascular Treatment for Acute ischaemic Stroke (MR CLEAN) was a prospective, randomised, open-label blinded-end point, two arm superiority trial that enrolled 500 patients with acute ischaemic stroke caused by a proximal intracranial occlusion in the anterior circulation (distal intracranial carotid artery, MCA M1 or M2, or anterior cerebral artery A1 or A2) determined by CTA, MRA or DSA, with a NIHSS ≥ 2, and for whom endovascular treatment within six hours of stroke onset was possible. Specific exclusion criteria were included for patients with coagulation abnormalities, previous ischaemic stroke, ICH, or severe head trauma depending on intra-arterial fibrinolysis was contemplated. Patients meeting national guidelines received IV tPA and those with little to no response were eligible. Patients were randomized 1:1 to standard care alone or IA treatment plus standard care. IA treatment consisted of arterial catheterisation with a microcatheter to the occlusion with the delivery of a fibrinolytic agent, mechanical thrombectomy, or both. 64% of patients presented with an M1 occlusion and an additional 27% presented with an M1 occlusion and ICA occlusion. Of 195 participants in the endovascular group of 233 receiving endovascular treatment, the stroke onset to groin puncture time was 260 minutes, a stent retriever was used in 81.5% and a TICI 2b/3 was achieved in 59%. There was an absolute difference of 13.5% in the rate of functional independence (mRS 0-2) in favor of intervention. There was no significant difference in mortality or the occurrence of sICH. The trial reported a stroke onset to reperfusion time of 332 minutes and demonstrated a significant decline in clinical benefit in such that the benefit may no longer be significant if reperfusion occurred after 6 hours and 19 minutes.[11]

ESCAPE

The Endovascular Treatment for Small Core and Anterior Circulation Proximal Occlusion with Emphasis on Minimizing CT to Recanalization Times (ESCAPE) was a prospective, randomized, open-label blinded-end point, two arm superiority trial that enrolled 316 patients with disabling acute ischaemic stroke (NIHSS > 5) with randomisation up to 12 hours post stroke onset. Groin puncture had to be possible within one hour of CT/CTA, therefore CT and CTA were performed rapidly with a target door-to-CT time of 25 minutes in order to identify patients with small infarct cores, occluded proximal intracranial artery in the anterior circulation (ICA, M1 MCA, or ≥M2s), and moderate to good collateral circulation (filling of 50% of the MCA pial arterial circulation on CTA). There were no exclusions for coagulation abnormalities, prior strokes, or head trauma. A total of 58 patients received IV tPA at a community hospital and were subsequently transferred to an ESCAPE endovascular center. Patients were randomized 1:1 to receive standard care alone or standard care plus endovascular treatment with the use of available thrombectomy devices. The use of retrievable stents and aspiration through a balloon-guided catheter during endovascular treatment was also recommended. Participants in both groups received IV tPA within four and a half hours after stroke onset if they met local guidelines. Of the 151 participants in the intervention group, retrievable stents were used in 130 (86.1%) and a TICI 2b/3 recanalisation was observed in 72.4%. The percentage of patients with a mRS 0-2 at 90 days was 53.0% in the intervention group and 29.3% in the standard care group. Mortality at 90 days was 10.4% in the intervention group and 19.0% in the standard care group. Clinically determined by the study sites, the rate of sICH in the intervention group was 3.6% and in the standard care group was 2.7%.[11]

SWIFT PRIME

A prospective, randomized, open-label blinded-end point trial, SWIFT PRIME, randomized 196 patients with acute ischaemic stroke and NIHSS 8-29, receiving IV tPA within 4.5 hours of stroke onset, and had CTA or MRA confirmation of intracranial ICA, M1, or carotid terminus occlusion. Groin puncture had to be possible within 6 hours of stoke onset. Specific exclusion criteria were included for coagulation abnormalities. Originally, enrollment required CT perfusion or multimodal MRI and was limited to patients with a target mismatch profile as defined by the ischaemic core lesion measuring ≤ 50ml, the volume of tissue with time to maximum delay of >10 seconds was ≤ 100ml, and the mismatch volume was at least 15 ml and the mismatch ratio was >1.8. In order to accommodate sites with limited perfusion imaging capability, the inclusion criteria was modified halfway through the study and sites without perfusion imaging used ASPECTS >6 when required. At total of 71 participants were enrolled under the initial imaging inclusion criteria and 125 patients were enrolled under the revised inclusion criteria. Perfusion imaging was used for enrollment in 82.6% of the participants. M1 occlusions were observed in 73% of the participants and 17% had ICA occlusions. IV tPA was administered at an outside hospital in 35% of the participants. Participants were randomized 1:1 to treatment with IV tPA alone or IV tPA followed by neurovascular thrombectomy with the use of a stent retriever. In an interim analysis, two simultaneous success criteria used for primary end point were both in favor or endovascular intervention: improved distribution of mRS at 90 days and increased proportion of mRS 0–2 (60% in the endovascular group and 35% in the non-endovascular group). TICI 2b/3 recanalisation was observed in 88% of the endovascular group and there were no significant differences in mortality or sICH.[11]

EXTEND-IA

Similar to the SWIFT PRMIE trial, The Extending the Time for Thrombolysis in Emergency Neurological Deficits-Intra-Arterial (EXTEND-IA) enrolled 70 participants determined eligible using standard criteria for IV tPA within four and half hours of stroke onset and the participants were randomized to receive either IV tPA only or IV tPA plus endovascular therapy with a stent retriever. Groin puncture had to be possible within six hours and endovascular treatment had to be completed within eight hours or stroke onset. Imaging, CT or MRI, had to be performed before commencing IV tPA. Occlusion of the ICA, M1 or M2 on CTA was also required. CT or MRI perfusion imaging had to show a mismatch ratio of > 1.2, an absolute mismatch volume of >10 ml, and an infarct core lesion volume of < 70 ml. There were additional specific exclusion criteria for coagulation abnormalities. About 31% of the participants presented with an ICA occlusion and 54% with a M1 occlusion. Co-primary outcomes were reperfusion at 24 hours and early neurologic improvement defined by a ≥8 point reduction on NIHSS or a score of 0–1 by day 3. The secondary outcome was mRS at 90 days. Results of an early interim analysis showed that the percentage of ischaemic territory having undergone reperfusion at 24 hours was greater in the endovascular therapy group than in the IV tPA only group. When initiated at a median time of 210 minutes from stroke onset, endovascular therapy increased neurologic improvement at three days. Functional independence was achieved in more endovascular therapy group participants than the IV tPA only group. There was no significant difference in the rates of mortality or sICH and a TICI 2b/3 recanalisation was achieved in 86% of participants in the endovascular group at a median of 248 minutes from stroke onset.[11]

Revascularisation with Solitaire Vs. Best Medical Therapy

REVASCAT

Endovascular Revascularization With Solitaire Device Versus Best Medical Therapy in Anterior Circulation Stroke Within 8 hours (REVASCAT) was a prospective, randomized, open-label, blinded-end point trial that randomized 206 patients with acute ischaemic stroke, NIHSS ≥6, who had intracranial ICA or M1 occlusion by CTA, MRA, or DSA. Patients who had received IV tPA were eligible if there was no significant neurological improvement at 30 minutes post-initiation of infusion and vascular imaging confirmed eligible occlusion. Groin puncture had to be possible within eight hours of stroke onset. There were additional exclusion criteria for coagulation abnormalities. The main exclusion criteria on imaging were ASPECTS <7 on non-enhanced CT or <6 on DWI-MRI. Patients presenting with ICA occlusion accounted for 26% and M1 occlusion accounted for 65% of enrolled. Participants were randomized 1:1 to either medical therapy alone or thrombectomy with a stent retriever. About

73% of participants received IV tPA. With the release of results from similar trials, the Data Safety Monitoring Board recommended stopping recruitment due to loss of equipoise although the interim data analysis results did not reach the pre-specified stopping boundaries. The primary outcome analysis showed an improvement in the distribution of the mRS score favouring endovascular treatment. In the intervention group, 43.7% of participants had a mRS of 0-2 at 90 days compared to only 28.2% in the control group. Of those in the endovascular group, 95% underwent thrombectomy with a TICI 2b/3 recanalisation observed in 66%. There were no significant differences in mortality or sICH.[11]

ANALYSIS AND CONCLUSION

SYNTHESIS, IMS III, and MR RESCUE evaluated the role of IV-rTPA versus endovascular therapy with intra-arterial tPA, mechanical clot disruption, clot retrieval or a combination of both. In these studies, however, stent retrievers were only used in 14% and 1.5%, in SYNTHESIS and IMS III, respectively, while MR RESCUE primarily utilized first generation embolectomy devices including MERCI and PENUMBRA. Using these methods, all three of these trials showed no significant benefit to endovascular treatment using IA tPA, clot disruption or embolectomy with first generation devices relative to IV tPA.[11]

Largely using stent retrievers, MR CLEAN, ESCAPE, SWIFT PRIME, EXTEND-IA, and REVASCAT, showed an overwhelming benefit to IV tPA plus endovascular treatment with stent retrieval vs IV tPA alone. In all five of these studies, enrolled participants were greater than 18 years of age, and stroke severity based on NIHSS ranged from 2 to 29. These trials did not provide sufficient data to show a benefit from endovascular treatment in patients with a NIHSS of less than 6.[11]

While REVASCAT and ESCAPE enrolled patients for endovascular therapy greater than 6 hours out, both studies had too little or no data to establish benefit in those who received therapy in that time frame. MR CLEAN, EXTEND IA, and SWIFT PRIME required that patient's undergo groin puncture within 6 hours of onset of symptoms with MR CLEAN investigators stating that there was a noted decline in benefit with increased time beyond 6 hours. Given such, recommended symptom onset to groin puncture for endovascular therapy is 6 hours or less.[11]

Four of the five trials used a baseline function evaluation for inclusion using either pre-stroke mRS of 0 to 1 (RESVASCAT and SWIFT PRIME), 0 to 2 (EXTEND-IA) or Barthel scores great than or equal to 90 (ESCAPE).[11]

All five studies required baseline non-enhanced CT or MRI, and four of the five studies evaluated ASPECT scores showing a benefit from endovascular therapy in patients with ASPECT scores greater than or equal to 6. In addition, all five studies used additional imaging in the form of CTA, MRA and in some cases DSA to identify large vessel occlusions. Because only a minority of patients gain recanalisation using IV tPA alone, noninvasive vascular imaging should be obtained as quickly as possible after the initiation of IV tPA to identify those patients who would benefit from endovascular therapy should imaging indicate its need.[11]

ESCAPE, EXTEND-IA, and SWIFT PRIME were initially designed to use additional imaging modalities for the evaluation of ischaemic core infarcts and salvageable brain tissue. ESCAPE utilized CTA in addition to CT with the calculation of ASPECT scores for determination of large vessel occlusion and small infarct cores in addition to good collateral circulation. EXTEND-IA patients underwent CT perfusion for demonstration of potentially salvageable tissue based on mismatch ratios and ischaemic core size while SWIFT PRIME excluded patients with infarcts greater than one-third of the MCA territory or involving greater than 100 ml of tissue. Despite the use of additional imaging for evaluation of endovascular intervention, none of these studies were designed to validate the utility of advanced imaging selection.[11]

A large majority of patients in the stent retriever trials had internal carotid artery or proximal M1 occlusions. The number of isolated M2 occlusions was small as ESCAPE, REVASCAT, and SWIFT PRIME only enrolled a small number of these patients despite initially setting out to exclude these patients. None of the stent retriever trials excluded patients on the basis of proximal cervical carotid stenosis. The numbers of patients with proximal cervical carotid stenosis or occlusion was noted to be significant in REVASCAT (18%) and MR CLEAN (32%). Many of the patients in both of these trials underwent stenting at the time of thrombectomy. Based on this data, thrombectomy following stenting in patients with cervical artery stenosis is indicated, though there may be a higher incidence of ICH given the need for aggressive antiplatelet therapy in stent patients.[11]

While the benefit of general anaesthesia with intubation versus conscious sedation for patients undergoing endovascular treatment was not directly addressed in these studies, the MR CLEAN trial showed that patients who had general anaesthesia with intubation did no better or worse compared to the non-endovascular control patients, whereas those endovascular patients who did not have general anaesthesia did better than the control group. A meta-analysis of 9 nonrandomized studies showed that of approximately 2000 patients, where roughly 800 received general anaesthesia and 1200 received conscious sedation, those who had general anaesthesia were shown to have lower odds of a favourable functional outcome, and higher odds of mortality. In addition, no significant difference was noted between mean groin puncture, mean procedure time, and mean symptom onset to revascularisation between the two methods of sedation. As a result, it is felt that conscious sedation may be safer and more effective than general anaesthesia in patients undergoing endovascular intervention.[11]

FUTURE OF ENDOVASCULAR STROKE TREATMENT

The rate of infarct development following blockage in the blood flow is highly variable and differs in individual patients. Salvageable brain tissue can be present in many patients beyond 6 hours from stroke onset. Identifying these patients and providing them appropriate endovascular therapy will have a major impact on stroke morbidity and stroke-related healthcare cost. Recently, Standford University in collaboration of National Institute of Neurological Disorders and stroke (NINDS), University of Cincinnati, Medical University of

South Carolina and NINDS Stroke Trials Network (StrokeNet) has initiated a study to evaluate the safety and efficacy of thrombectomy in carefully selected patients with ischaemic stroke who are treated with thrombectomy between 6-16 hours from stroke onset. The study has been named as **"Endovascular Therapy Following Imaging Evaluation for ischaemic Stroke (DEFUSE 3)"**. The information provided in this section is a *Courtesy* of Dr Gregory Albers who is the Director of Stanford Stroke Center and also the lead sponsor for this study.

DEFUSE 3 is an NIH funded, prospective, randomized, phase III, multicentre, controlled, adaptive and open label trial. The purpose of the study is to assess the safety and efficacy of thrombectomy in patients with acute anterior circulation ischaemic stroke who can be treated with thrombectomy between 6-16 hours from stroke onset. The study will shift the patient selection from time-based to imaging-based.[12]

According to the proposed protocol of the study, patients will be first screened for the following clinical criteria. Once they clear the screening criteria, the next step will be to order a CT perfusion with IV contrast or an MRI along with CTA or MRA. The neuroimaging inclusion and exclusion criteria are provided separately below. Once the patient meets both clinical and neurological criteria, the next step would be a randomization in a 1:1 ratio to treatment group (endovascular therapy plus standard medical therapy) versus standard medical therapy alone. Only FDA cleared thrombectomy devices such as Trevo Retriever, Solitaire FR Revascularisation Device, Penumbra thrombectomy system [Penumbra Aspiration Pump 115v, Penumbra System Separator Flex (026, 032, 041, 054), Penumbra System MAX, Penumbra Pump MAX] or Covidien MindFrame Capture Revascularization Device can be used in this study. The individual endovascular therapist can select any of these devices for the procedure. Enrollment of a maximum of 476 patients (238 in each arm) is planned over the four year duration from April 2016 to June 2020. A novel adaptive design will identify the group with the best prospect for showing maximum positive effect from endovascular treatment, based on baseline DWI lesion volumes and the times since stroke onset. The team will also perform an Interim analysis at 200th and 340th patients to determine if the study needs to be continued or stopped based on the efficacy or futility. The primary end point of the study is the modified Rankin Score (mRS) at 90 days from stroke onset. DEFUSE 3 will be a very important breakthrough in the future ischaemic stroke management by determining if endovascular treatment, performed within 16 hours from stroke symptom onset or last known normal, improves functional outcome in patients meeting below mentioned clinical and neuroimaging criteria. The study has a potential to offer endovascular treatment to a large number of stroke patients which can subsequently result in a reduction in stroke morbidity and stroke-related healthcare costs.[12]

Clinical Inclusion Criteria

- Signs and symptoms consistent with the diagnosis of acute anterior circulation ischaemic stroke

- Age 18–90 years
- Baseline NIHSSS is ≥6 and remains ≥6 immediately prior to randomization.
- Endovascular treatment can be initiated (femoral puncture) between 6 and 16 hours of stroke onset. Stroke onset is defined as the time the patient was last known to be at their neurologic baseline (wake-up strokes are eligible if they meet the above time limits).
- Modified Rankin Scale less than or equal to 2 prior to qualifying stroke (functionally independent for all ADLs).
- Patient/Legally Authorized Representative has signed the Informed Consent form.

Clinical Exclusion Criteria

- Other serious, advanced, or terminal illness (investigator judgment) or life expectancy is less than 6 months.
- Pre-existing medical, neurological or psychiatric disease that would confound the neurological or functional evaluations.
- Pregnant
- Unable to undergo a contrast brain perfusion scan with either MRI or CT.
- Known allergy to iodine that precludes an endovascular procedure.
- Treated with tPA >4.5 hours after time last known well.
- Treated with tPA 3–4.5 hours after last known well AND any of the following; age >80, current anticoagulant use, history of diabetes or prior stroke, NIHSS >25.
- Known hereditary or acquired haemorrhagic diathesis, coagulation factor deficiency; recent oral anticoagulant therapy with INR >3 (recent use of one of the new oral anticoagulants is not exclusion if estimated GFR >30 ml/min).
- Seizures at stroke onset if it precludes obtaining an accurate baseline NIHSS.
- Baseline blood glucose of <50 mg/dl (2.78 mmol) or >400 mg/dl (22.20 mmol).
- Baseline platelet count <50,000/µl
- Severe, sustained hypertension (Systolic BP >185 mmHg or diastolic BP >110 mmHg).
- Current participation in another investigational drug or device study.
- Presumed septic embolus; suspicion of bacterial endocarditis.
- Clot retrieval attempted using a neurothrombectomy device prior to 6 hours from symptom onset.

Neuroimaging Inclusion Criteria

- ICA or MCA-M1 occlusion (carotid occlusions can be cervical or intracranial; with or without tandem MCA lesions) by MRA or CTA AND.
- Target mismatch profile on CT perfusion or MRI (ischaemic core volume is <70 ml, mismatch ratio is ≥/= 1.8 and mismatch volume* is ≥15 ml).

Alternative Neuroimaging Inclusions Criteria (if Perfusion imaging or CTA/MRA is technically inadequate)

A. If CTA (or MRA) is technically inadequate:
Tmax >6s perfusion deficit consistent with an ICA or MCA-M1 occlusion AND Target Mismatch Profile (ischaemic core volume is <70 ml, mismatch ratio is >1.8 and mismatch volume is >15 ml as determined by RAPID software).
B. If MRP is technically inadequate:
ICA or MCA-M1 occlusion (carotid occlusions can be cervical or intracranial; with or without tandem MCA lesions) by MRA (or CTA, if MRA is technically inadequate and a CTA was performed within 60 minutes prior to the MRI) AND DWI lesion volume <25 ml.
C. If CTP is technically inadequate:
Patient can be screened with MRI and randomized if neuroimaging criteria are met.

Neuroimaging Exclusion Criteria

- ASPECTS score <6 on non-contrast CT (if baseline non-contrast CT was performed).
- Evidence of intracranial tumor (except small meningioma) acute intracranial haemorrhage, neoplasm, or arteriovenous malformation.
- Significant mass effect with midline shift.
- Evidence of internal carotid artery dissection that is flow limiting or aortic dissection.
- Intracranial stent implanted in the same vascular territory that precludes the safe deployment/removal of the neurothrombectomy device.
- Occlusions in multiple vascular territories (e.g., bilateral anterior circulation, or anterior/posterior circulation).

RAPID Software

DEFUSE 3 study will use the images processed by the RAPID software for the selection of 100% of the patients. RAPID is cleared by FDA for clinical and research use. RAPID is actually a medical image software package that is useful for viewing, processing and analysis of brain images. It processes CT or MRI brain images quickly, accurately and efficiently. It is fast and easy to use. The results can be viewed on any computer. The hospital only requires a computer connected with the CT/MRI scanner. It is compatible with CT and MRI machines from all major manufactures in the market.[13]

RAPID Features

The RAPID program produces high-quality perfusion maps from dynamic contrast MRI or CT perfusion scans. It computes brain image maps with volumes of interest from diffusion and perfusion MRI scans and CT perfusion scans. CT or MRI technologist sends the CTP or MRI images from the scanner to the processing system where the data are processed automatically using the pre-specified parameters. The final output becomes available in minutes on hospital DICOM devices such as PACS and can be viewed along with the patient's clinical images. The software provides a real time view of brain perfusion that is easy to interpret which allows physicians to determine accurate volume of core infarct and penumbra.[13]

Understanding CT Images

- No perfusion (Fig. 1)
- Reperfusion (Fig. 2)
- Large CBF Lesion (Fig. 3).

Understanding MRI Images:

- No reperfusion (Fig. 4)
- Reperfusion (Fig. 5).

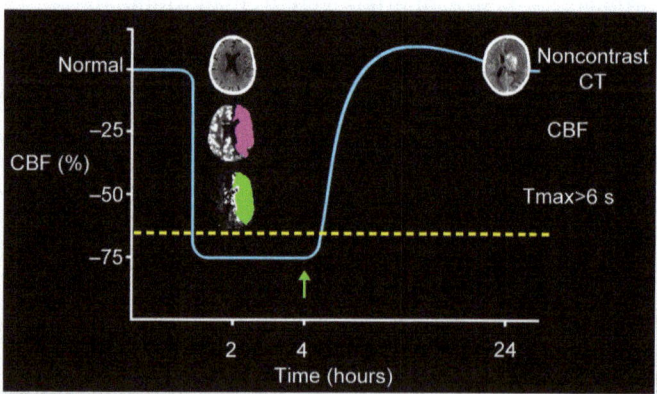

Figure 1: Patient with a persistent left middle cerebral artery (MCA) occlusion: 2 hours after symptom onset the non-contrast CT (NCCT) is normal. Cerebral blood flow (CBF) is reduced by >70% in a small region of the left hemisphere (pink on the RAPID CBF map). Perfusion is substantially delayed (>6 seconds) in a much larger region of the left hemisphere (green on the RAPID Tmax >6 s map). By 8 hours the early ischaemic lesion is now visible on the NCCT and the volume of the lesion with > 70% reduction in CBF has grown (pink on the RAPID CBF map). The degree of perfusion delay (green on the RAPID Tmax map) is unchanged. Despite the persistent MCA occlusion, at 24 hours the CBF values within the ischaemic lesion have increased, due to improved collateral flow, and are now reduced by less than 70% and therefore no longer visible as pink on the RAPID CBF map. The full ischaemic lesion is now clearly seen on the NCCT. CBF (0.3): regions with CBF reduced by >70% are pink on CBF maps. Regions with perfusion delay >6 seconds are green on Tmax >6 s maps

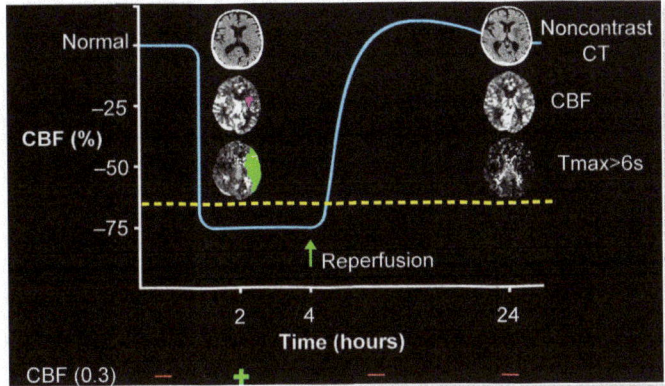

Figure 2: Patient with a left middle cerebral artery (MCA) occlusion and early reperfusion: 2 hours after symptom onset the noncontrast CT (NCCT) is normal. Cerebral blood flow (CBF) is reduced by >70% in a small region of the left hemisphere (pink on the RAPID CBF map). Perfusion is substantially delayed (>6 seconds) in a much larger region of the left hemisphere (green on the RAPID Tmax >6 s map). Early reperfusion occurs at 4 hours (green arrow) resulting in a sudden rise in CBF values. At 24 hours the CBF values within the ischaemic lesion are normal; therefore the lesion is no longer visible on the CBF map. A small ischaemic lesion is now clearly seen on the NCCT in the same region as the initial CBF lesion. Regions with CBF reduced by >70% are pink on CBF maps. Regions with a perfusion delay >6 seconds are green on Tmax > 6 s maps

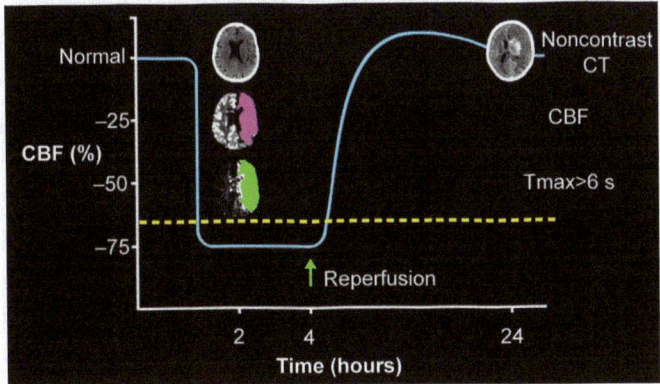

Figure 3: Patient with a left middle cerebral artery (MCA) occlusion and large lesion with low cerebral blood flow (CBF): 2 hours after symptom onset the noncontrast CT (NCCT) is normal. CBF is reduced by >70% in a large region of the left hemisphere (pink on the RAPID CBF map). Perfusion is substantially delayed (> 6 seconds) in the same region of the left hemisphere (green on the RAPID Tmax map) that has low CBF. Despite reperfusion at 4 hours no tissue salvage occurs. A large ischaemic lesion with haemorrhagic transformation and substantial oedema is seen on the 24 hour NCCT. Regions with CBF reduced by >70% are pink on CBF map. Regions with a perfusion delay >6 seconds are green on Tmax >6 s map

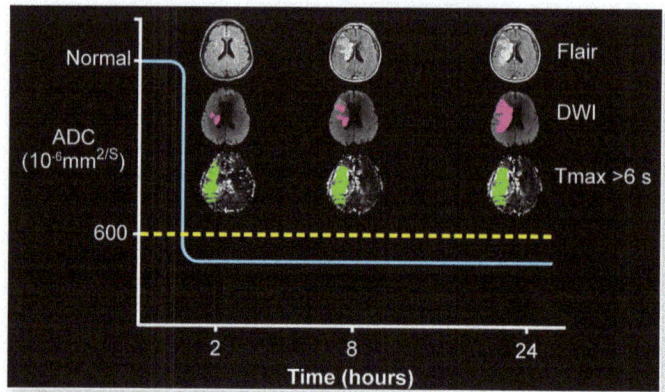

Figure 4: Patient with a persistent right middle cerebral artery (MCA) occlusion: 2 hours after symptom onset the FLAIR sequence is normal. The apparent diffusion coefficient (ADC) values are substantially reduced in a small region of the right hemisphere (pink on the RAPID DWI map). Perfusion is substantially delayed (>6 seconds) in a much larger region of the right hemisphere (green on the RAPID Tmax map). By 8 hours the early ischaemic lesion is now visible on the FLAIR and the volume of the lesion with a severed reduction in ADC has grown (pink on DWI map). The degree of perfusion delay (green on Tmax map) is unchanged. At 24 hours, the full ischaemic lesion is now clearly seen on both the DWI and FLAIR. Regions with apparent diffusion coefficient (ADC) reduced <600 are pink on DWI maps. Regions with perfusion delay >6 seconds are green on Tmax >6 s maps

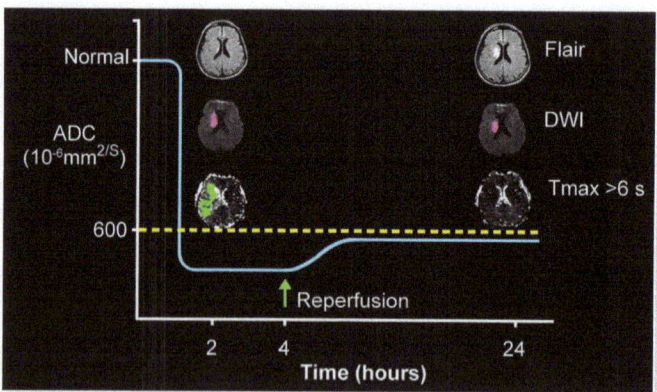

Figure 5: Patient with a right middle cerebral artery (MCA) occlusion and early reperfusion: 2 hours after symptom onset the FLAIR sequence is normal. The apparent diffusion coefficient (ADC) values are substantially reduced in a small region of the right hemisphere (pink on the RAPID DWI map). Perfusion is substantially delayed (>6 seconds) in a much larger region of the right hemisphere (green on the RAPID Tmax map). Early reperfusion occurs resulting in complete resolution of the green perfusion lesion and an increase in ADC values. The ischaemic lesion remains pink on the RAPID DWI map because the ADC values are still below 600. At 24 hours, a small ischaemic lesion is now clearly seen on both the FLAIR and the DWI in the same region as the initial DWI lesion. Regions with apparent diffusion coefficient (ADC) reduced <600 are pink on DWI maps. Regions with perfusion delay >6 seconds are green on Tmax >6 s maps

RECOMMENDATIONS FROM GUIDELINES

Endovascular Interventions

1. Patients eligible for intravenous r-tPA should receive intravenous r-tPA even if endovascular treatments are being considered (Class I; Level of Evidence A).
2. Patients should receive endovascular therapy with a stent retriever if they meet all of the following criteria (Class I; Level of Evidence A).
   a. Pre-stroke mRS score 0 to 1
   b. Acute ischaemic stroke receiving intravenous r-tPA within 4.5 hours of onset according to guidelines from professional medical societies,
   c. Causative occlusion of the internal carotid artery or proximal MCA (M1),
   d. Age ≥18 years,
   e. NIHSS score of ≥6,
   f. ASPECTS of ≥6, and
   g. Treatment can be initiated (groin puncture) within 6 hours of symptom onset
3. As with intravenous r-tPA, reduced time from symptom onset to reperfusion with endovascular therapies is highly associated with better clinical outcomes. To ensure benefit, reperfusion to TICI grade 2b/3 should be achieved as early as possible and within 6 hours of stroke onset (Class I; Level of Evidence B-R).
4. When treatment is initiated beyond 6 hours from symptom onset, the effectiveness of endovascular therapy is uncertain for patients with acute ischaemic stroke who have causative occlusion of the internal carotid artery or proximal MCA (M1) (Class IIb; Level of Evidence C). Additional randomized trial data are needed.
5. In carefully, selected patients with anterior circulation occlusion who have contraindications to intravenous r-tPA, endovascular therapy with stent retrievers completed within 6 hours of stroke onset is reasonable (Class IIa; Level of Evidence C). There are inadequate data available at this time to determine the clinical efficacy of endovascular therapy with stent retrievers for those patients whose contraindications are time-based or nontime-based (e.g. prior stroke, serious head trauma, haemorrhagic coagulopathy, or receiving anticoagulant medications).
6. Although the benefits are uncertain, use of endovascular therapy with stent retrievers may be reasonable for carefully selected patients with acute ischaemic stroke in whom treatment can be initiated (groin puncture) within 6 hours of symptom onset and who have causative occlusion of the M2 or M3 portion of the MCAs, anterior cerebral arteries, vertebral arteries, basilar artery, or posterior cerebral arteries (Class IIb; Level of Evidence C).
7. Endovascular therapy with stent retrievers may be reasonable for some patients <18 years of age with acute ischaemic stroke who have demonstrated large vessel occlusion in whom treatment can be initiated (groin puncture) within 6 hours of symptom onset, but the benefits are not established in this age group (Class IIb; Level of Evidence C).

8. Although the benefits are uncertain, use of endovascular therapy with stent retrievers may be reasonable for patients with acute ischaemic stroke in whom treatment can be initiated (groin puncture) within 6 hours of symptom onset and who have pre-stroke mRS score of >1, ASPECTS <6, or NIHSS score <6 and causative occlusion of the internal carotid artery or proximal MCA (M1) (Class IIb; Level of Evidence B-R). Additional randomised trial data are needed.
9. Observing patients after intravenous r-tPA to assess for clinical response before pursuing endovascular therapy is not required to achieve beneficial outcomes and is not recommended. (Class III; Level of Evidence B-R).
10. Use of stent retrievers is indicated in preference to the MERCI device. (Class I; Level of Evidence A). The use of mechanical thrombectomy devices other than stent retrievers may be reasonable in some circumstances (Class IIb, Level B-NR).
11. The use of proximal balloon guide catheter or a large bore distal access catheter rather than a cervical guide catheter alone in conjunction with stent retrievers may be beneficial (Class IIa; Level of Evidence C). Future studies should examine which systems provide the highest recanalisation rates with the lowest risk for nontarget embolization.
12. The technical goal of the thrombectomy procedure should be a TICI 2b/3 angiographic result to maximize the probability of a good functional clinical outcome (Class I; Level of Evidence A). Use of salvage technical adjuncts including intra-arterial fibrinolysis may be reasonable to achieve these angiographic results, if completed within 6 hours of symptom onset (Class IIb; Level of Evidence B-R).
13. Angioplasty and stenting of proximal cervical atherosclerotic stenosis or complete occlusion at the time of thrombectomy may be considered but the usefulness is unknown (Class IIb; Level of Evidence C). Future randomised studies are needed.
14. Initial treatment with intra-arterial fibrinolysis is beneficial for carefully selected patients with major ischaemic strokes of < 6 hours' duration caused by occlusions of the MCA (Class I; Level of Evidence B-R). However, these data derive from clinical trials that no longer reflect current practice, including use of fibrinolytic drugs that are not available. A clinically beneficial dose of intra-arterial r-tPA is not established, and r-tPA does not have FDA approval for intra-arterial use. As a consequence, endovascular therapy with stent retrievers is recommended over intra-arterial fibrinolysis as first-line therapy (Class I; Level of Evidence E).
15. Intra-arterial fibrinolysis initiated within 6 hours of stroke onset in carefully selected patients who have contraindications to the use of intravenous r-tPA might be considered, but the consequences are unknown (Class IIb; Level of Evidence C).
16. It might be reasonable to favor conscious sedation over general anaesthesia during endovascular therapy for acute ischaemic stroke. However, the ultimate selection of anaesthetic technique during endovascular therapy for acute ischaemic stroke should be individualised based on patient risk factors, tolerance of the procedure, and other clinical characteristics. Randomised trial data are needed (Class IIb; Level of Evidence C).[11]

REFERENCES

1. Borhani NO. Changes and geographic distribution of Mortality from cerebrovascular disease. Am J Public Health Nations Health. 1965;55:673-81.
2. "What Is Stroke?" Stroke.org. National Stroke Association, 16 July 2014. Available at: http://www.stroke.org/understand-stroke/what-stroke. Accessed Feb. 3, 2015.
3. Sen S, Sumner R, et al. Periodontal disease and recurrent vascular events in stroke/transient ischaemic attack patients. J Stroke Cerebrovasc Dis. 2013; 22(8):1420-7.
4. You Z, Cushman M, Jenny NS, Howard G. Tooth loss, systemic inflammation, and prevalent stroke among participants in the reasons for geographic and racial difference in stroke (REGARDS) study. Atherosclerosis. 2009;203(2):615-9.
5. Sfyroeras GS, Roussas N, Saleptsis VG, Argyriou C, Giannoukas AD. Association between periodontal disease and stroke. J Vasc Surg. 2012;55(4):1178-84.
6. "About Stroke" American Heart Association & American Stroke Association http://www.strokeassociation.org/STROKEORG/AboutStroke/TypesofStroke/TIA/TIA-Transient-Ischemic-Attack_UCM_310942_Article.jsp.
7. Whiteley, William et al. "The Association of Circulating Inflammatory Markers with Recurrent Vascular Events after Stroke: A Prospective Cohort Study." Stroke; a journal of cerebral circulation 42.1 (2011): 10–16. PMC. Web. 29 Aug. 2016.
8. "Stroke Treatments." American Heart Association/American Stroke Association. 23 May 2013. Web.
9. Johansson A, Johansson I, et al. Systemic antibodies to the leukotoxin of the oral pathogen Actinobacillus actinomycetemcomitans correlate negatively with stroke in women. Cerebrovasc Dis. 2005;20(4):226-32.
10. Diaz J, Sempere AP. Cerebral ischemia: new risk factors. Cerebrovasc Dis. 2004; 17 Suppl 1:43-50.
11. Powers WJ, Derdeyn CP, et al. 2015 American Heart Association/American Stroke Association Focused Update of the 2013 Guidelines for the Early Management of Patients With Acute ischaemic Stroke Regarding Endovascular Treatment: A Guideline for Healthcare Professionals From the American Heart Association/American Stroke Association. Stroke. 2015;46(10):3020-35.
12. Endovascular Therapy Following Imaging Evaluation for ischaemic Stroke 3 (DEFUSE 3). Endovascular Therapy Following Imaging Evaluation for ischaemic Stroke 3. US National Institutes of Health, 21 Oct. 2015. Web. 29 July 2016.
13. ISchema View RAPID - RAPID Features. ISchemaView RAPID - RAPID Features. ISchemaView, 2016. Web. 29 July 2016.

CHAPTER

11

Protection Devices in Endovascular Practice

WNDP Chinthaka Appuhamy, Sundeep Punamiya

INTRODUCTION

Endovascular therapy has gained acceptance as a highly successful primary treatment modality for atherosclerotic vascular diseases. Distal embolisation of thromboembolic material generated during endovascular recanalisation can potentially lead to obstruction of the microvascular bed or larger feeding arteries with significant clinical implications.[1,2]

This often necessitates the use of additional bail-out interventions, such as thrombectomy or thrombolysis, resulting in longer procedure times, greater volumes of contrast used, increased cost and higher radiation exposure.

To overcome this potential complication, mechanical embolic protection devices (EPDs) have been developed and tested in different vascular territories. Initially used during angioplasty of carotid arteries and coronary saphenous venous bypass grafts to protect against intervention stroke and myocardial ischaemia respectively, their usage has expanded to endovascular recanalisation of renal and peripheral arteries.[3]

DISTAL EMBOLISATION

During manipulation within a diseased artery, a variety of plaque and vessel wall components may embolise into the distal vasculature, including cholesterol-rich particles, extracellular matrix, endothelial cells, and platelet-thrombus.[3] Although predominantly microscopic in nature, this phenomenon of distal embolism and its affection of distal microvascular bed has been detected consistently with transcranial Doppler, magnetic resonance imaging, peripheral Doppler and myocardial contrast echocardiography. Lam et al used a 4-MHz Doppler probe for continuous monitoring in the ipsilateral popliteal artery during proximal lower limb endovascular treatments, and registered embolic signals in every patient during critical portions of the procedure: guidewire crossing, balloon angioplasty, stent deployment and/or atherectomy.[4] In other series, embolic capture by filters positioned distal to the treated segment confirmed the incidence of embolism in every patient undergoing carotid angioplasty. Direct analysis of captured debris revealed emboli to be most often microscopic and invisible to the naked eye, with size of debris ranging from 10 microns to 8.57 mm; larger macroscopic emboli were noted in almost 25% of patients. Not surprisingly, symptomatic patients were associated with larger volume and bigger size of embolic debris.[5]

EMBOLIC PROTECTION DEVICES

While distal embolisation is inevitable during angioplasty, it becomes essential to prevent emboli, especially the larger ones, from occluding important vascular beds and producing clinical sequelae. Embolic protection devices (EPDs) provide effective mechanical protection from emboli, and has been used in various arterial beds with success. Many devices are currently in use, using either filtration or flow cessation as the method of protection. Devices are categorised into three classes:
A. Distal protection devices
   1. Filter devices
   2. Distal occlusion devices
B. Proximal occlusion devices
   1. With flow reversal
   2. Without flow reversal
C. Proximal and distal occlusion devices.

Distal Protection Devices

Distal protection devices need to cross the target lesion and are deployed in the distal artery, where they trap the embolic debris before they can be removed. Available in the form of filters or occlusive balloons.

Filter Devices

Distal filter EPDs are small baskets deployed distal to the lesion to catch any debris that may be produced by manipulation during angioplasty and stent placement, while allowing blood to continue flowing through its pores. (Tables 1 and 2) (Fig. 1). Most devices have filter pore sizes of around 100–150 microns.

There are essentially two types of filter devices: (a) Fixed-wire devices: this is a single-piece system where the filter is fixed at the distal end of a 0.014" wire, with a leading floppy tip; (b) Bare-wire devices: where the guiding wire and filter device are independent and not attached to each other. A guidewire is used to cross the lesion, over which the filter is advanced.

The base of the filter cone may be eccentric or concentric on the wire tip (Figs 2 and 3). It is believed that eccentric filters engage the vessel wall more firmly than concentric EPDs, thereby providing better protection, but this has not been substantiated. Regardless of which type of filter is used, the technique broadly remains the same (Fig. 4). The filter is constrained in a delivery sheath and advanced through the lesion. The filter is then deployed in a disease-free

Table 1: Commercially available distal filter protection devices.

Name	Company	Crossing Profile	Pore size	Design	Wire Technique
Angioguard RX	Cordis	3.2 – 3.9 F	100 µm	Concentric	Fixed wire
Emboshield NAV6	Abbott Vascular	3.7 – 3.9 F	140 µm	Concentric	Bare wire
Fiber Net	Medtronic	1.7 – 2.9 F	40 µm	Concentric	Fixed wire
Filter Wire EZ	Boston Scientific	3.2 F	110 µm	Eccentric	Fixed wire
GARDEX EPD	Gardia Medical	3.4 F	120 µm	Concentric	Fixed wire
Gore Embolic Filter	W.L. Gore & Associates	3.2 F	100 µm	Concentric	Fixed wire
RX Accunet	Abbott Vascular	3.5 – 3.7 F	125 µm	Concentric	Fixed wire
Rubicon	Rubicon Medical	< 2 F	100 µm	Concentric	Fixed wire
Spider FX	ev3	3.2 F	Variable 50 – 300 µm	Eccentric	Bare wire
Wirion EPD System	Gardia Medical	3.2 F	120 µm	Eccentric	Fixed wire

Table 2: Advantages and disadvantages of distal filter devices

Advantages	*Disadvantages*
• Flow preservation • Angiography possible during protection • Less spasm in distal artery than with distal occlusion devices	• Larger crossing profile • Difficulties to pass tight/tortuous lesion with fixed-wire system • Potential thrombus or occlusion of filter with debris • Risk of embolisation long side the filter due to incomplete coverage of the vessel if an undersized filter is used • Risk of microinfarcts as most of the filters can generally retrieve debris >100 µm.

segment of the target vessel several centimeters past the lesion. Angioplasty/stenting is performed, following which a retrieval catheter is used to close the filter and remove it from the artery. All equipment exchanges are routinely performed under fluoroscopic visualization to monitor the position of the EPD and ensure that there is no proximal or distal migration during the procedure.

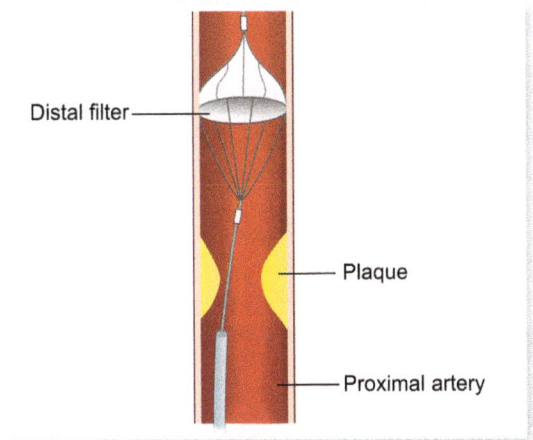

Figure 1: Schematic diagram of distal filter device

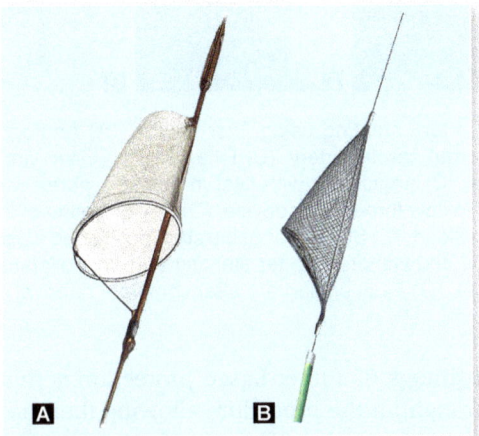

Figure 2: Eccentric distal filter devices (A) EV3 SpiderFX (Ev3), (B) FilterWire EZ (Boston Scientific). (Sources: www.ev3.net; www.bostonscientific.com)

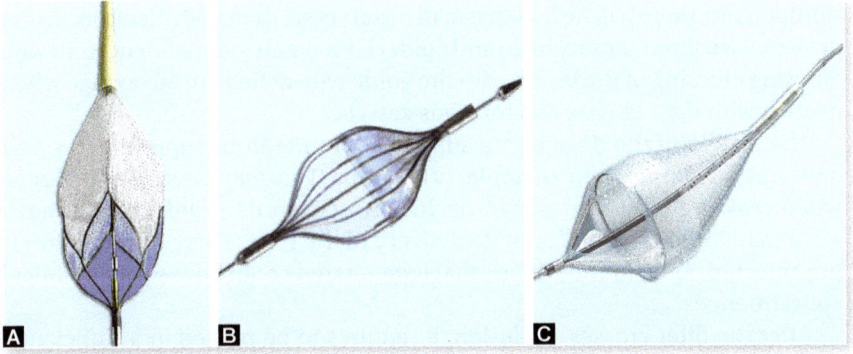

Figure 3: Concentric distal filter devices (A) RX Accunet Embolic Protection (Abbott Vascular), (B) AngioGuard (Cordis Endovascular), (C) Emboshield NAV6 (Abbott Vascular). (Sources: www.cordislabeling.com; www.abbottvascular.com)

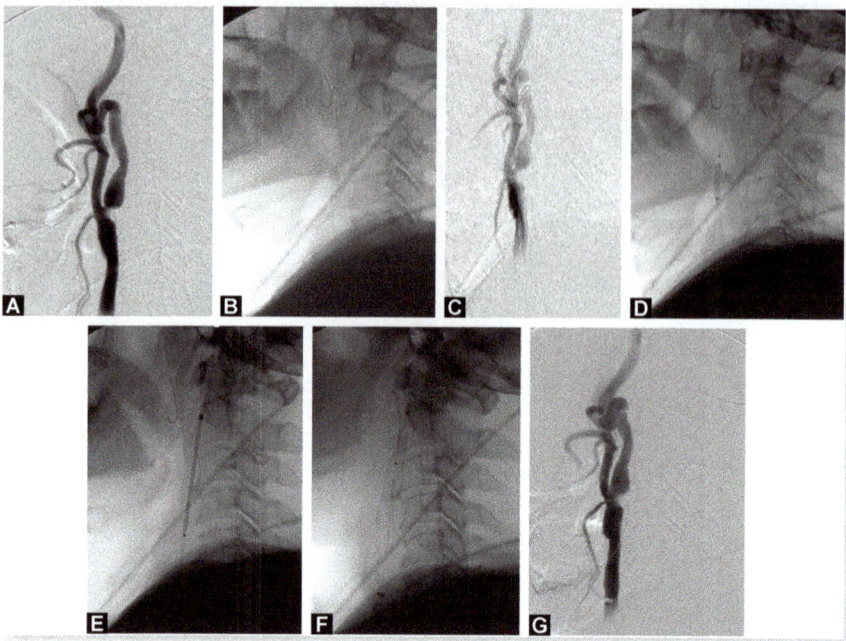

Figure 4: Carotid artery stenting using filter device: (A) Angiography sowing ostial stenosis of left internal carotid artery, (B) Filter device (FilterWire EZ) parked in ICA above the stenosis, (C) Angiogram with filter in position; pores within the filter allows blood and contrast to flow through the device, (D) Pre-dilatation of the ICA stenosis with 3 mm angioplasty balloon, (E) Self-expandable stent positioned across the ICA stenosis, (F) Filter recaptured and withdrawn after stenting and post-dilatation; captured device seen within the stent, (G) Final angiogram after complete removal of the filter device

The major advantage of a filter-based protection is that distal perfusion is maintained throughout the procedure allowing their use in patients with poor collateral circulation, e.g. during carotid artery stenting in patients total contralateral internal carotid artery (ICA) occlusion, severe contralateral ICA stenosis, intracranial stenosis, or a poor circle of Willis. Secondly, angiography is possible during protection allowing accurate placement of the stent. Additionally, there will be less spasm in distal vessel than with distal occlusion devices. Two filters, Emboshield and Spider FX have an independent guidewire allowing crossing of the lesion with the guide wire at first, an advantage when dealing with tight lesions and tortuous vessels.

The profile of the devices are supported on medium support wires and have a profile larger than angioplasty balloons. This may present a challenge when crossing tight stenoses or occlusions. Given its profile, tight lesions need to be predilated to facilitate delivery of the EPD. This pre-dilatation is unprotected, and embolic debris that is generated could have serious clinical consequences.

After the filter crosses the lesion, it requires to be parked in a sufficiently long and healthy landing zone. In patients with diffuse atherosclerosis, it may be difficult to find such an area. The risks of deployment in a diseased vessel include dissection or spasm, usually related to device motion during the procedure. The operator should be aware of the size of the footprint of the device being used to ensure that an appropriate implantation zone be chosen.

After the angioplasty/stenting is completed, the filter needs to be recaptured before removal. If there are large amounts of macroscopic debris is captured, this can lead to the device being completely filled with debris. A filled EPD may lead to loss of antegrade flow past the target lesion. When this occurs, it is imperative to ensure that the device is retrieved expeditiously to restore the distal flow. Additionally, this can be further complicated by the inability to capture the filled filter system with the manufacturer's capture catheter. In this instance, a guide catheter (at least 5F or 6F) needs to be advanced past the target lesion to capture the EPD. The device should not be retrieved without being captured in order to minimise the risk of embolic debris escaping during retrieval.

Distal Occlusion Devices

Distal occlusion devices use a balloon catheter inflated beyond the lesion to temporarily arrest antegrade flow while angioplasty/stenting is being performed (Tables 3 and 4). The debris mobilized at the time of intervention is removed with an aspiration catheter prior to balloon retrieval and antegrade flow restoration (Figs 5 to 7).

Unlike filter devices, these have a lower crossing profile, are more flexible and require a shorter landing zone. However, it necessitates cessation of flow within the distal circulation; this transient interruption in flow may not be well tolerated in patients undergoing carotid artery stenting (CAS) with contralateral

Table 3: Commercially available distal occlusion devices

Name	Company
Guard dog	Possis Medical-MEDRAD
GuardWire	Medtronic
TriActiv	Kensey Nash
Twin One	Minvasys

Table 4: Advantages and disadvantages of distal occlusion devices

Advantages	Disadvantages
• Complete protection of distal artery • Low crossing profile • Highly flexible • One size fits all	• Blood flow interrupted during protection resulting unusable in patients with contralateral occlusion in carotid interventions • Angiography impossible during protection • Potential arterial spasm • During ICA balloon occlusion, blood flow is redirected to the ECA with the potential for cerebral and retinal embolisation through large collaterals

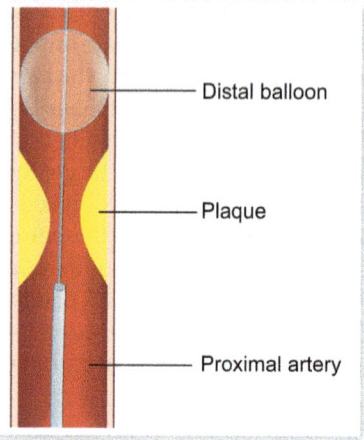

Figure 5: Schematic diagram of flow arrest by distal balloon inflation

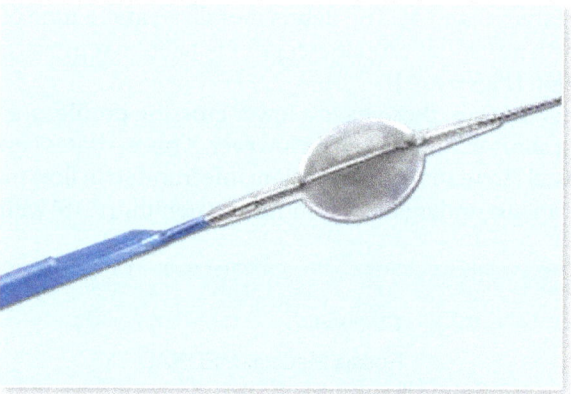

Figure 6: PercuSurge GuardWire device

stenosis/occlusion. Also, once inflated, the index lesion is not well seen on angiograms, and one needs to rely on landmarks or road-mapping for accurate stent placement.

Proximal Occlusion Devices

These devices have been designed exclusively for carotid revascularisation procedures (Tables 5 and 6). They are based on producing flow stasis at the treatment site by balloon occlusion of the proximal carotid artery, with either aspiration of debris or flow reversal at the treatment site to prevent debris from embolising distally. Unlike other EPDs, proximal occlusion offers a major advantage in providing embolic protection before there is any wire/device manipulation across the ICA stenosis. Two types of devices using this principle have been developed:

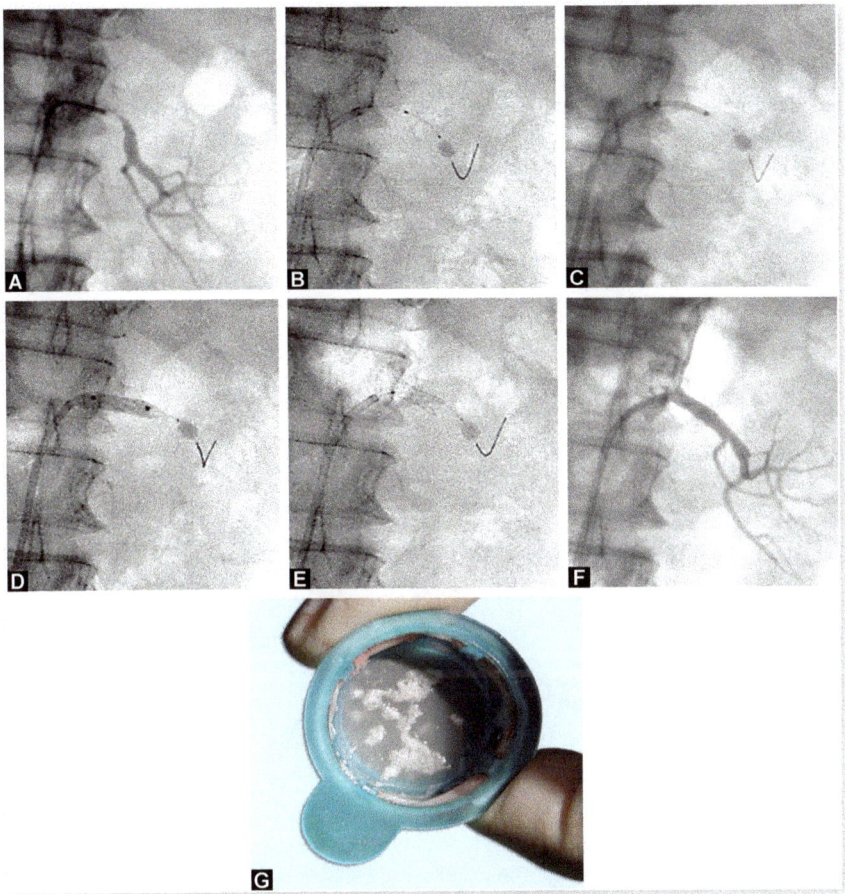

Figure 7: Left renal artery stenting using distal balloon occlusion: (A) Angiography showing ostial stenosis left renal artery, (B) PercuSurge balloon inflated in renal artery distal to stenosis, (C) Balloon-expandable stent positioned across stenosis, (D) Renal stent deployed, (E) Export aspiration catheter being advanced through the stent, opaque marker of tip in proximal stent, (F) Post-stenting angiogram after aspiration of debris and removal of occlusion device, (G) Debris aspirated from Export catheter

Table 5: Commercially available proximal flow occlusion devices		
Name	Company	Mechanism
Mo. Ma. Ultra	Medtronic	Proximal flow blockage
Gore flow reversal system	W.L. Gore and Associates	Proximal flow reversal
MICHI neuroprotection system	Silk Road Medical	Proximal flow reversal

Flow Arrest and Aspiration

The Mo.Ma device produces flow stasis within the ICA by balloon occlusion of the common and external carotid arteries. Once stasis is achieved, angioplasty

Table 6: Advantages and disadvantages of proximal occlusion devices	
Advantages	*Disadvantages*
• Complete protection before lesion passage • Tight/tortuous lesions are treatable • Ability to use any guide wire	• Blood flow interrupted during protection resulting unusable in patients with contra lateral carotid occlusion • Large introducer size • Potential for arterial spasm

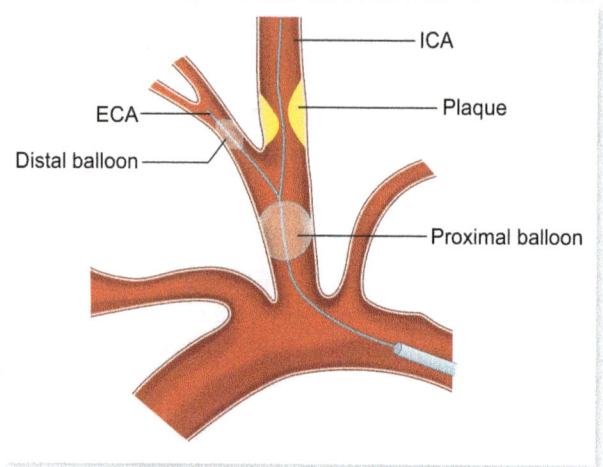

Figure 8: Schematic diagram showing inflation of the Mo.Ma distal and proximal balloons

and stenting of the ICA is performed, followed by aspiration of the debris-laden blood. Antegrade flow is then restored by deflation of the occlusion balloons (Fig. 8). This approach appears to parallel the effectiveness of clamping during a carotid endarterectomy procedure, but with the advantage of being minimally invasive.

Proximal Occlusion and Dynamic Flow Reversal

The Parody antiembolisation catheter (PAEC) is similar to the Mo.Ma device, but uses a flow reversal system instead of aspiration for removal of debris (Fig. 9). The arterial guiding sheath that contains the occlusion balloon is externally connected to a femoral venous sheath to create a temporary arteriovenous shunt. This shunt creates reversal of flow in the ICA during angioplasty/stenting, actively removing particulate matter of all sizes and capturing them by a filter placed at the arteriovenous connection (Table 7).

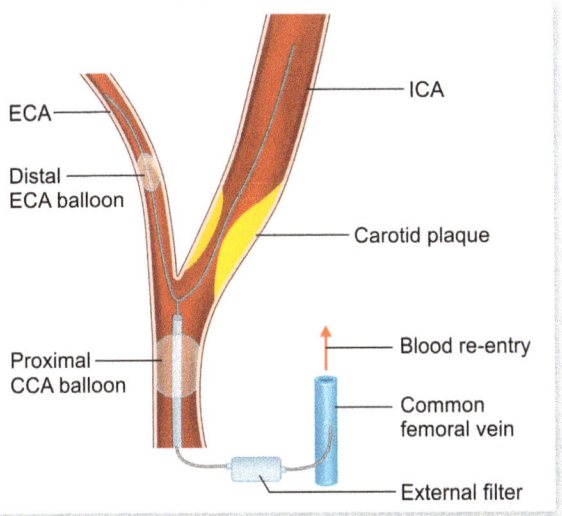

Figure 9: Schematic diagram of flow arrest by proximal balloon inflation and dynamic flow reversal

Table 7: Advantages of Parody antiembolisation catheter

Advantages	Disadvantages
• The lesion can be crossed with any guide wire of choice under protection • Complete protection achieved before manipulating the lesion • Embolisation to the brain is not possible during reversed flow • Particles of all sizes can be captured • Tight, tortuous lesions, and stenosis with limited landing zones can be treated • The technique avoids flushing through the ECA with the risk of brain embolisation in the case of collateral circulation between the ECA and ICA or vertebral artery • Complications associated with filter retrieval and filter related vasospasm in the ICA are eliminated	• The interruption of flow during protection may not be tolerated in some patients (5%) • Need a 9-French introducer • The technique has the potential to cause spasm or dissection in the ECA or CCA • A brain embolism may occur during placement of the catheter in the CCA. This step cannot be protected

Combined Proximal and Distal Protection

The main drawback of the proximal occlusion system is its inability to be used in patients with contralateral carotid occlusion or an interrupted circle of Willis. To overcome this, Parody et al. described the use of the PAEC with a distal filter. The technique involves use of proximal occlusion and flow reversal with the PAEC as described above. Once flow reversal is initiated, an E Trap Filter (MSD) is delivered to the distal ICA. Flow reversal is discontinued after filter deployment by deflating the occlusion balloons. The angioplasty/stenting is then performed under distal filter protection. This technique theoretically combines the advantages of all device systems, but is cumbersome to use.

CLINICAL APPLICATIONS

Carotid Interventions

The overall 30-day risk of stroke or death after CAS is approximately 5%, contributed significantly by plaque disruption and intracranial embolisation during endovascular intervention. EPDs were introduced into clinical practice by Theron in 1990 in an attempt to reduce the incidence of embolisation. Since then, EPDs have been evaluated in numerous studies of CAS[6-11] (Table 8). Despite the heterogeneity in patient population, operator experience, choice of stent and protection device, and lack of absolute evidence demonstrating its efficacy, it is almost universally agreed that use of embolic protection is mandatory in CAS. This is based on the fact that ex-vivo and clinical studies show definite release of embolic debris during CAS, large percentage of which are macro-emboli, and that clinical effects correlate with the size and volume of debris. Registry, summary and meta-analysis data also seem to support this intuitive practice.[12-14]

While there is little evidence that demonstrates superiority of any specific device, there is justification for use of a proximal occlusion device in complex lesions and limited cerebral reserve, and a filter device when treating patients with contralateral carotid occlusion and poor intracranial collateral circulation.[15]

Table 8: Safety of EPDs in carotid stenting

Device	Trial and year	No of patients	30-d stroke	30-d MI/stroke/death
Angioguard	SAPPHIRE[6] (2008)	167	3.6%	4.8%
Accunet	ARCHeR[7] (2006)	581	5.5%	8.3%
GuardWire	MAVErIC I/II[8] (2004)	498	4.2%	5.4%
Mo.Ma Ultra	ARMOUR[9] (2010)	262	2.3%	2.7%
Gore Flow Reversal	EMPIRE[10] (2011)	245	2.9%	2.7%
FiberNet	EPIC[11] (2010)	237	2.1%	3%

Coronary Interventions

Periprocedural major adverse cardiac events following saphenous vein bypass graft (SVG) interventions occurs in approximately 20% of the patients, mainly from distal embolisation of soft and friable plaques from degenerative grafts. In a pivotal trial of SVG graft angioplasty, a 42% relative risk reduction of major adverse cardiac events was achieved with protection using distal balloon occlusion.[16] The use of EPDs has since become standard practice in SVG interventions, but not recommended for arterial bypass grafts and native coronary arteries due to lower risk of distal embolism from arterial plaques.

Renal Artery Interventions

Almost 30% of patients have decline in function after renal artery stenting, and it is widely believed that cholesterol embolisation is one of the major factors causing deterioration in renal function.[17] While patients with normal renal function can tolerate the embolic shower, those with diminished renal reserve can progress to overt renal failure. Initial non-randomized studies demonstrated the ability of the EPDs to trap embolic particles in 44–100% of revascularised renal arteries, reducing the risk of renal functional decline to <5% of patients (Table 9).[18-21] Hence, the use of EPD for revascularisation of only high-risk patients could be justifiable. Holden et al. published a cohort study using EPDs in a high-risk group of patients with moderate-to-severe renal impairment and reported stabilised or improved renal function in 97% patients, suggesting the efficacy of EPDs in patients with preexisting renal impairment.[21]

There are unique demands on an EPD in the renal artery circulation. As most atherosclerotic renal artery stenosis occur at the ostium, only filters and distal occlusion balloons can be used.[22] Maneuvering a fixed-type filter wire across a stenotic renal ostium that takes off at an acute angle from the aorta can be a technical challenge. Also, renal arteries are often short; early branching of the renal artery would require the filter to be parked in a more dominant branch, limiting the extent of renal parenchymal protection. Filter designs that use short landing zones (e.g. PercuSurge GuardWire, FiberNet EPS) are hence preferred (Fig. 10).

Table 9: Results of EPDs in renal revascularisation								
Author and year	No of pts/ RAs	Device	Technical success	Debris retrieval	Renal outcome measure	Improved	Stabilised	Decline
Henry[18] (2003)	56/65	Distal balloon	100%	100%	SCr 6 m	18%	82%	0
Holden[19] (2003)	37/46	Filter	100%	65%	CrCl 6 m	38%	57%	5%
Edwards[20] (2006)	26/32	Distal balloon	88%	44%	eGFR 4–6 w	50%	50%	0
Holden[21] (2006)	63/63	Filter	100%	60%	eGFR 6 m	40%	57%	3%

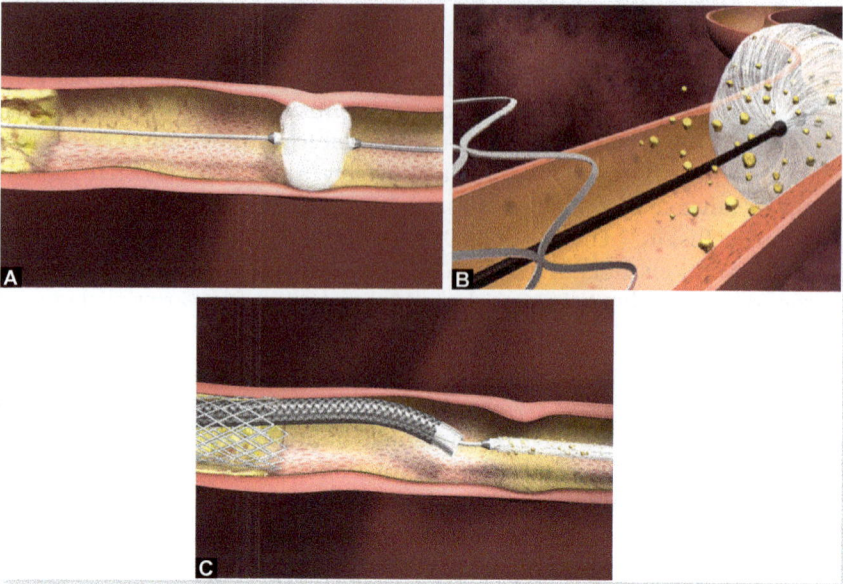

Figure 10: Diagram of the FiberNet system: (A) Deployment of device distal to the stenosis; (B) Debris captured by the fibres of the device during intervention; (C) Aspiration debris prior to withdrawal of device. (Source: www.peripheral.medtronicendovascular.com)

Lower Extremity Interventions

Distal embolisation occurs in 1.6-2.4% of patients undergoing peripheral interventions, the rate climbing higher to almost 24% in case of intra-arterial thrombolysis.[23] The PROTECT registry reported macroscopic debris being captured in 55% of patients, with higher rates among patients being treated by atherectomy (100%).[24] Another study by Muller-Hulsbeck et al. demonstrated macroscopic debris in 90% of cases.[25] Despite this extensive embolic shower, clinical impact is at best minimal, likely due to an extensive collateral network in the lower limb. Hence, there has been very little evidence to support its routine use in peripheral angioplasty. Data, however, suggest the use of EPD to be beneficial in peripheral interventions when using mechanical atherectomy, mechanical thrombectomy, intra-arterial thrombolysis, and in patients with limited runoff.[24,26,27]

Transcatheter Aortic Valve Implantation

Cerebral injuries during transcatheter aortic valve implantation (TAVI) can result from embolic debris originating from the valve implantation site and the passage of large-caliber catheters through a diseased and calcified aortic arch. Initial randomized clinical trials showed a high rate of neurological complications, ranging between 5.5% and 6.7%.[28] These rates have declined appreciably, and are currently ranging between 1.7% and 3.4%. However, in one series positive DWI signal was recorded up to 80% of cases after TAVI

Table 10: Commercially available EPDs used in transcatheter aortic valve implantation (TAVI)

Device	Manufacturer	Design	Access	Delivery	Deployment
Sentinel	Claret Medical Inc.	Filter	Radial/brachial	6F	2 filters to brachiocephalic trunk and left common carotid
Embol-X	Edwards Lifesciences	Filter	Surgical	14F	Ascending aorta
Embrella	Edwards Lifesciences	Deflector	Radial/brachial	6F	Aortic arch
TriGuard	Keystone Heart Ltd,	Deflector	Femoral	9F	Aortic arch

irrespective of the access strategy used.[29] EPDs has shown promise in reducing the risk of TAVI-related stroke and currently four devices are available for this purpose that either deflect or capture emboli (Table 10).

CONCLUSION

The EPD is an important tool for the interventionist. It can be used in a various vascular territories to prevent clinical sequelae secondary to embolisation of disrupted plaque and debris. While it is well established in SVG and carotid artery interventions, it does have an expanded, although specific usage in providing better outcomes during coronary, renal, peripheral and aortic interventions.

REFERENCES

1. Topol EJ, Yadav JS. Recognition of the importance of embolization in atherosclerotic vascular disease. Circulation. 2000;101(5):570-80.
2. Karnabatidis D, Katsanos K, Kagadis GC, Ravazoula P, Diamantopoulos A, Nikiforidis GC, et al. Distal embolism during percutaneous revascularisation of intra-aortic occlusive disease an underestimated phenomenon. J Endovasc Ther. 2006;13(3):269-80.
3. Roffi M. Current role of emboli protection devices in percutaneous coronary and vascular interventions. Am Heart J. 2009;157(2):263-70.
4. Lam RC, Shah S, Faries PL, McKinsey JF, Kent KC, Morrissey NJ. Incidence and clinical significance of distal embolization during percutaneous interventions involving the superficial femoral artery. J Vasc Surg. 2007;46(12):1155-9.
5. Yang M, Yu Y, Walsh WR, Yang JL, Baker L, Lennox AF, et al. A microscopic and biomarker evaluation of embolic filter debris collected during carotid artery stenting. J Endovasc Ther. 2016;23(2):275-84.
6. Gurm HS, Yadav JS, Fayad P, Batzen BT, Mishkel GJ, Bajwa TK, et al. Long-term results of carotid stenting versus endarterectomy in high-risk patients. N Engl J Med. 2008;358:1572-9.

7. Gray WA, Hopkins LN, Yadav S, Davis T, Wholey M, Atkinson R, et al. Protected carotid stenting in high-surgical-risk patients: the ARCHeR results. J Vasc Surg. 2006;44(2):258-68.
8. Higashida RT, Popma JJ, Apruzzese P, Zimetbaum P, MAVErIC I and II Investigators. Evaluation of the Medtronic exponent self-expanding carotid stent system with the Medtronic Guardwire temporary occlusion and aspiration system in the treatment of carotid stenosis: combined from the MAVErIC (Medtronic AVE Self-expanding CaRotid Stent System with distal protection In the treatment of Carotid stenosis) I and MAVErIC II trials. Stroke. 2010;41(2):e102-9.
9. Ansel GM, Hopkins LN, Jaff MR, Rubino P, Bacharach JM, Scheinert D, et al. Investigators for the ARMOUR Pivotal Trial. Safety and effectiveness of the INVATEC MO.MA proximal cerebral protection device during carotid artery stenting: results from the ARMOUR pivotal trial. Catheter Cardiovasc Interv. 2010;76(1):1-8.
10. Clair DG, Hopkins LN, Mehta M, Kasirajan K, Schermerhorn M, Schonholz C, et al. EMPIRE Clinical Study Investigators. Neuroprotection during carotid artery stenting using the GORE flow reversal system: 30-day outcomes in the EMPIRE Clinical Study. Catheter Cardiovasc Interv. 2011;77(3):420-9.
11. Myla S, Bacharach JM, Ansel GM, Dippel EJ, McCormick DJ, Popma JJ. Carotid artery stenting in high surgical risk patients using the FiberNet embolic protection system: the EPIC trial results. Catheter Cardiovasc Interv. 2010;75(6):817-22.
12. Garg N, Karagiorgos N, Pisimisis GT, et al. Cerebral protection devices reduce periprocedural strokes during carotid angioplasty and stenting: a systematic review of the current literature. J Endovasc Ther. 2009;16:412-27.
13. Touze E, Trinquart L, Chatellier G. et al. Systematic review of the perioperative risks of stroke or death after carotid angioplasty and stenting. Stroke. 2009; 40:e683-93.
14. Kastrup A, Groschel K, Krapf H, Brehm BR, Dichgans J, Schulz JB. Early outcome of carotid angioplasty and stenting with and without cerebral protection devices: a systematic review of the literature. Stroke. 2003;34(3):813-9.
15. Schneider PA, Ansel G. How to I select cerebral protection devices today? J Cardiovasc Surg. 2010;51:873-83.
16. Baim DS, Wahr D, George B, Leon MB, Greenberg J, Cutlip DE, et al. Randomized trial of a distal embolic protection device during percutaneous intervention of saphenous vein aorto-coronary bypass grafts. Circulation. 2002;105(11):1285-90.
17. Leertouwer TC, Gussenhoven EJ, Bosch JL, et al. Stent placement for renal arterial stenosis: Where do we stand? A meta-analysis. Radiology. 2000;216:78-85.
18. Henry M, Henry I, Klonaris C, et al. Renal angioplasty and stenting under protection: The way for the future? Catheter Cardiovasc Interv. 2003;60:299-312.
19. Holden A, Hill A. Renal angioplasty and stenting with distal protection of the main renal artery in ischemic nephropathy: Early experience. J Vasc Surg. 2003; 38:962-8.
20. Edwards MS, Craven BL, Stafford J, et al. Distal embolic protection during renal artery angioplasty and stenting. J Vasc Surg. 2006;44:128-35.
21. Holden A, Hill A, Jaff MR, Pilmore H. Renal artery stent revascularization with embolic protection in patients with ischemic nephropathy. Kidney Int. 2006; 70:948-55.
22. Holden A. Is there an indication for embolic protection in renal artery intervention? Tech Vasc Interv Radiol. 2011;14(2):95-100.

23. Karnabatidis D, Katsanos K, Kagadis GC, Ravazoula P, Diamantopoulos A, Nikiforidis GC, et al. Distal embolism during percutaneous revascularization of infra-aortic arteries: an underestimated phenomenon. J Endovasc Ther. 2006;13:269-80.
24. Shammas NW, Dippel EJ, Coiner D, Shammas GA, Jerin M, Kumar A. Preventing lower extremity distal embolization using embolic filter protection: results of the PROTECT registry. J Endovasc Ther. 2008;15(3):270-6.
25. Muller-Hulsbeck S, Humme TH, Philippp Schafer J, Charalambous N, Paulsen F, Heller M, et al. Final results of the protected superficial femoral artery trial using the FilterWire EZ system. Cardiovasc Interv Radiol. 2010;33(6):1120-7.
26. Siablis D, Karnabatidis D, Katsanos K, Ravazoula P, Kraniotis P, Kagadis GC. Outflow protection filters during percutaneous recanalization of lower extremities' arterial occlusions: a pilot study. Eur J Radiol. 2005;55:243-49.
27. Wholey MH, Toursarkissian B, Postoak D, Natarajan B, Joiner D. Early experience in the application of distal protection devices in treatment of peripheral vascular disease of the lower extremities. Catheter Cardiovasc Intervent. 2005;64:227-35.
28. Steinvil A, Benson RT, Waksman R. Embolic protection devices in transcatheter aortic valve replacement. Circ Cardiovasc Interv. 2016;9(3):e003284.
29. Van Mieghem NM, El Faquir N, Rahhab Z, Rodriques-Olivares R, Wilschut J, Ouhlous M, et al. Incidence and predictors of debris embolizing to the brain during transcatheter aortic valve implantation. JACC Cardiiovasc Interv. 2015;8(5):718-24.

CHAPTER 12

Status of CEA in an Endovascular Era

Dovile Gudzinskaite-Brar, Raghvinder Pal Singh Gambhir

INTRODUCTION

Stroke is a major cause of the death and disability. Carotid artery atherosclerotic emboli account for 10% ischaemic strokes and pose a significant risk of recurrent strokes.[1]

Carotid endarterectomy (CEA) and carotid artery stenting (CAS) are both accepted modalities of treatment, for prevention of stroke in patients with carotid artery atherosclerotic disease, along with best medical therapy.

Three major randomised controlled trials: North American Symptomatic Carotid Endarterectomy (NASCET) Trial, the Veterans Affairs Cooperative Study (VACS), the European Carotid Surgery Trial (ECST) clearly demonstrated the benefits of Carotid Endarterectomy (CEA) in prevention of stroke in symptomatic patients with >70% ipsilateral carotid stenosis.[2-4]

GUIDELINES

Based on these landmark studies most international guidelines have recommended CEA as the treatment of choice for patients with symptomatic carotid stenosis.[1,5-9] Table 1 summarises the current guidelines with the level of evidence and class of recommendations for each intervention.

TIMING OF INTERVENTION

The timing of intervention is critical. The published risk of recurrent stroke within the first 2 weeks after the index neurological event has been reported as 5-8% at 48 hours, 17% at 72 hours, 8-22% at 7 days and 11-25% at 14 days.[10] The annual risk of a further ischaemic stroke is estimated to be 3-4%.[11] CEA after 12 weeks will prevent only 8 strokes per 1000 CEA performed.[12]

The existing American Heart Association (AHA) and European Society for Vascular Surgery (ESVS) guidelines recommend CEA within 2 weeks.[13] This 2

Table 1: Summary of current guidelines based on level of evidence and class of recommendation

Patient Status	Ipsilateral internal carotid artery status	Recommendation	Qualifying remark	Class of recommendation/ Level of evidence
Symptomatic patient: Transient Ischaemic attacks (TIA), non-disabling strokes (Modified Rankin Scale ≤2) or amaurosis fugax within last 6 months	>70% stenosis on Duplex >50% on catheter angiography	CEA	If anticipated rate of perioperative stroke or mortality is less than 6%	Class I Benefit>>>Risk Level A evidence
		CAS is an alternative	In those with low risk of endovascular procedures and anticipated rate of peri-procedural stroke or mortality is less than 6%	Class IIa Benefit>>Risk Level B evidence
	50–69% stenosis	CEA	Patient-specific decision, based on age, comorbidities, if anticipated perioperative stroke or mortality is less than 6%	Class I Benefit>>>Risk Level B evidence
	<50% stenosis	Neither CEA/CAS	Except in exceptional circumstances	Class III No Benefit Level A evidence
Asymptomatic	>70% stenosis by Duplex	CEA	Treat based on patient life expectancy and comorbid conditions, if the risk of perioperative stroke, myocardial infarction, and death is low	Class IIa Benefit>>Risk Level A evidence
		CEA preferable over CAS	In patients >70 years old, when arterial anatomy is unfavourable for endovascular intervention	Class IIa, Benefit>>Risk Level B evidence
		CAS over CEA	When neck anatomy unfavourable for arterial surgery	Class IIa, Benefit>>Risk Level B evidence
	>60% by Catheter angiography >70% stenosis by Duplex	CAS	Effectiveness compared with medical therapy alone is not proven	Class IIb, Benefit ≥Risk Level B evidence
Symptomatic or asymptomatic	Complete occlusion of ICA	Neither CEA /CAS	Medical therapy alone	Class III (No Benefit) Level C evidence
	Severely disabled after stroke Modified Rankin Scale of ≥3	Neither CEA /CAS	Medical therapy alone	Class III (No Benefit) Level C evidence

week period is being increasingly challenged and future guidelines are likely to change this to 1 week. A large number of reports have been published regarding CEA during the hyper-acute phase. The need for an expedited CEA within 48 hours is not universally accepted and is not always feasible. The slightly higher risk of complications will deter its universal acceptance in spite of some good results by some groups.[14-18]

TECHNIQUE

Duplex ultrasound and computed tomography angiography (CTA) remain the investigations of choice to assess carotid artery stenosis. The technique of carotid endarterectomy—eversion or conventional is a matter of individual preference among surgeons. Both offer similar freedom from neurologic morbidity, death, and reintervention.[19] Similarly though many surgeons swear by the advantages of loco-regional anaesthesia the GALA study failed to show any benefit of CEA performed under local anaesthesia.[20] It does however allow ideal neurological monitoring, selective shunting with better haemodynamic stability.

BEST MEDICAL THERAPY

Besides carotid revascularisation, all patients require optimal medical management and vascular risk factor modifications. Medical management has evolved since the time patients were recruited into those initial landmark trials. Early initiation of antiplatelet agent and statins after the initial neurological event reduces the risk of recurrent stroke significantly.[8,10,21] Lifestyle modifications, smoking cessation, diet and exercise regimen and optimal treatment of coexisting hypertension, atrial fibrillation, hyperlipidaemia and diabetes are all essential components of management of these patients. After 2–3 years the annual stroke risk declines to that of asymptomatic patients if the patients remain on best medical therapy.[8]

CAROTID ARTERY STENTING

CAS has been around since 1990s and numerous trials using combined end point of peri-procedural stroke, death, and MI, have attempted to show either equivalence/non-inferiority to CEA.[22-26]

CAS as a less invasive technique. The risk of peri-procedural stroke is however higher than in CEA, but in contrast the risk of perioperative MI is higher with CEA.[27,28] Advocates for CEA have argued that the long-term effect of sequel of stroke on quality of life is worse than that of perioperative MI while the advocates for CAS argue that long-term mortality is higher in patients who had an MI during CEA.[27-30]

The debate remains inconclusive and historically stenting has been reserved for those considered high risk for CEA: either because of medical comorbidities, but more commonly because of loco-regional anatomical factors as mentioned in Table 2.

Table 2: Current recommended indications for CAS as the first choice for carotid revascularisation

	CAS	Class of recommendation/ Level of evidence
Symptomatic	Uncorrectable coronary artery disease, congestive heart failure, or chronic obstructive pulmonary disease	Class II, Level C Evidence
	In presence of tracheal stoma, Situations where local tissues are scarred and fibrotic from prior ipsilateral surgery (block dissection of neck) or external beam radiotherapy, Prior cranial nerve injury, Contralateral recurrent laryngeal nerve injury, Severe cervical spine arthritis, Surgically inaccessible carotid stenosis (e.g. obesity, high carotid bifurcation, tandem lesions) Lesions that extend proximal to the clavicle or distal to the C2 vertebral body, Contralateral internal carotid occlusion Recurrent stenosis following previous CEA	Class II; Level B evidence
Asymptomatic (minimum 60% by angiography, 70% by validated Doppler ultrasound)	In highly selected patients, in high-volume centres with documented death or stroke rate <3%	Class IIb; Level B Evidence

With increasing use of CAS over the last decade, the technique, the stent design, the role of cerebral protection devices and the pre-procedural medication regimen have become more defined. Use of dual anti-platelets prior to CAS, and continued post-procedure is now an accepted practice. There is benefit of using closed cell stent designs in comparison to open cell stent design which have been associated with a higher risk of stroke. Cerebral protection devices, though intuitively ideal in all CAS to reduce embolism during the procedure, have not always shown consistent results. There is enough evidence now to show that stenting is associated with higher risks in patients aged 70 or more.[8,24,26]

ASYMPTOMATIC CAROTID DISEASE

Cerebrovascular emboli from asymptomatic atherosclerotic carotid disease do carry a risk of stroke, the risk however is small. Two randomised controlled trials: the Asymptomatic carotid atherosclerosis study (ACAS), asymptomatic

Table 3: Suggested algorithm for managing carotid disease				
Patient status	Carotid scan	1st choice	2nd choice	Time frame
Symptomatic within last 3 months	50–99% stenosis	CEA + BMT if the operator stroke risk is <6%	CAS + BMT if the operator stroke risk is <6%	Within 1 week of index event
	<50%	BMT alone No intervention unless an ulcerated plaque		
Asymptomatic (Decision to treat based on comorbidity and life expectancy)	60–99% stenosis	BMT alone	CEA or CAS + BMT if the operator stroke risk is <3%	

carotid surgery trial (ACST) reported benefits of CEA in reducing the stroke risk from 2 to 1% in these patients.[31,32]

The management of asymptomatic disease remains controversial. The long-term benefits of intervention are debated.[33] It is estimated that greater than 90% of revascularisation are unwarranted and subject the patient to a peri-procedural stroke risk of greater than 3%.[34,35]

There is no biological marker or proven imaging characteristic that can categorically predict plaque rupture in these patients. There is therefore a case for managing these patients with best medical therapy and vascular risk factor modification. CREST 2 and ECST 2 trials are currently recruiting asymptomatic patients and may in future clarify the role of best medical management. SPACE 2 trial could have provided an answer to the role of best medical management alone when compared with CEA or CAS, but unfortunately the trial had to close due to poor recruitment.[36]

The debate as to the best modality of treatment is still not over,[37] but based on present evidence and understanding of the disease, carotid endarterectomy is preferred over carotid stenting. The risks of either form of management need to be discussed with the patient and informed decision made with patient. A simplified algorithm for management is as suggested in Table 3.

CONCLUSION

Management of carotid disease is based on evidence from a number of randomised trials over 5 decades. The techniques of carotid endarterectomy and now carotid stenting have been refined over years and medical therapy has become well defined. Symptomatic patients will continue to need carotid endarterectomy or stenting within a week of the index event, to be performed by experienced operators with peri-intervention stroke rates of less than 3%. Ongoing trials will further delineate the role of medical therapy in asymptomatic patients.

REFERENCES

1. Chaturvedi S, Sacco RL. How recent data have impacted the treatment of internal carotid artery stenosis. J Am Coll Cardiol. 2015;65(11)1134-43.
2. North American Symptomatic Carotid Endarterectomy Trial collaborators. Beneficial effect of carotid endarterectomy in symptomatic patients with high-grade stenosis. N Engl J Med. 1991;325:445-53.
3. Mayberg MR, Wilson SE, Yatsu F, Weiss DG, Messina L, Hershey LA, et al. Veterans Affairs Cooperative Studies Program 309 Trialist Group. Carotid endarterectomy and prevention of cerebral ischemia in symptomatic carotid stenosis. JAMA. 1991;266:3289-94.
4. European Carotid Surgery Trialists' Collaborative Group. Randomised trial of endarterectomy for recently symptomatic carotid stenosis: final results of the MRC European Carotid Surgery Trial (ECST). Lancet. 1998;351:1379-87.
5. Brott TG, Halperin JL, Abbara S, Bacharach JM, Barr JD, Bush RL et al., ASA/ACCF/AHA/AANN/AANS/ACR/ASNR/CNS/SAIP/SCAI/SIR/SNIS/SVM/SVS guideline on the management of patients with extracranial carotid and vertebral artery disease: executive summary. Stroke. 2011;42:e420-e63.
6. Timaran CH, McKinsey JF, Schneider PA, Littooy F. Reporting standards for carotid interventions from the Society for Vascular Surgery. J Vasc Surg. 2011;53:1679-95.
7. American Heart Association Statistics Committee and Stroke Statistics Subcommittee. Heart disease and stroke statistics—2015 Update. Circulation. 2015;131:e169-e77.
8. Kernan WN, Ovbiagele B, Black HR, Bravata DM, Chimowitz MI, Ezekowitz MD et al., on behalf of the American Heart Association Stroke Council, Council on Cardiovascular and Stroke Nursing, Council on Clinical Cardiology, and Council on Peripheral Vascular Disease. Guidelines for the prevention of stroke in patients with stroke and transient ischemic attack: a guideline for healthcare professionals from the American Heart Association/American Stroke Association. Stroke. 2014;45:2160-236.
9. Rerkasem K, Rothwell PM. Carotid endarterectomy for symptomatic carotid stenosis. Cochrane Database Syst Rev. 2011;CD001081.
10. Batchelder A, Hunter J, Cairns V, Sandford R, Munshi A, Naylor AR. Dual antiplatelet therapy prior to expedited carotid surgery reduces recurrent events prior to surgery without significantly increasing peri-operative bleeding complications. Eur J Vasc Endovasc Surg. 2015;50:412-9.
11. Dhamoon MS, Sciacca RR, Rundek T, Sacco RL, Elkind MS. Recurrent stroke and cardiac risks after first ischemic stroke: the Northern Manhattan Study. Neurology. 2006;66:641-6.
12. Rothwell PM, Eliasziw M, Gutnikov SA, Warlow CP, Barnet HJM. Sex Difference in the effect of time from symptoms to surgery on benefit from carotid endarterectomy for transient ischaemic attack and non-disabling stroke. Stroke. 2004;35:2855-61.
13. Liapis CD, Bell PRF, Mikhailidis D, Sivenius J, Nicolaides A, Fernandes J, et al. ESVS Guidelines. Invasive treatment for carotid stenosis: indications, techniques. Eur J Vasc Endovasc Surg. 2009;37:S1-19.
14. Stromberg S, Gelin J, Osterberg T, Bergstrom GM, Karlstrom L, Osterberg K. Swedish vascular registry (SwedVasc) steering committee. Very urgent endarterectomy confers increased procedural risk. Stroke. 2012;43:1331-5.

15. Sharpe R, Sayers RD, London NJ, Bown MJ, McCarthy MJ, Nasim A, et al. Procedural risk following carotid endarterectomy in the hyperacute period after onset of symptoms. Eur J Vasc Endovasc Surg. 2013;46:519-24.
16. Rantner B, Schmidauer C, Knoflach M, Fraedrich G. Very urgent carotid endarterectomy does not increase the procedural risk. Eur J Vasc Endovasc Surg. 2015;49:129-36.
17. Naylor AR. Carotid endarterectomy is safer than stenting in the hyperacute period after onset of symptoms. Eur J Vasc Endovasc Surg. 2015;49:623-27.
18. Rerkasem K, Rothwell PM. Systematic review of the operative risks of carotid endarterectomy for recently symptomatic stenosis in relation to the timing of surgery. Stroke. 2009;40:e564-72.
19. Schneider JR, Helenowski IB, Jackson CR, Verta MJ, Zamar KC, Patel NH, et al. A comparison of results with eversion versus conventional carotid endarterectomy from the Vascular Quality Initiative and the Mid-America Vascular Study Group. Society for Vascular Surgery Vascular Quality Initiative and the Mid-America Vascular Study Group. J Vasc Surg. 2015;61(5):1216-22.
20. GALA Trial Collaborative Group. General Anaesthesia versus Local Anaesthesia for carotid surgery (GALA): a multicenter, randomized controlled trial. Lancet. 2008;372:2132-42.
21. Sillesen H, Amarenco P, Hennerici MG, et al., on behalf of the SPARCL Investigators. Atorvastatin reduces the risk of cardiovascular events in patients with carotid atherosclerosis: a secondary analysis of the Stroke Prevention by Aggressive Reduction in Cholesterol Levels (SPARCL) Trial. Stroke. 2008;39:3297-302.
22. CAVATAS Investigators. Endovascular versus surgical treatment in patients with carotid stenosis in the Carotid and Vertebral Artery Transluminal Angioplasty Study (CAVATAS): a randomised trial. Lancet. 2001;357:1729-37.
23. Yadav JS, Wholey MH, Kuntz RE, Fayad P, Katzen BT, Mishkel GJ, et al., for the Stenting and Angioplasty with Protection in Patients at High Risk for Endarterectomy Investigators. Protected carotid-artery stenting versus endarterectomy in high-risk patients. N Engl J Med. 2004;351:1493-501.
24. Cohen DJ, Stolker JM, Wang K, Magnuson EA, Clark WM, Demaerschalk BM, et al., on behalf of the CREST Investigators. Health-related quality of life after carotid stenting versus carotid endarterectomy: results from CREST (Carotid Revascularization Endarterectomy Versus Stenting Trial). J Am Coll Cardiol. 2011;58:1557-65.
25. Liu ZJ, Fu WG, Guo ZY, Shen LG, Shi ZY, Li JH. Updated systematic review and meta-analysis of randomized clinical trials comparing carotid artery stenting and carotid endarterectomy in the treatment of carotid stenosis. Ann Vasc Surg. 2012;26:576-90.
26. Doig D, Turner EL, Dobson J, Featherstone RL, Lo RTH, Gaines PA, et al., Investigators. Predictors of Stroke, Myocardial Infarction or Death within 30 Days of Carotid Artery Stenting: Results from the International Carotid Stenting Study p327-334 Published online: October 23 2015.
27. Macdonald S. Carotid artery stenting trials: conduct, results, critique, and current recommendations. Cardiovasc Intervent Radiol. 2013;35:15-29.
28. Brott TG, Hobson RW 2nd, Howard G, Roubin GS, Clark WM, Brooks W, et al. Stenting versus endarterectomy for treatment of carotid artery stenosis. N Engl J Med. 2010;363:11-23.

29. Cohen DJ, Stolker JM, Wang K, Magnuson EA, Clark WM, Demaerschalk BM, et al. Health-related quality of life after carotid stenting versus carotid endarterectomy: results from the CREST Trial. J Am Coll Cardiol. 2011;58:1557-65.
30. Hye RJ, Voeks JH, Malas MB, Tom M, Longson S, Blackshear JL, Brott TG. Anesthetic type and risk of myocardial infarction after carotid endarterectomy in the Carotid Revascularization Endarterectomy versus Stenting Trial (CREST). J Vasc Surg. 2016;64(1):3-8.e1.
31. Executive committee for the asymptomatic carotid atherosclerosis study. Endarterectomy for asymptomatic carotid stenosis. JAMA. 1995;273:1421-8.
32. Halliday A, Mansfield A, Marro J, Peto C, Peto R, Potter J, et al. MRC Asymptomatic Carotid Surgery Trial (ACST) Collaborative Group. Prevention of disabling and fatal strokes by successful carotid endarterectomy in patients without recent neurological symptoms: randomized controlled trial. Lancet. 2004;363:1491-502.
33. Halliday A, Harrison M, Hayter E, Kong X, Mansfield A, Marro J, et al. 10-year stroke prevention after successful carotid endarterectomy for asymptomatic stenosis (acst-1): a multicentre randomised trial. Lancet. 2010;376:1074-84.
34. Pini R, Faggioli G, Longhi M, Vacirca A, Gallitto E, Freyrie A, Gargiulo M, Stella A. The detrimental impact of silent cerebral infarcts on asymptomatic carotid endarterectomy outcome J Vasc Surg. 2016;64(1):15-24.
35. Naylor AR. Why is the management of asymptomatic carotid disease so controversial?. Surgeon. 2015;13:34-43.
36. Eckstein HH, Reiff T, Ringleb P, Jansen O, Mansmann U, Hacke W, on behalf of the SPACE-2 Steering Committee. SPACE-2: a missed opportunity to compare carotid endarterectomy, carotid stenting, and best medical treatment in patients with asymptomatic carotid stenoses. Eur J Vasc Endovasc Surg. 2016;51:761-5.
37. The Advisory Board Company. Medicare panel says current clinical evidence insufficient to determine best treatment for carotid atherosclerosis. Available at: https://www.advisory.com/research/service-line-strategy-advisor/the-pipeline/2012/01/medicare-panel-says-current-clinical-evidence-insufficient-to-determine-best-treatment [accessed 15.07.16].

CHAPTER

13

Role of Interventions in Acute Lower Limb Deep Venous Thrombosis: Current Options

Krishna Gummalla, Sundeep Punamiya

INTRODUCTION

Deep venous thrombosis (DVT) of the lower limbs is a common medical problem that is associated with significant morbidity and mortality despite improvement in diagnosis and treatment over the last 60 years. Early complications of DVT include painful limb swelling that can progress to venous ischaemia and phlegmasia cerulea dolens, pulmonary embolism (PE) and death. Anticoagulation has been the standard of therapy for acute DVT since the 1940s. Although it have proven to be effective in preventing further clot propagation and PE, it is ineffective in lysing the clot, relying on the body's endogenous fibrinolytic mechanism, collateralisation and recanalisation to improve symptoms. The ensuing persistent/residual thrombosis and valvular incompetence causes long-standing venous hypertension and stasis, producing a constellation of symptoms like chronic limb oedema, pain, varicosities, skin hyperpigmentation and venous ulcers.[1] This spectrum of findings, termed post-thrombotic syndrome (PTS), occurs in 25-50% of patients with proximal DVT that has been treated with standard anticoagulation therapy.[2] Active removal of thrombus results in improved luminal patency of the vein, restoration of venous flow and valvular function, which in turn reduces the risk of DVT recurrence and severity of PTS. [3,4]

Various endovascular techniques for thrombus removal have been described, including catheter-directed thrombolysis and mechanical thrombectomy, used alone or in combination, along with adjunct procedures like IVC filter placement to prevent pulmonary emboli, and balloon angioplasty and/or stent placement to increase the luminal calibre of the affected segment or to treat the stenosis which may be the causative factor for thrombosis. There have been many trials with reasonable evidence showing the efficacy of these procedures.

In this chapter, we will discuss about various diagnostic modalities to detect DVT as well as various medical, surgical and endovascular treatment options for DVT.

TRIAGING PATIENTS WITH DVT

Validated clinical predictive rules (e.g. Well's score) are used to estimate the probability of DVT[5] (Table 1). In patients with low to intermediate probability of DVT, a D-dimer test is usually recommended due to its high negative predictive value; a negative D-dimer nearly excludes a DVT, while a positive D-dimer warrants imaging to confirm DVT. In patients with intermediate to high probability, Duplex ultrasonography is recommended to rule out DVT.[6]

Once DVT is confirmed, therapeutic anticoagulation is immediately commenced in the form of low-molecular-weight heparin (e.g. enoxaparin, nadroparin), unfractionated heparin or factor Xa inhibitors (e.g. rivaroxaban). LMWH is preferred over unfractionated heparin, except in patients with renal failure due to primarily renal excretion of the latter. Anticoagulation is administered for 3–12 months, depending on the site of thrombosis and ongoing presence of risk factors. Although anticoagulation is most often successful in resolving the acute symptoms of DVT, reducing risk of PE and preventing further propagation of thrombus, it does not exclude absolute risk of PE and PTS. Hence, some of these patients have to be referred to a vascular specialist as these patients may benefit from aggressive interventional management for DVT.

INTERVENTIONS FOR ACUTE DVT

Management of acute lower limb DVT depends on the location and extent of the thrombus. Calf vein DVT or distal DVT usually does not require percutaneous intervention as the risk of life threatening PE and incidence of PTS are very low owing to their small calibre and presence of companion veins.[7,8] Intervention in calf-vein DVT may be considered if there is extensive and severely symptomatic thrombosis from ankle to groin. Iliofemoral or proximal DVT, on the other hand, rarely recanalises on anticoagulation alone and has a higher the risk of PTS fatal PE; therefore removing the thrombus becomes proportionately more important.[9]

Table 1: Well's criteria /scoring for prediction of DVT

Clinical characteristic	Score
Active cancer (treatment or palliation within 6 months)	+1
Paralysis, paresis or recent cast immobilisation of lower extremity	+1
Bedridden for ≥3 days, or major surgery within 12 weeks	+1
Localised tenderness along deep venous system	+1
Entire leg swelling	+1
Calf swelling >3 cm more than asymptomatic side	+1
Pitting oedema confined to symptomatic leg	+1
Collateral non-varicose superficial veins	+1
Previously documented DVT	+1
Alternative diagnosis to DVT at least as likely	–2

–2–0: low probability; 1–2 points: moderate probability; 3–8 points: high probability

There are several treatment options for patients with proximal DVT with the main aim of early thrombus removal and restoring venous patency.[9-12]

Surgical Thrombectomy

Surgical thrombectomy involves a venotomy in the common femoral vein and use of a thrombectomy catheter to remove the clot, often accompanied with a post-procedure arteriovenous fistula to maintain flow and prevent rethrombosis. It is more invasive compared to equally efficacious endovascular procedures, requires general anaesthesia, and associated with longer immobilisation time and recovery time.[10] It may also delay stenting of obstructive venous lesions and hence is no longer a preferred option. Surgical thrombectomy can however be considered when thrombolysis is contraindicated or has failed, if the thrombus is secondary to tumour, or if there is no available endovascular expertise.[13]

Systemic Thrombolysis

Numerous studies have shown that thrombolysis is more effective than anticoagulation alone in acute DVT. Watz and Savidge did a randomised trial of streptokinase versus heparin and reported that complete lysis and preservation of valvular function were seen in 44% and 92% patients with thrombolysis compared to with 6% and 13% of patients with heparin.[14] Another randomised trial done by Turpie et al. with recombinant tissue plasminogen activator (rtPA) reported 58% of lysis compared to none with heparin.[15] Since the thrombolytic agent is dispersed throughout the blood pool and little concentration available at the thrombus site, systemic thrombolysis requires high dose infusion for long periods, eventually leading to higher risk of bleeding.[9,10,16] This was reflected in a pooled analysis review of 6 studies of systemic thrombolysis that reported thrombolysis to be 3.7 times more often effective than anticoagulation, but with 2.9 times increased incidence of bleeding complications.[17] Due to its systemic effect, its use can only be justified in patients with concomitant significant, massive PE.

Flow-directed Thrombolysis

In flow directed thrombolysis, the drug is injected into the pedal vein of the affected leg, with or without the use of tourniquets to direct the drug towards the deep veins. (Fig. 1) This however was not proved to be superior to systemic thrombolysis and is only recommended to be used in severely symptomatic extensive lower limb DVT to treat the thrombus segment in the calf region.[12,18]

Catheter-directed Therapy

Catheter-directed therapies were introduced on an effort to improve the efficacy and safety profile of endovascular DVT treatment by reducing the dose and duration of lytic therapy, accelerating clot removal, and producing early symptomatic relief. Various forms of thrombolysis, thromboaspiration

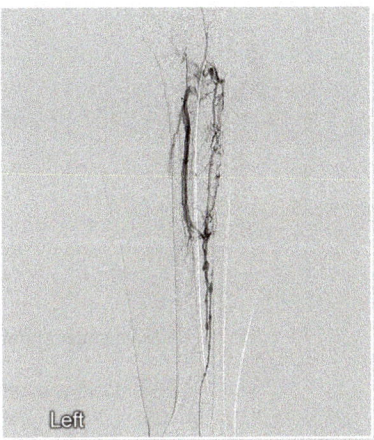

Figure 1: Venography from pedal puncture showing extensive infrapopliteal venous thrombosis, requiring lytic infusion through the peripheral venous cannula while intermittently applying tourniquets to direct infusion towards the thrombosed veins

and mechanical thrombectomy are being used currently, either alone or in combination. These procedures diminish but do not mitigate the risk of bleeding complications, and are hence offered only after considering the risk-benefit of aggressive DVT management. Broadly, endovascular DVT therapy is offered to younger, fully functional patients with proximal DVT and highly symptomatic patients. Indications for catheter directed therapy are summarised in Table 2.

Catheter-directed Thrombolysis (CDT)

In catheter directed thrombolysis, a multi side-hole infusion catheter is placed across the thrombus and fibrinolytic infusion is delivered directly into the thrombus (Fig. 2). This delivers a higher local intrathrombic drug concentration (enhancing efficacy) with reduced systemic effect and lower drug dose (enhancing safety). It also enables restoration of venous valvular function by lysing the clot adherent to the valves.[19] The thrombolytic therapy is more effective in the treatment of acute thrombus (<3 days old) and becomes increasing less effective in thrombus older than 4 weeks.

Table 2: Indications for catheter directed therapy[21]
Young or highly functional patients with acute iliofemoral DVT
Phlegmasia cerulea dolens
Extensive thrombus burden
Venous gangrene
Extension to IVC
Symptomatic IVC thrombosis after IVC filter placement
High risk of fatal PE
Propagation of DVT despite conventional therapy

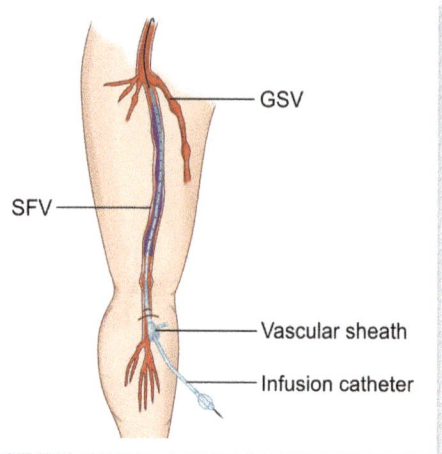

Figure 2: CDT diagram: Infusion catheter is positioned across the entire thrombus. (Source: Sharafuddin MJ, et al. J Vasc Interv Radiol. 2003;14:405-23)

Multiple studies have shown CDT to be more effective than systemic thrombolysis or anticoagulation. Laiho et al. in their study of 32 patients with iliofemoral DVT, reported 56% venous patency with CDT, compared to 19% with systemic thrombolysis. A randomised controlled trial comparing CDT with standard medical therapy also demonstrated iliofemoral patency in 65.9% with CDT compared to 47.4% with anticoagulation. Importantly, a 14.4% absolute risk reduction of PTS was noted with CDT on long-term follow up.[19] Baldwin et al. did a pooled review of literature of more than 600 patients with catheter directed thrombolysis and found decreased PTS, improved quality of life, and some evidence for reduced incidence of recurrent DVT.[20]

CDT procedure involves ultrasound guided access of the vein with a micropuncture set, usually below the thrombosed segment. The popliteal vein is mostly accessed owing to its size, easy antegrade advancement of wire/catheter, as well as the ability to achieve hemostasis with compression following the procedure. If the popliteal vein is thrombosed, then the short saphenous near its insertion into the popliteal vein or the proximal posterior tibial vein can be accessed. Access from the jugular vein or contralateral femoral vein can also be utilised, but is usually not preferred as retrograde passage of catheters and wires past the femoro-popliteal venous valves can be challenging. Additionally longer length of equipment is required, to be able to reach the knee joint level from a jugular access. Once accessed, a multi-hole infusion catheter is parked across the thrombosed segment. If the thrombosis extends over a long length, the catheter is placed at the distal-most segment of the thrombus, advanced sequentially during subsequent check angiograms.

The commonly used thrombolytic agents in clinical practice are recombinant tissue plasminogen activators: alteplase (0.01 mg/kg/hour upto maximum 1.0 mg/hour), reteplase (0.25-0.50 units/hour) and tenecteplase (0.25 mg/hour). There are different infusion strategies: bolus and wait, continuous overnight infusion, partial bolus and partial continuous overnight infusion and daily single dosing.[21] The bolus can be delivered either by simple lacing of the lytic agent into the thrombus, by brief high-pressure sprays of the agent via a multi-side-hole catheter (pulse spray technique), or using ultrasound (acoustic pulse technique). During the infusion, the patient is strictly monitored for bleeding complications. Close monitoring with complete blood count, partial thromboplastin time, plasma fibrinogen level every 6 hours is recommended. A low dose heparin (100-500 IU/hour) is also administered through a peripheral vein. In minor bleeding episodes and pericatheter oozing, the dose of the thrombolysis can be adjusted according to the laboratory values.[12]

Check venography is performed after overnight catheter directed infusion. If there is large persistent clot burden, the infusion can be continued for an additional day with strict monitoring in an ICU setting. If there is satisfactory reduction in clot burden, the residual clots can be macerated with balloon angioplasty to increase surface area for thrombolysis. If there is any obstructive lesion, it may be treated with balloon angioplasty and/or stent placement.

The limitations to CDT are long infusion time to obtain complete lysis of extensive DVT (1-3 days) and the healthcare resources used, including the ICU stay (Fig. 3). In a large multicentre registry, major bleeding was reported in 11% of patients, neurologic complications in 0.4% and minor bleeding complication in 16% of patients.[16]

Contraindications to the use of this pharmacologic thrombolytic therapy are related to the factors that increase the risk of haemorrhagic complications, which include recent major surgery, active internal bleeding, pregnancy, intracranial or intraspinal pathology, presence of varices or aneurysms and coagulopathic conditions.[21]

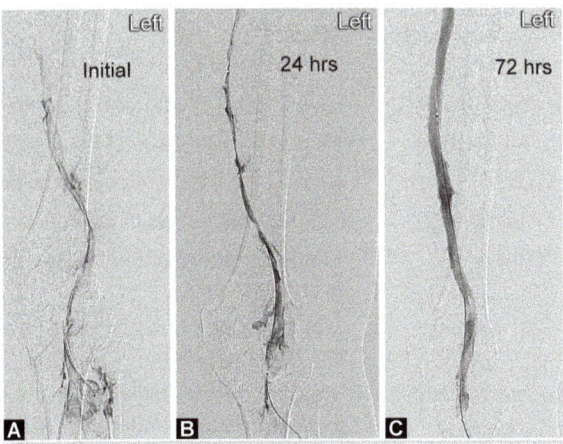

Figure 3: CDT: A 70-year-old female presented with phlegmasia cerulea dolens secondary to femoropopliteal and infrapopliteal DVT. (A) Initial venogram after SSV access demonstrating extensive femoropopliteal DVT. A 4F Fountain infusion catheter was parked in the popliteal vein thrombus and overnight thrombolysis was performed; (B) 24 hours check venogram showing partial resolution of thrombus. The infusion catheter was advanced further in the SFV and thrombolysis was continued; (C) Venogram done after 72 hours of initiation of thrombolysis shows significant resolution of the clots with good flow

Percutaneous Thrombectomy

Percutaneous thrombectomy refers to removal of clot through an endovascular approach and is a popular adjunct to CDT. Although it does not usually removed the thrombus completely, it is effective in reducing clot burden and lowering mean lytic infusion dose and duration, thereby reducing the morbidity and hospital stay with overall cost benefit. Thrombectomy devices may be purely mechanical, using aspiration or motorised mechanical techniques, or pharmacomechanical, using lytic agents to augment mechanical clot removal (Table 3).

Mechanical Thrombectomy

Percutaneous mechanical thrombectomy (PMT) involves maceration of the thrombus and removal of the thrombus fragments, thereby increasing the surface area of the residual thrombus and improving the efficiency of the endogenous thrombolysis. The disadvantages of the mechanical thrombectomy include increased procedure time, potential for embolism, and damage to the venous valves and endothelium.[12, 21]

1. Aspiration devices: With aspiration thrombectomy, a large bore catheter is used for aspiration of the thrombus using a manual or vacuum suction pressure. Guiding catheters and modified sheaths up to 11F have been used for manual aspiration of thrombus; the Indigo system uses vacuum suction through an 8F catheter system (Fig. 4). These catheters need to be advanced several times to aspirate the clot completely; residual thrombus requires thrombolytic drug infusion for complete clearance.

Table 3: Devices used for catheter-directed therapy

Name of device	Company name	Mode of operation
Uni Fuse	Angio Dynamics	Pulse spray infusion of lytic within thrombus
Fountain	Merit Medical	Pulse spray infusion of lytic within thrombus
Eko Sonic	BTG	Ultrasonic dispersion of lytic within thrombus
Indigo	Penumbra	Vacuum aspiration of thrombus
Trerotola	Arrow	Motor-driven rotating basket producing clot fragmentation
Cleaner	Argon	Motor-driven sinusoidal wire tip producing clot fragmentation
AngioJet	Boston Scientific	Venturi effect by high-velocity water jets enclosed in catheter, producing microfragmentation
Aspirex	Straub Medical	High-speed rotational coil within catheter creates suction and maceration of thrombus
Trellis	Medtronic Inc.	Selective infusion and dispersion of lytic followed by aspiration of lysed thrombus
Omniwave	Omnisonics	Ultrasonic dissolution of thrombus

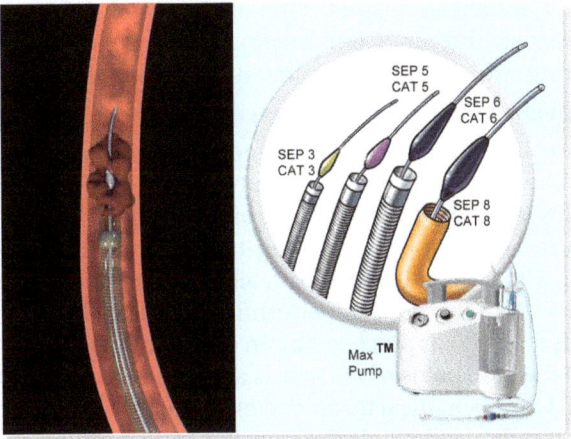

Figure 4: Indigo system. For treatment of DVT, the largest catheter (CAT8) is used

Park et al. retrospectively evaluated the efficacy of single session aspiration thrombectomy using 11F catheters without pharmacologic thrombolysis to treat acute and subacute lower limb DVT in 74 patients. Angioplasty and stent placement were performed when needed. They recorded initial success rate of 89.2%. The failures were due to underlying chronic thrombi and stent failure due to large pelvic mass. They concluded that single session aspiration thrombectomy for acute and subacute lower extremity DVT using large introducer catheters without pharmacologic thrombolysis is feasible with acceptable immediate and midterm results, without any complications related to pharmacologic thrombolysis.[22]

A recently introduced Angiovac device (Angiodynamics) uses a large bore 22F suction catheter to remove clots from larger vessels, such as IVC and iliac veins.

2. Mechanical thrombectomy devices: Broadly these devices can be categorised into three depending on the mechanism of their clot removal: microfragmentation (rotational), hydrodynamic (rheolytic) and ultrasound-enhanced.

The rotational thrombectomy devices employ a high speed rotating basket or impeller to macerate the thrombus into smaller particles which are cleared through the pulmonary circulation.[21,23,24] Currently available devices include the Trerotola (Arrow), Aspirex (Straub Medical) and cleaner device (Argon Medical). The Trellis device uses a rotating sinusoidal nitinol wire that disengages and aspirates lytic-laden thrombus isolated between two occlusion balloons. This category of devices carry risk of endothelial damage, although there is no conclusive evidence that it leads to recurrent DVT in future.

The hydrodynamic or rheolytic thrombectomy devices rely on the Venturi effect through retrogradely directed high speed saline jets (350–450 km/hour) for thrombus fragmentation. The fragmented thrombus is then aspirated into the device. The AngioJet (Boston Scientific) is the only currently available device using this mechanism and it theoretically produces less valvular or endothelial damage than rotational thrombectomy devices.

Ultrasound-enhanced devices, such as the Omniwave, uses ultrasound energy to dissipate thrombus into microparticles, 90% 0f which are smaller than 10 microns, which are then aspirated from the body.

Pharmacomechanical Catheter-directed Thrombectomy

Pharmacomechanical catheter-directed thrombolysis (PCDT) involves combined use of mechanical thrombectomy and CDT. Mechanical thrombectomy increases the surface area of thrombus thereby accelerating the pharmacological thrombolysis, reducing the dose and duration of subsequent lytic infusion, with resultant reduction in bleeding complications and ICU stay.

There are various methods in performing PCDT: (i) Multi-session PCDT: where PMT is followed or preceded by an overnight CDT infusion; (ii) Single session PCDT: where bolus of the lytic is administered within the thrombus, to be followed by mechanical thrombectomy after 30–60 minutes.

Two commonly used single session PCDT techniques involve use of Angiojet (Boston Scientific) and Trellis (Medtronic) devices.[18] Initial experience with these techniques suggested 80–90% efficacy in acute DVT treatment, although the impact of these techniques in the prevention of PTS has not yet been determined.[12] The Acute Venous Thrombosis: Thrombus Removal with Adjunctive Catheter-Directed Thrombolysis (ATTRACT) trial is an ongoing multicentre randomised trial to evaluate PCDT for the prevention of PTS in patients with proximal DVT, where 692 patients with DVT are being randomized to receive PCDT plus standard therapy versus standard DVT therapy alone.[25]

COMMONLY USED THROMBECTOMY DEVICES

Angiojet System

Angiojet rheolytic system (Boston Scientific) is the most commonly used mechanical thrombectomy system for standalone mechanical thrombectomy or in conjunction with pharmacological thrombolysis. This device is based on Bernoulli's principle. Rapidly flowing saline jets within the catheter generate a vacuum force which draws the thrombus into the catheter and fragmenting it. The disintegrated thrombus is subsequently aspirated into the device.

To enhance its efficiency, a "power pulse" technique is used to spray a bolus dose of thrombolytic drug forcefully into the thrombus using the Angiojet catheter. The drug is allowed to disperse within the thrombus for 15–30 minutes, following which thrombectomy is carried out with the Angiojet catheter (Fig. 5). As there is no rotational component, there is no risk of vascular wall damage. However, uncontrolled fragmentation of red blood cells releases adenosine, often producing bradycardia and haemoglobinuria with prolonged use of the system.

In one of the earliest study using Angiojet, Kasirajan et al. reported the efficacy of the Angiojet system in clot removal, venous patency restoration and clinical improvement. In their study, approximately 24% had venographic evidence of greater than 90% thrombus removal, 35% demonstrated 50–90% thrombus removal and 41% had less than 50% removed. Adjunctive CDT was required in 9 of 13 patients with less than 90% thrombus extraction by PMT.

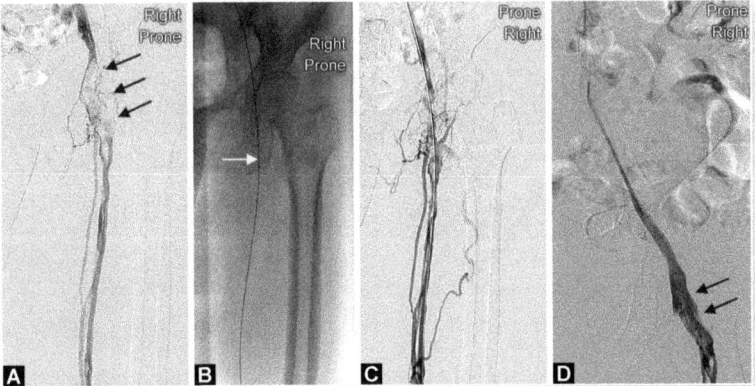

Figure 5: Angiojet power pulse thrombectomy: A 71-year-old female presented with worsening right lower limb DVT since 10 days. (A) Venogram through popliteal vein access in prone position showing short segment CFV thrombus (arrows); (B) Power pulse Angiojet thrombectomy was performed; Atleplase was delivered into the clot using Angiojet device (white arrow); (C) Venogram after 30 minutes of power pulse; (D) Final venogram showing >90% resolution after Angiojet thrombectomy. No underlying stenosis was noted on venography and IVUS

Significant clinical improvement was demonstrated in 82% of patients. No complication was seen related to the Angiojet catheter.[11]

Lin et al. in their comparative study of 52 DVT patients treated with Angiojet and 46 patients treated with CDT reported similar treatment success in terms of thrombus resolution and clinical improvement, and reported reduced treatment time and reduced ICU stay in patients treated with Angiojet.[26]

PEARL Registry (Peripheral Use of AngioJet Rheolytic Thrombectomy with a Variety of Catheter Lengths) is the largest registry for Angiojet study in which 329 patients were enrolled in 32 sites in the USA and Europe. The patients were divided into four treatment approaches using the Angiojet device: Angiojet without lytic in 4% of patients (13 of 329), Power Pulse Angiojet in 35% (115 of 329), Power Pulse Angiojet with CDT in 52% of patients (172 of 329) and Angiojet with CDT in 9% patients (29 of 329). Procedures were completed in <24 hours for 73% of patients, 86% of cases were completed in ≤2 sessions, and a mean of 18.7 mg alteplase was used. More than 95% of patients had substantial lysis at end of treatment, and the 3-, 6- and 12-month recurrence-free survival was 94%, 87% and 83%, respectively. Significant bleeding events occurred in 12 patients (3.6 %), but none were related to Angiojet procedure.[27]

Trellis Peripheral Infusion System

The Trellis (Medtronics) is a novel device for segmental and controlled PCDT. It consists of a catheter with proximal and distal occlusion balloons to isolate the thrombosed segment with drug infusion holes in between the balloons (Fig. 6). The thrombolytic agent is delivered locally between the occluding balloons as a bolus directly into the thrombus. Mechanical thrombectomy is performed by active spinning of sinusoidal dispersion wire which is inserted into the catheter at 1500–3000 rpm. The combined effect of vibration and

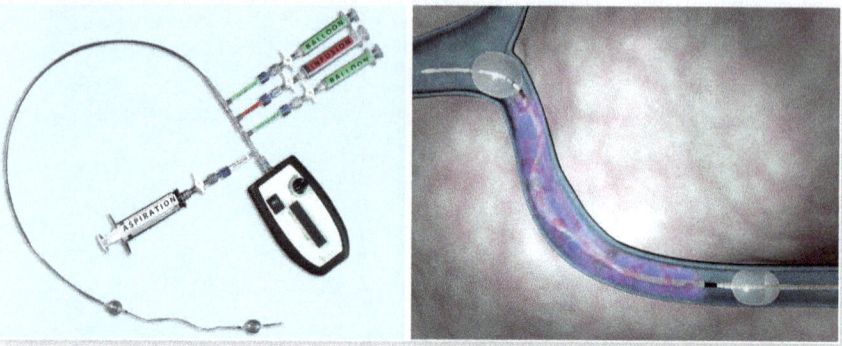

Figure 6: Trellis device: It consists of a catheter with proximal and distal occlusion balloons that are positioned on either side of the thrombus. The thrombolytic agent is delivered locally between the occluding balloons, following which mechanical thrombectomy is performed by active spinning of sinusoidal dispersion wire

thrombolytic dispersion leads to rapid clot lysis. After 20-30 minutes, the lysed thrombus is aspirated.[28, 29]

The occlusive balloons of the Trellis ensures that the lytic drug is confined within the treated segment, thus reducing the systemic bleeding complications. The risk of embolisation during aspiration of thrombus is also minimised with distal balloon occlusion. As the thrombolytic infusate is aspirated along with the clot debris, this procedure can be performed even in patients in whom thrombolytic therapy is contraindicated.

Arko et al. published a series of 18 patients with iliofemoral DVT undergoing successful venous thrombectomy with the Trellis device. In their study, iliofemoral patency was achieved in a single setting in 80% of these patients and that 88% of treated veins remained patent during follow up period of 6 months. The amount and duration of the thrombolytic agent administered was limited and they observed that the decreased requirement of thrombolytic agent represents a clinical advantage in reducing potential haemorrhagic complications.[30]

O'Sullivan et al. in their study of 10 patients with acute DVT treated with Trellis-8 thrombectomy combined with low-dose thrombolysis reported achievement of venous patency with flow in all the cases. The thrombus removal was at least 95% in 14% patients and 50-95% in 82% patients. No major complication was reported. Primary patency rate of the treated venous segments at 2 days was 86% and primary assisted patency rate was 100% at 30 days. They opined that the Trellis system can achieve single session PMT in patients with acute DVT.[28]

EkoSonic System

Rosenshein et al. were the first to report that ultrasonic energy is effective in disrupting the fibrin matrix within the thrombus. The EkoSonic endovascular system (BTG) is a novel ultrasound accelerated thrombolytic system, which generates a localised acoustic field that accelerates lytic dispersion by driving the drug deeper into the clot (Fig. 7). This therapy achieves its effect by first

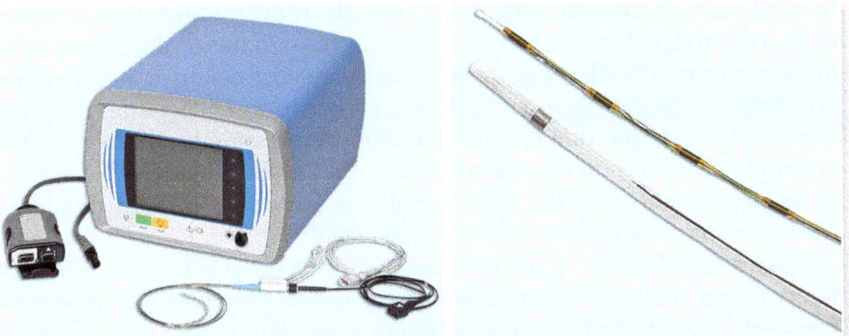

Figure 7: EkoSonic system

dissociating the fibrin mesh to increase surface area of the thrombus to the thrombolytic drug. The acoustic streaming caused by the ultrasound waves drives the thrombolytic agent into the loosened clot. The ultrasound energy can penetrate the venous valves and dissolve the thrombi located behind the venous valves. As the entire thrombosed venous segment can be exposed to ultrasound energy, it potentially reduces the infusion time as well as dosage of the thrombolytic agent.

Grommes et al. conducted a prospective non-randomised study with ultrasound accelerated CDT for DVT. 12 patients (7 cavoileofemoropopliteal, 3 iliofemoropopliteal, 1 femoropopliteal and 1 superior caval) receiving standard anticoagulant and compression therapy, were treated with additional ultrasound accelerated CDT (13 procedures) using the EKOS endowave system. Thrombolysis was successful in 85% (11/13), with complete clot lysis. No pulmonary embolism was seen. There was one case of bleeding at the catheter insertion site. 4 patients developed early recurrent thrombosis due to untreated residual venous obstruction. The authors concluded that ultrasound accelerated CDT is a safe and promising treatment in patients with DVT and residual venous obstruction should be treated with angioplasty and stent insertion to avoid early rethrombosis.[31]

Parikh et al. in their study evaluated the success of lysis and clinical improvement in patients treated with ultrasound accelerated thrombolysis for DVT. 47 patients with 53 cases of DVT were treated with US-accelerated thrombolysis at eight centres in United States. Complete lysis (>90%) was seen in 37 of 53 (70%) and overall lysis (complete + partial) was seen in 48 (91%). No lysis was seen in 5 cases, 4 of which were chronic DVT. Significant bleeding complication (hematoma at prior operative site) was seen in only 2 patients (3.8%). No intracranial or retroperitoneal haemorrhage is seen. The study showed comparable or better lysis with lower average drug dose and duration than reported in studies with standard catheter directed thrombolysis.[32]

Adjunctive Venous Angioplasty and Stenting

After the completion of thrombolytic or thrombectomy therapy, balloon angioplasty may be required to trawl away or macerate any residual thrombus.

In most cases there is an underlying stenosis or obstructive disease in the central or proximal vein, which is usually due to stenotic/occlusive sequelae from a previous thrombotic occlusion, malignant obstruction or May-Thurner syndrome.[33,34] In May-Thurner syndrome, patients have left proximal iliac vein stenosis, web or spur due to long-standing compression on the vein by the crossing right common iliac artery against the vertebral body. It is believed to be quite prevalent in the adult population (around 20%), and should be suspected in young patients with left sided DVT.[35]

Regardless of cause, if any residual venous stenosis is found, additional intervention such as balloon angioplasty and/or venous stenting will be required[19] (Fig. 8). Self-expanding nitinol stents (10-16 mm diameter) are preferred in the iliac veins because of their conformability to the iliac vein curvature and lower risk of migration. Predilatation with an angioplasty balloon is usually performed before stent deployment. Post deployment the stent may be dilated using an appropriate angioplasty balloon, the diameter of which is best assessed with intravascular ultrasound (IVUS). Post-procedure all the patients are prescribed oral anticoagulant for 6 months to maintain INR in the range of 2.0-3.0.

Several studies have shown the efficacy of these adjuvant procedures in DVT treatment, with reported 79-100% primary patency rates of iliac vein stents at 1-2 years.[36-39] There is a 73% recurrence of iliofemoral DVT if the underlying obstructive lesion is not treated.[40]

IVC Filters

IVC filters are effective in preventing PE and are inserted in select patients with DVT (contraindication, failure or complication of anticoagulation). However, their long-term safety is questionable. Decousus et al. performed a prospective multicenter randomized controlled trial of IVC filters that showed the use of IVC filters was associated with significant decrease in the occurrence of PE compared with use of anticoagulation alone (1.1% vs. 4.8%). However, this difference was not statistically significant at 2-year follow-up and there was significant increase in risk of recurrent DVT in patients treated with IVC filters compared with anticoagulation alone (20.8% vs. 11.6%).[41] Due the long-term implications of caval filtration, permanent filters have given way to retrievable filters. These filters are used as adjunctive treatment before endovascular DVT intervention to prevent likelihood of clot fragments embolising to the lungs during mechanical thrombectomy. Although thrombectomy related PE is most often minor and silent, filter insertion should be considered in the following situations before treating DVT: (i) preexisting pulmonary hypertension, (ii) preexisting PE, (iii) iliocaval thrombosis, and (iv) contraindication to anticoagulation.

The IVC filters are mostly placed below the renal veins to avoid renal vein thrombosis. Suprarenal placement can be considered if there is thrombus extension to the level of the renal veins. When performing endovascular treatment for DVT, one must ensure wires/catheters do not dislodge the IVC filter. Filters are retrieved after 6 weeks while the patient is fully anticoagulated to avoid long term complications associated with them.[42] Venacavography is

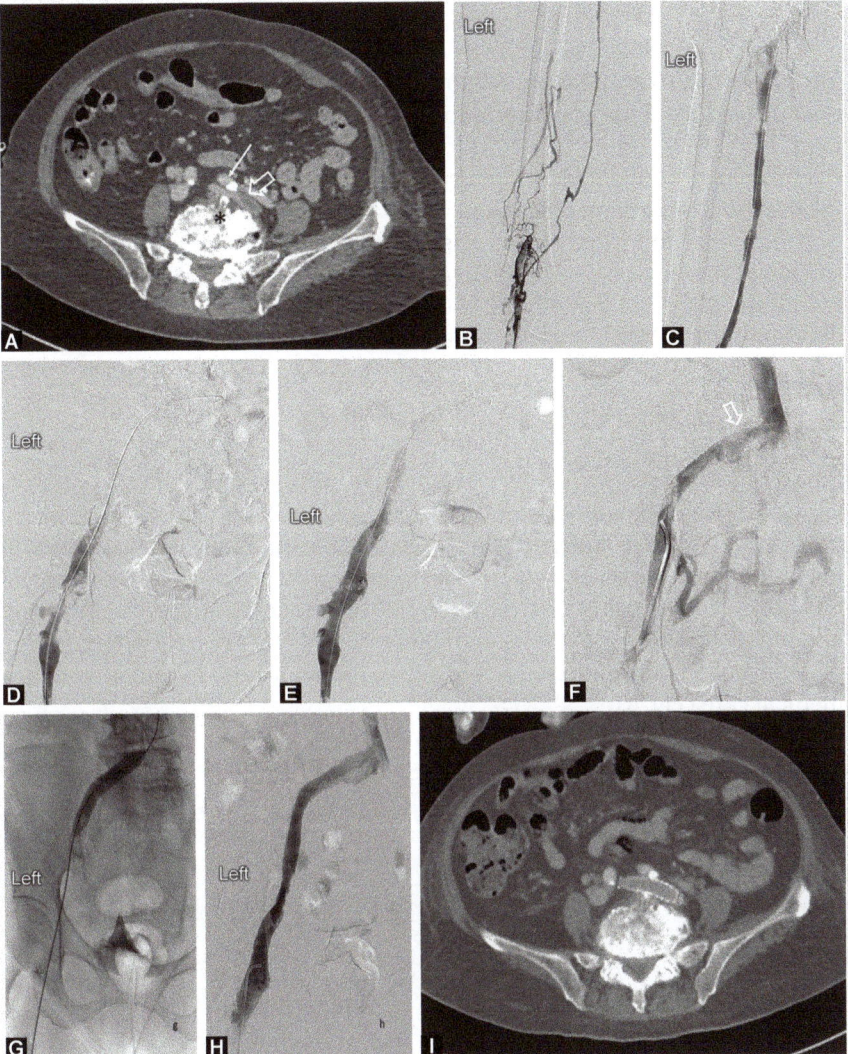

Figure 8: A 76-year-old female presenting with extensive left lower limb DVT. (A) CT done showing May-Thurner syndrome, with compression of left common iliac vein between vertebral body spur (asterisk) and left common iliac artery (arrow) and iliac vein thrombosis below the level of compression (thick arrow); (B and C) Venogram through left popliteal access showing iliofemoral venous thrombosis. Pharmacomechanical thrombectomy with Angiojet catheter was performed over wire with significant reduction in femoral clots; (D to F) Iliac vein thrombosis was treated with further thrombectomy and overnight CDT, uncovering the iliac vein compression (thick arrow); (G and H) Stenosis of the left common iliac vein is unmasked for which iliac venous stenting was performed; (I) CT done after 12 months showing good patency of the stented iliac vein

to be performed before filter retrieval to document any presence of residual vein thrombus. If there is significant residual thrombus, thrombolysis should be considered before filter removal.

POST-PROCEDURE MANAGEMENT

Thrombotic venous disease needs to be medically managed more aggressively post procedure than non-thrombotic disease due to higher rethrombosis rates. For post thrombotic lesions long-term therapy with warfarin or newer rivaroxaban are indicated. Antiplatelet agents such as aspirin and clopidogrel are used following stent placement.[11]

It is also important that patient gets utmost supportive care with compression stockings, pneumatic compression and wound care post-procedure not only to improve the patient symptoms but also to prevent recurrence of DVT and development of PTS.

SUMMARY

Endovascular therapy for DVT is effective in restoring venous patency, alleviating acute symptoms and reducing risk of PTS. It has shown to be more effective than anticoagulation and safer than systemic infusion of thrombolytics. However, it is not completely risk free, and in the absence of well-designed trials it is only offered to select patient groups: young and highly functional patients with iliofemoral DVT, severely symptomatic patients not responding to standard anticoagulation, and failure of standard medical care (Fig. 9).

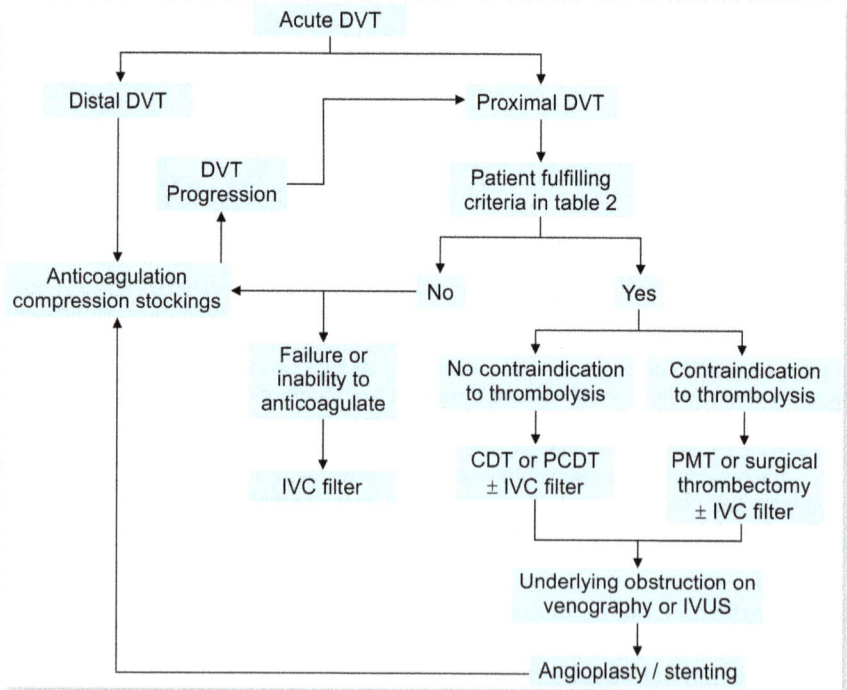

Figure 9: An algorithmic approach for endovascular treatment of DVT

Amongst the various methods to treat DVT, pharmacomechanical catheter-directed thrombolysis (PCDT) seems to be the most preferred method due to its efficacy, safety profile and ability to provide single-session treatment. Adjunctive balloon dilatation and stenting of central veins is often required to improve the long-term results of endocascular treatment.

REFERENCES

1. Young L, Ockelford P, Milne D, Rolfe-Vyson V, Mckelvie S, Harper P. Post-treatment residual thrombus increases the risk of recurrent deep vein thrombosis and mortality. J Thromb Haemost. 2006;4(9):1919-24.
2. Vedantham S. Interventions for deep vein thrombosis: re-emergence of a promising therapy. Am J Med. 2008;121(11):S28-39.
3. Enden T, Haig Y, Kløw NE, Slagsvold CE, Sandvik L, Ghanima W, et al. Long-term outcome after additional catheter-directed thrombolysis versus standard treatment for acute iliofemoral deep vein thrombosis (the CaVenT study): a randomised controlled trial. The Lancet. 2012;379(9810):31-8.
4. Pianta MJ, Thomson KR. Catheter-directed thrombolysis of lower limb thrombosis. Cardiovasc Intervent Radiol. 2011;34(1):25-36.
5. Wells PS, Anderson DR, Bormanis J, et. al. Value of assessment of pretest probability of deep-vein thrombosis in clinical management. Lancet. 1997;350(9094):1795-8.
6. Snow V, Qaseem A, Barry P, Hornbake ER, Rodnick JE, Tobolic T, et al. Management of venous thromboembolism: a clinical practice guideline from the American College of Physicians and the American Academy of Family Physicians. Ann Intern Med. 2007;146(3):204-10.
7. Righini M, Bounameaux H. Clinical relevance of distal deep vein thrombosis. Curr Opin Pulm Med. 2008;14(5):408-13.
8. Vedantham S, Thorpe PE, Cardella JF, Grassi CJ, Patel NH, Ferral H, et al. Quality improvement guidelines for the treatment of lower extremity deep vein thrombosis with use of endovascular thrombus removal. J Vasc Interv Radiol. 2006;17(3):435-48.
9. O'Sullivan GJ. The role of interventional radiology in the management of deep venous thrombosis: advanced therapy. Cardiovasc Intervent Radiol. 2011;34(3):445-61.
10. Kearon C, Kahn SR, Agnelli G, Goldhaber S, Raskob GE, Comerota AJ. Antithrombotic therapy for venous thromboembolic disease: American College of Chest Physicians evidence-based clinical practice guidelines. CHEST Journal. 2008;133(Suppl):454S-545S.
11. Kasirajan K, Gray B, Ouriel K. Percutaneous AngioJet thrombectomy in the management of extensive deep venous thrombosis. J Vasc Interv Radiol. 2001;12(2):179-85.
12. Sista AK, Vedantham S, Kaufman JA, Madoff DC. Endovascular interventions for acute and chronic lower extremity deep venous disease: state of the art. Radiology. 2015;276(1):31-53.
13. Augustinos P, Ouriel K. Invasive approaches to treatment of venous thromboembolism. Circulation 2004;110(Suppl 1):I27-I34.
14. Watz R, Savidge GF. Rapid thrombolysis and preservation of valvular venous function in high deep vein thrombosis. Acta Med Scand. 1979;205:293-8.

15. Turpie AG, Levine MN, Hirsh J, Ginsberg JS, Cruickshank M, Jay R, Gent M. Tissue plasminogen activator (rt-PA) vs heparin in deep vein thrombosis: results of a randomized trial. CHEST Journal. 1990;97(Suppl):172S-5S.
16. Mewissen MW, Seabrook GR, Meissner MH, Cynamon J, Labropoulos N, Haughton SH. Catheter-directed Thrombolysis for Lower Extremity Deep Venous Thrombosis: Report of a National Multicenter Registry 1. Radiology. 1999;211(1):39-49.
17. Goldhaber SZ, Buring JE, Lipnick RJ, Hennekens CH. Pooled analyses of randomized trials of streptokinase and heparin in phlebographically documented acute deep venous thrombosis. Am J Med. 1984;76(3):393-7.
18. Schwieder G, Grimm W, Siemens HJ, Flor B, Hilden A, Gmelin E, et al. Intermittent regional therapy with rt-PA is not superior to systemic thrombolysis in deep vein thrombosis (DVT)--a German multicenter trial. J Thromb Haemost. 1995;74(5):1240-3.
19. Lin PH, Ochoa LN, Duffy P. Catheter-directed thrombectomy and thrombolysis for symptomatic lower-extremity deep vein thrombosis: review of current interventional treatment strategies. Perspect Vasc Surg Endovasc Ther. 2010;22(3):152-63.
20. Baldwin ZK, Comerota AJ, Schwartz LB. Catheter-directed thrombolysis for deep venous thrombosis. Vasc Endovascular Surg. 2004;38(1):1-9.
21. Nazir SA, Ganeshan A, Nazir S, Uberoi R. Endovascular treatment options in the management of lower limb deep venous thrombosis. Cardiovasc Intervent Radiol. 2009;32(5):861-76.
22. Park SI, Lee M, Lee MS, Kim MD, Won JY, Lee DY. Single-session aspiration thrombectomy of lower extremity deep vein thrombosis using large-size catheter without pharmacologic thrombolysis. Cardiovasc Intervent Radiol. 2014;37(2):412-9.
23. Delomez M, Beregi JP, Willoteaux S, Bauchart JJ, d'Othée BJ, Asseman P, Perez N, Thery C. Mechanical thrombectomy in patients with deep venous thrombosis. Cardiovasc Intervent Radiol. 2001;24(1):42-8.
24. Molan GS, Fitt G, Brooks DM. Mechanical thrombectomy in acute venous thrombosis using an Amplatz thrombectomy device. Australas Radiol. 1999;43(4):456-60.
25. Vedantham S, Goldhaber SZ, Kahn SR, Julian J, Magnuson E, Jaff MR, et al. Rationale and design of the ATTRACT Study: a multicenter randomized trial to evaluate pharmacomechanical catheter-directed thrombolysis for the prevention of postthrombotic syndrome in patients with proximal deep vein thrombosis. Am Heart J. 2013;165(4):523-30.
26. Lin PH, Zhou W, Dardik A, Mussa F, Kougias P, Hedayati N, et al. Catheter-direct thrombolysis versus pharmacomechanical thrombectomy for treatment of symptomatic lower extremity deep venous thrombosis. Am J Surg. 2006;192(6):782-8.
27. Garcia MJ, Lookstein R, Malhotra R, Amin A, Blitz LR, Leung DA, et al. Endovascular Management of Deep Vein Thrombosis with Rheolytic Thrombectomy: Final Report of the Prospective Multicenter PEARL (Peripheral Use of AngioJet Rheolytic Thrombectomy with a Variety of Catheter Lengths) Registry. J Vasc Interv Radiol. 2015;26(6):777-85.
28. O'Sullivan GJ, Lohan DG, Gough N, et al. Pharmacomechanical thrombectomy of acute deep vein thrombosis with the Trellis-8 isolated thrombolysis catheter. J Vasc Interv Radiol. 2007;18(6):715-24.

29. Hilleman DE, Razavi MK. Clinical and economic evaluation of the Trellis-8 infusion catheter for deep vein thrombosis. J Vasc Interv Radiol. 2008;19(3):377-83.
30. Arko FR, Davis CM, Murphy EH, Smith ST, Timaran CH, Modrall JG, et al. Aggressive percutaneous mechanical thrombectomy of deep venous thrombosis: early clinical results. Arch Surg. 2007;142(6):513-9.
31. Grommes J, Strijkers R, Greiner A, et al. Safety and feasibility of ultrasound-accelerated catheter-directed thrombolysis in deep vein thrombosis. Eur J Vasc Endovasc Surg. 2011;41(4):526-32.
32. Parikh S, Motarjeme A, McNamara T, Raabe R, Hagspiel K, Benenati JF, et al. Ultrasound-accelerated thrombolysis for the treatment of deep vein thrombosis: initial clinical experience. J Vasc Interv Radiol. 2008;19(4):521-8.
33. Bjarnason H, Kruse JR, Asinger DA, Nazarian GK, Dietz CA, Caldwell MD, et al. Iliofemoral deep venous thrombosis: safety and efficacy outcome during 5 years of catheter-directed thrombolytic therapy. J Vasc Interv Radiol. 1997;8(3):405-18.
34. Johnson BF, Manzo RA, Bergelin RO, Strandness DE. Relationship between changes in the deep venous system and the development of the postthrombotic syndrome after an acute episode of lower limb deep vein thrombosis: a one-to six-year follow-up. J Vasc Surg. 1995;21(2):307-13.
35. Lamont JP, Pearl GJ, Patetsios P, Warner MT, Gable DR, Garrett W, et al. Prospective evaluation of endoluminal venous stents in the treatment of the May–Thurner syndrome. Ann Vasc Surg. 2002;16(1):61-4
36. Patel NH, Stookey KR, Ketcham DB, Cragg AH. Endovascular management of acute extensive iliofemoral deep venous thrombosis caused by May-Thurner syndrome. J Vasc Interv Radiol. 2000 Dec 31;11(10):1297-302.
37. O'Sullivan GJ, Semba CP, Bittner CA, Kee ST, Razavi MK, Sze DY, Dake MD. Endovascular management of iliac vein compression (May-Thurner) syndrome. J Vasc Interv Radiol. 2000;11(7):823-36.
38. Neglen P, Berry MA, Raju S. Endovascular surgery in the treatment of chronic primary and post-thrombotic iliac vein obstruction. Eur J Vasc Endovasc Surg. 2000;20(6):560-71.
39. Hurst DR, Forauer AR, Bloom JR, Greenfield LJ, Wakefield TW, Williams DM. Diagnosis and endovascular treatment of iliocaval compression syndrome. J Vasc Surg. 2001;34(1):106-13.
40. Binkert CA, Schoch E, Stuckmann G, Largiader J, Wigger P, Schoepke W, Zollikofer CL. Treatment of pelvic venous spur (May-Thurner syndrome) with self-expanding metallic endoprostheses. Cardiovasc Intervent Radiol. 1998;21(1):22-6.
41. Decousus H, Leizorovicz A, Parent F, Page Y, Tardy B, Girard P, et al. A clinical trial of vena caval filters in the prevention of pulmonary embolism in patients with proximal deep-vein thrombosis. N Engl J Med. 1998;338(7):409-16.
42. Crowther MA. Inferior vena cava filters in the management of venous thromboembolism. Am J Med. 2007;120(10):S13-7.

CHAPTER
14

Current Concepts in Management of Pulmonary Embolism

R Sekhar, Simit Vora, Pranav Thusay

INTRODUCTION

Pulmonary embolism (PE) is an under diagnosed yet important cause of morbidity and mortality in patients worldwide. Though Indian data is sparse on incidence, an autopsy study on 1,000 medical patients at the Postgraduate Institute of Medical Education and Research (PGIMER), Chandigarh revealed that PE was present in 159 (16%) of 1,000 patients who died in the hospital—it was a fatal embolus in 36 and was a major contributor to death in 90 patients; in 30 patients, the embolus was an incidental finding at autopsy as death occurred due to some other cause. A clinical (pre-mortem) suspicion of PE was recorded in 30% of patients and a diagnosis of PE could be made in <10%; >80% of 159 patients with PE were young (<50 years).[1] Despite awareness about this potentially fatal condition continuing to increase in India, management protocols are varied, often depending on which speciality gets to treat the patient.

This chapter will be an attempt to standardize the diagnosis and management of PE in a streamlined manner, with an emphasis on triaging and using evidence-based modalities.

Acute PE is the most serious clinical presentation of VTE. Acute PE interferes with both the circulation and gas exchange. Pulmonary artery pressure increases only if more than 30–50% of the total cross-sectional area of the pulmonary arterial bed is occluded by thromboemboli.[2] The association between elevated circulating levels of biomarkers of myocardial injury and an adverse early outcome indicates that right ventricular ischaemia is of pathophysiological significance in the acute phase of PE.[3] Right ventricular (RV) failure due to pressure overload is the primary cause of death in severe PE.[4]

TRIAGING OF PULMONARY EMBOLISM IN THE ACCIDENT AND EMERGENCY DEPARTMENT (FIG. 1 AND TABLE 1)

Triaging for severity of an episode of acute PE is based on the estimated PE-related early mortality risk defined by in-hospital or 30-day mortality.[4] This triaging, which has important implications both for the diagnostic and therapeutic strategies, is based on the patient's clinical condition while presenting to the treating physician, **High risk** PE being labelled if in shock or persistent arterial hypotension (BP <90 mmHg) and **Not high risk** PE in the absence of this sign (Table 1).[5]

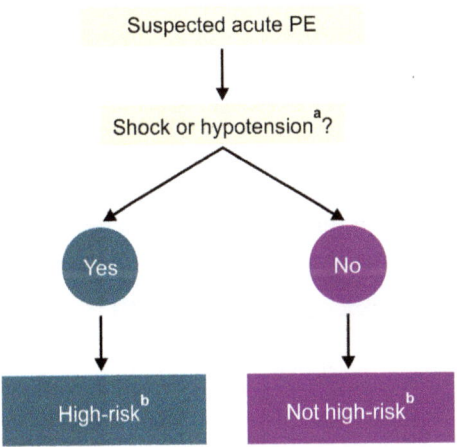

PE = pulmonary embolism
[a]Defined as systolic blood pressure <90 mmHg, or a systolic pressure drop by ≥40 mmHg, for >15 minutes, if not caused by new-onset arrhythmia, hypovolaemia, or sepsis
[b]Based on the estimated PE-related in-hospital or 30-day mortality

Figure 1: Initially triaging in PE[4]

Table 1: Characteristics of suspected PE patients presenting in an emergency department (Pollock et al 2011)[5]

Feature	PE confirmed (n = 1880)	PE not confirmed (n = 528)
Dyspnoea	50%	51%
Pleuritic chest pain	39%	28%
Cough	23%	23%
Substernal chest pain	15%	17%
Fever	10%	10%
Haemoptysis	8%	4%
Syncope	6%	6%
Unilateral leg pain	6%	5%
Signs of DVT (unilateral swelling)	24%	18%

Figure 2 summarizes the plan of action in **high risk** patients for PE. Suspected high-risk PE is an immediately life-threatening situation, and patients presenting with shock or hypotension have a serious clinical problem. The clinical probability is usually high, and the differential diagnosis includes acute valvular dysfunction, tamponade, acute coronary syndrome (ACS), and aortic dissection.[4] The most useful initial test in this situation is bedside transthoracic echocardiography, which will yield evidence of acute pulmonary hypertension and RV dysfunction if acute PE is the cause of the patient's haemodynamic decompensation. In a highly unstable patient, echocardiographic evidence of RV dysfunction is sufficient to prompt immediate reperfusion without further testing. This decision may be strengthened by the (rare) visualisation of right heart thrombi.[6-8] Ancillary bedside imaging tests include trans-oesophageal echocardiography which, though not easily available in an ER in most centres, might allow direct visualization of thrombi in the pulmonary artery and its main branches,[9-11] and bedside CUS (Compression Ultrasound), which can detect proximal DVT. As soon as the patient can be stabilized by supportive treatment, final confirmation of the diagnosis by CT angiography should be sought.

For unstable patients admitted directly to the catheterization laboratory with suspected ACS, pulmonary angiography may be considered as a diagnostic

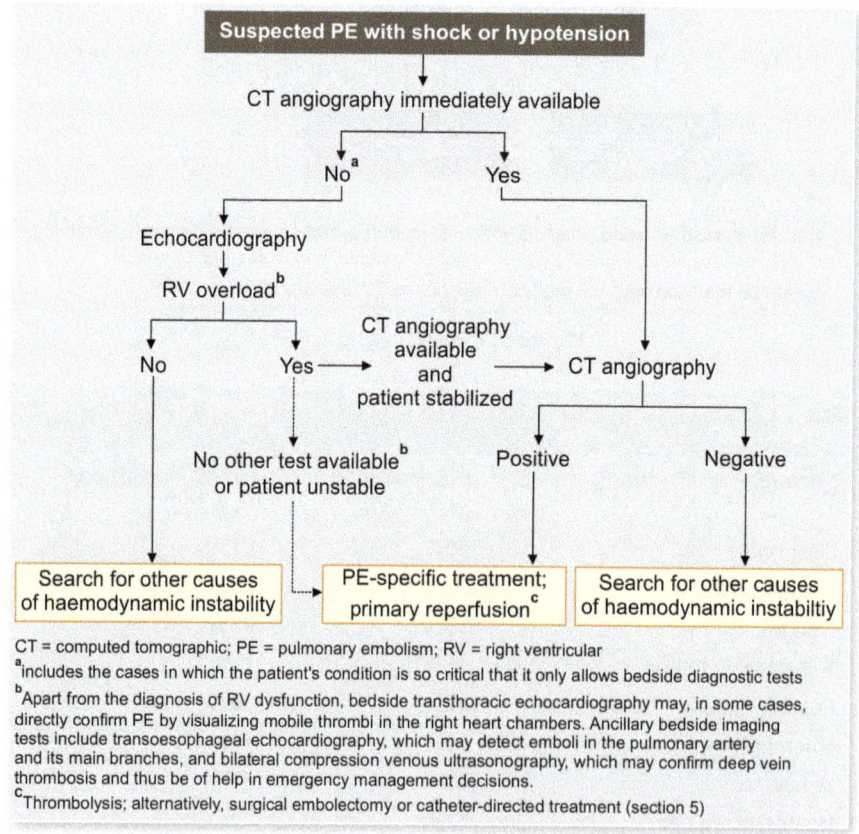

Figure 2: Plan of action for PE with shock/hypotension[4]

procedure after the ACS has been excluded, provided that PE is a probable diagnostic alternative and particularly if percutaneous catheter-directed treatment is a therapeutic option.

All patients in the high risk group should be subjected to a CT Angiogram where facilities are available. The PIOPED II trial (Prospective Investigation on Pulmonary Embolism Diagnosis) observed a sensitivity of 83% and a specificity of 96% for MDCT (multi-detector computed tomographic). PIOPED II also highlighted the influence of clinical probability on the predictive value of MDCT.[12]

Once acute PE has been diagnosed, the traditional management of this condition is systemic thrombolysis. The FDA-approved regimen of alteplase for an acute, massive pulmonary embolism is 100 mg administered by intravenous infusion over 2 hours.[13] Overall, >90% of patients appear to respond favourably to thrombolysis, as judged by clinical and echocardiographic improvement within 36 hours.[14] The greatest benefit is observed when treatment is initiated within 48 hours of symptom onset, but thrombolysis can still be useful in patients who have had symptoms for 6-14 days.[15] Strong positive evidence is available for use of thrombolytics in the management of acute PE. A meta-analysis of 11 randomised studies in patients with acute PE, thrombolytic therapy was associated with significant reduction in recurrent PE or death in high risk hemodynamically unstable patients.[16] Other studies ICOPER (1999)[17] RIETE (2007),[18] EMPEROR (2008)[19] have also shown benefits with thrombolytics in significantly reducing the mortality rate in acute massive PE.[20] Alteplase should be preferred over streptokinase and urokinase based on the current evidence on efficacy, safety and clinical experience[20] (Table 2). rt-PA rapidly improves right-ventricular function and pulmonary perfusion among patients with PE and may lead to lower rate of adverse clinical outcomes.[21] Recently published results of MOPETT trial[22] showed that <50% of the standard dose of tPA is safe and effective in the treatment of moderate PE.

A presentation of 100 cases at the ACC 2014 recommended, that when the clinician is undecided about thrombolysis or complete evaluation cannot be done due to unavailability of tests or cost constraints, half dose tPA (10 mg bolus and 40 mg infusion over two hours) can be administered along with weight-adjusted unfractionated heparin. This reduces the chance of bleeding,

Table 2: Contraindications to alteplase[20,38]

Absolute contraindications	Relative Contraindications
Internal bleeding	Age >75
Previous intracranial haemorrhage	Currant use of anticoagulants
History of CVA within 3 months	Non compressible vascular punctures
Recent intracranial or intraspinal surgery or trauma	Prolonged CPR>10 min
Intracranial neoplasm	Severe uncontrolled hypertension
AV malformation or aneurysms	Dementia
Known bleeding diathesis	Recent GI bleed within 2-3 weeks

but remains effective as pulmonary thrombi respond differently from arterial thrombi. However, this half dose therapy is currently not an approved dose for thrombolysis.[22]

A review of randomised trials performed before 2004 indicated that thrombolysis may be associated with a reduction in mortality or recurrent PE in high-risk patients who present with haemodynamic instability.[16] In a recent epidemiological report, in-hospital mortality attributable to PE was lower in unstable patients who received thrombolytic therapy, compared with those who did not (RR 0.20; 95% CI 0.19–0.22; P<0.0001).[23] In the absence of haemodynamic compromise at presentation, the clinical benefits of thrombolysis have remained controversial for many years. In a randomized comparison of heparin vs. alteplase in 256 normotensive patients with acute PE and evidence of RV dysfunction or pulmonary hypertension—obtained by clinical examination, echocardiography, or right heart catheterization—thrombolytic treatment (mainly secondary thrombolysis) reduced the incidence of escalation to emergency treatment (from 24.6% to 10.2%; P = 0.004), without affecting mortality.[24] More recently, the Pulmonary Embolism Thrombolysis (PEITHO) trial was published.[25] This was a multicentre, randomized, double-blind comparison of thrombolysis with a single weight-adapted intravenous bolus of tenecteplase plus heparin vs. placebo plus heparin. Patients with acute PE were eligible for the study if they had RV dysfunction, confirmed by echocardiography or CT angiography, and myocardial injury confirmed by a positive troponin I or -T test. A total of 1006 patients were enrolled. The primary efficacy outcome, a composite of all-cause death or haemodynamic decompensation/collapse within 7 days of randomization, was significantly reduced with tenecteplase (2.6% vs. 5.6% in the placebo group; P = 0.015; OR 0.44; 95% CI 0.23–0.88). The benefit of thrombolysis was mainly driven by a significant reduction in the rate of haemodynamic collapse (1.6% vs. 5.0%; P = 0.002); all-cause 7-day mortality was low: 1.2% in the tenecteplase group and 1.8% in the placebo group (P = 0.43).[25] Thrombolytic treatment carries a risk of major bleeding, including intracranial haemorrhage. Analysis of pooled data from trials using various thrombolytic agents and regimens reported intracranial bleeding rates between 1.9% and 2.2%.[26,27] Increasing age and the presence of comorbidities have been associated with a higher risk of bleeding complications.[28] Major non-intracranial bleeding events were also increased in the tenecteplase group, compared with placebo (6.3% vs. 1.5%; P < 0.001).[25] These results underline the need to improve the safety of thrombolytic treatment in patients at increased risk of intracranial or other life-threatening bleeding. A strategy using reduced-dose rtPA appeared to be safe in the setting of 'moderate' PE in a study that included 121 patients,[22] and another trial on 118 patients with haemodynamic instability or 'massive pulmonary obstruction' reported similar results.[29] Although studies have demonstrated the effectiveness of this approach, it is also associated with an approximate 20% risk of significant haemorrhage and a 3% to 5% risk of intracranial haemorrhage.[30] Heparin therapy should be stopped during the alteplase infusion and reinstituted after the infusion when the activated partial thromboplastin time (aPTT) or thrombin time returns to twice normal or less.[4] In addition, supportive treatment is vital in patients with PE and RV failure. Experimental studies indicate that aggressive volume expansion is of no benefit and may even worsen RV function by causing mechanical overstretch, or by reflex mechanisms that depress contractility.[31] On the other hand, modest (500 ml) fluid challenge may help to increase cardiac index in patients with PE, low cardiac index, and normal BP.[32]

Use of vasopressors is often necessary, in parallel with (or while waiting for) pharmacological, surgical, or interventional reperfusion treatment. Norepinephrine appears to improve RV function via a direct positive inotropic effect, while also improving RV coronary perfusion by peripheral vascular alpha-receptor stimulation and the increase in systemic BP. Its use should probably be limited to hypotensive patients. Based on the results of small series, the use of dobutamine and/or dopamine may be considered for patients with PE, low cardiac index, and normal BP; however, raising the cardiac index above physiological values may aggravate the ventilation–perfusion mismatch by further redistributing flow from (partly) obstructed to unobstructed vessels.[33] Epinephrine combines the beneficial properties of norepinephrine and dobutamine, without the systemic vasodilatory effects of the latter. It may therefore exert beneficial effects in patients with PE and shock.

Vasodilators decrease pulmonary arterial pressure and pulmonary vascular resistance, but the main concern is the lack of specificity of these drugs for the pulmonary vasculature after systemic (intravenous) administration. According to data from small clinical studies, inhalation of nitric oxide may improve the haemodynamic status and gas exchange of patients with PE.[34,35] Preliminary data suggest that levosimendan may restore right ventricular–pulmonary arterial coupling in acute PE by combining pulmonary vasodilation with an increase in RV contractility.[36]

Hypoxaemia and hypocapnia are frequently encountered in patients with PE, but they are of moderate severity in most cases. A patent foramen ovale may aggravate hypoxaemia due to shunting when right atrial- exceeds left atrial pressure.[37] Hypoxaemia is usually reversed with administration of oxygen. When mechanical ventilation is required, care should be taken to limit its adverse haemodynamic effects. In particular, the positive intrathoracic pressure induced by mechanical ventilation may reduce venous return and worsen RV failure in patients with massive PE; therefore, positive end-expiratory pressure should be applied with caution. Low tidal volumes (approximately 6 ml/kg lean body weight) should be used in an attempt to keep the end-inspiratory plateau pressure <30 cm H_2O.

On completion of thrombolysis, the patient is started on anticoagulation as per Table 3.

CATHETER-BASED MANAGEMENT OF HIGH RISK PE

Systemic thrombolysis for acute pulmonary embolism (PE) carries up to a 20% risk of major bleeding, including a 2% to 5% risk of haemorrhagic stroke.[4] Catheter-directed therapy has evolved to directly remove the clot burden and rapidly restore systemic blood pressure.

Table 3: Dosage and interval of anticoagulants		
	Dosage	Interval
Enoxaparin	1.0 mg/kg or	Every 12 hours
	1.5 mg/kg	Once daily
Tinzaparin	175 U/kg	Once daily
Dalteparin	100 IU/kg or	Every 12 hours
	200 IU/kg	Once daily
Nadroparin	86 IU/kg or	Every 12 hours
	171 IU/kg	Once daily
Fondaparinux	5 mg (body weight <50 kg); 7.5 mg (body weight <50–100 kg); 10 mg (body weight >100 kg);	Once daily

Catheter-based techniques include fragmentation with a pigtail catheter, balloon maceration, or use of a rheolytic mechanism like EKOSONIC, an ultrasound based catheter. Additional local, intraclot delivery of thrombolytics can be performed at a fraction of the systemic dose typically used for PE.[4]

The PERFECT[39] *(Pulmonary Embolism Response to Fragmentation, Embolectomy, and Catheter Thrombolysis)* registry (Dr. William Kuo at Stanford University) is evaluating the safety and effectiveness of catheter-directed therapy (CDT) as an alternative treatment of acute PE. One hundred one consecutive patients receiving CDT for acute PE were prospectively enrolled in a multicenter registry, 28 of these being **High risk** (Massive PE). Patients were treated with immediate catheter-directed mechanical or pharmacomechanical thrombectomy and/or catheter-directed thrombolysis through low-dose hourly drug infusion with tissue plasminogen activator (tPA) or urokinase. Clinical success was defined as meeting all the following criteria: stabilization of haemodynamics; improvement in pulmonary hypertension, right-sided heart strain, or both; and survival to hospital discharge. Primary safety outcomes were major procedure-related complications and major bleeding events.

Clinical success was achieved in 24 of 28 patients with **High risk** massive PE. Among patients monitored with follow-up echocardiography. There were no major procedure-related complications, major hemorrhages, or haemorrhagic strokes. What is significant in the PERFECT trial is that 64% cases a standard catheter rather than the EKOSONIC ultrasonic device was used for treatment, thus making this method an option in countries where EKOSONIC is not yet available for use. This registry may provide adequate support for a randomized clinical trial and a stronger level of recommendation for catheter-based treatment by the ACCP.

Percutaneous Catheter-directed Treatment

The objective of interventional treatment is the removal of obstructing thrombi from the main pulmonary arteries to facilitate RV recovery and improve symptoms and survival.[40] For patients with absolute contraindications to thrombolysis, interventional options include (a) thrombus fragmentation with pigtail or balloon catheter, (b) rheolytic thrombectomy with hydrodynamic catheter devices, (c) suction thrombectomy with aspiration catheters and (d) rotational thrombectomy (e) ultrasound driven catheters. On the other hand, for patients without absolute contraindications to thrombolysis, catheter-directed thrombolysis or pharmacomechanical thrombolysis are preferred approaches. A review on interventional treatment included 35 non-randomized studies covering 594 patients.[41] Clinical success, defined as stabilization of haemodynamic parameters, resolution of hypoxia, and survival to discharge, was 87%. The contribution of the mechanical catheter intervention per se to clinical success is unclear because 67% of patients also received adjunctive local thrombolysis. Publication bias probably resulted in underreporting of major complications (reportedly affecting 2% of interventions), which may include death from worsening RV failure, distal embolisation, pulmonary artery perforation with lung haemorrhage, systemic bleeding complications, pericardial tamponade, heart block or bradycardia, haemolysis, contrast-induced nephropathy, and puncture-related complications.[40]

While anticoagulation with heparin alone has little effect on improvement of RV size and performance within the first 24–48 hours,[42] the extent of early RV recovery after low-dose catheter-directed thrombolysis appears comparable to that after standard-dose systemic thrombolysis.[43,44] In a randomized, controlled clinical trial of 59 intermediate-risk patients, when compared with treatment by heparin alone, catheter-directed ultrasound-accelerated thrombolysis—administering 10 mg tPA per treated lung over 15 hours—significantly reduced the subannular RV/LV dimension ratio between baseline and 24-hour follow-up without an increase in bleeding complications.[45]

Contemporary Catheter Techniques

Thrombus Fragmentation

The aim of this technique is to reduce pulmonary vascular resistance by mechanically disrupting thrombus into smaller fragments. Thrombus fragmentation can be achieved by manual rotation of a pigtail catheter[46] or with peripheral balloon angioplasty catheters[47]. One disadvantage of this technique is the risk of macroembolisation causing haemodynamic deterioration when fragments from a large nonobstructive thrombus embolize.[47] Fragmentation techniques are often combined with other mechanical manoeuvres[48,49] or with CDT (Fig. 3).[46,50]

Rheolytic Thrombectomy

A high-pressure saline jet within the AngioJet® device generates a pressure gradient by Bernoulli's principle, enabling the removal of thrombus

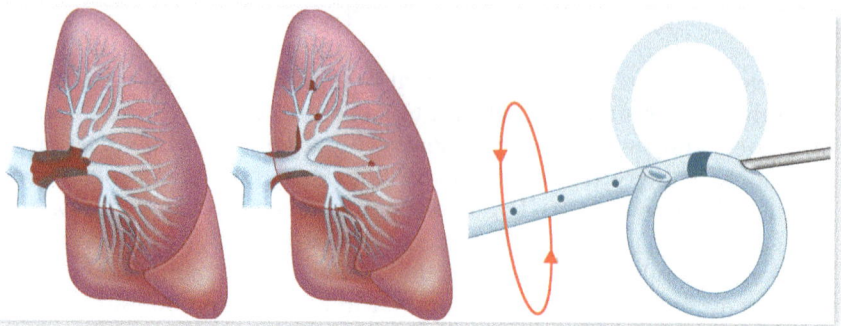

Figure 3: Fragmentation of embolus using rotational movement of a pigtail catheter

fragments.[51] This device also permits local injection of thrombolytic agents by the Power Pulse spray technique, forcing the drug into the thrombus. Bradycardia is a device-specific side effect and is possibly caused by transient release of bradykinin, adenosine, or potassium secondary to haemolysis. It usually occurs with prolonged thrombectomy runs >20 seconds and may result in heart block or asystole.[52] Hemoglobinuria is also caused by haemolysis and is usually reversible without clinical sequelae.[41]

Penumbra Indigo system is FDA 510(k) approved for the removal of thrombi from pulmonary vasculature (Fig. 4).

Suction Thrombectomy

Suction of thrombus through large-lumen catheters (8-9 F) is achieved by either manually applying negative pressure with an aspiration syringe or through various mechanical pumps. Conventional vascular access sheaths are not suitable for aspiration of large thrombus because it usually gets trapped within the sheath during suction thrombectomy because of the hemostatic valve. Therefore, this technique requires the use of a dedicated aspiration sheath with a detachable hemostatic valve, permitting percutaneous removal of thrombus without the need for surgical cut down (Figs 5 and 6).[53]

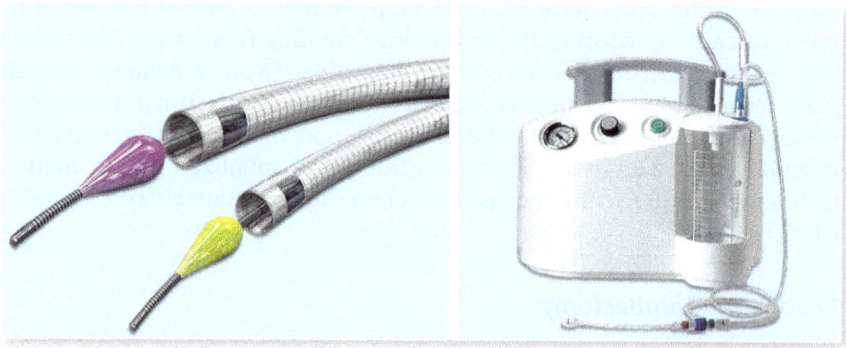

Figure 4: The Penumbra Indigo Vacuum assisted thrombectomy system

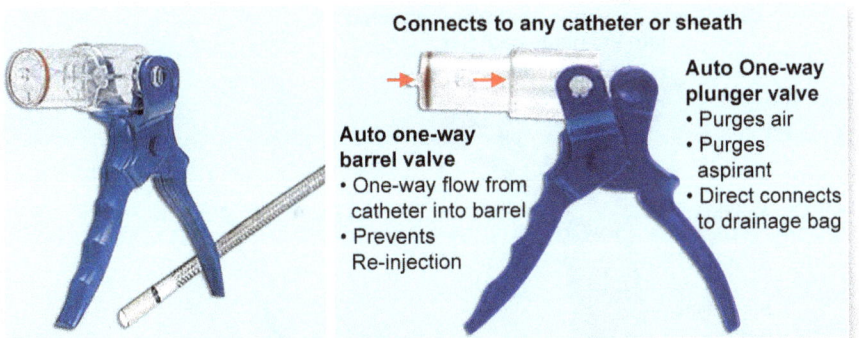

Figure 5: Aspire max mechanical aspiration system

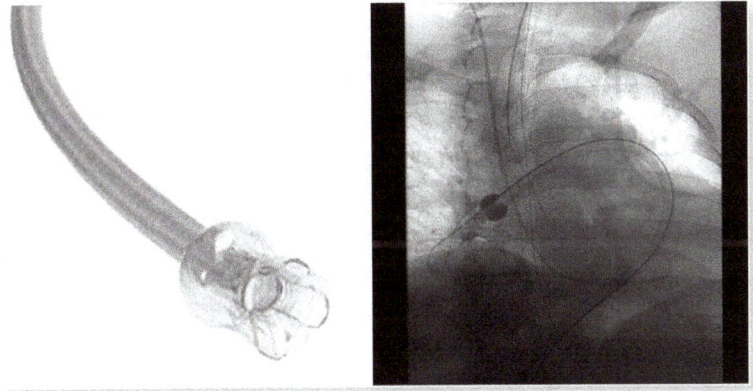

Figure 6: The AngioVac VORTEX device for suction thrombectomy

Rotational Thrombectomy

The central part of the Aspirex catheter is a protected, high-speed rotational coil that creates negative pressure through an L-shaped aspiration port at the catheter tip, resulting in maceration and aspiration of the thrombus.[54] This technique may be combined with other mechanical interventions, such as thrombus fragmentation (Fig. 7).[49]

Ultrasound Accelerated Catheter-directed Thrombolysis

Ultrasound-accelerated catheter-directed thrombolysis is a novel treatment in which pulmonary artery thrombolytic therapy is delivered through an infusion catheter that emits ultrasound energy to accelerate the thrombolytic cascade.[55] This treatment is achieved using the EkoSonic® Endovascular System (EKOS Corporation; Bothell, WA), which is approved by the US Food and Drug Administration for pulmonary artery infusion. It is currently the only device FDA approved for use in PE. The system uses a 5.2-French multilumen sideport infusion catheter, with infusion lengths of 6–50 cm depending on the length of the thrombotic occlusion. Once the EkoSonic catheter is positioned in the

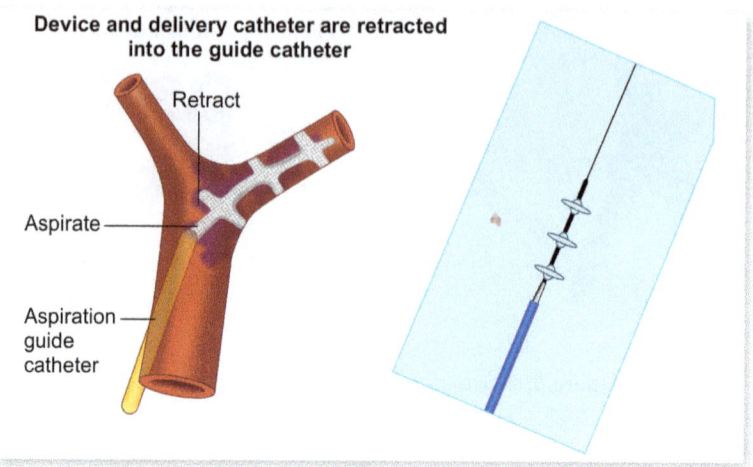

Figure 7: FlowTriever device for mechanical thrombectomy

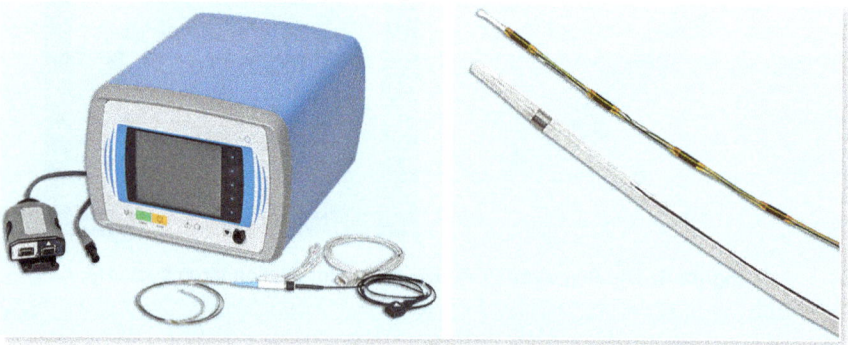

Figure 8: EkoSonic pulmonary embolism system

pulmonary artery, an ultrasound core wire containing a series of ultrasound transducer elements (2.2 MHz, 0.45 W) is positioned within the infusion catheter (Fig. 8). The ultrasound catheter is then connected to a control unit that provides continuous monitored variables, including temperature and ultrasound energy power output in the treatment zone by means of thermocouples incorporated in the catheter, and automatically adjusts power to optimize lysis of the intravascular thrombosis. The acoustic streaming energy dissociates the fibrin and increases the fibrin porosity without causing distal embolization, which also facilitates the penetration of thrombolytic agents into the thrombus for receptor binding.[55]

Conventional Catheter-directed Thrombolysis

Because bleeding complications seem to occur less frequently with catheter-directed than with full-dose systemic thrombolysis, this approach is often performed in patients with PE in the presence of relative contraindications to systemic thrombolysis.[56] Fibrinolytic agents are usually administered as a continuous infusion; a bolus can be considered at the time of catheter placement in patients who are haemodynamically unstable. Various drug regimens have been used, for example, recombinant tissue plasminogen activator at a dose of 0.5–2.0 mg per hour per catheter for less than 24 hours (bolus dose of 2–5 mg per catheter).

Practical Aspects for Catheter Interventions

Patients undergoing invasive pulmonary angiography and catheter intervention require continuous haemodynamic and electrocardiographic monitoring. Duplex ultrasonography of the common femoral vein is useful to rule out suspected concomitant iliofemoral DVT.

In our opinion, it is important to obtain complete right heart haemodynamic measurements before and after completion of the procedure for monitoring the treatment effect. The amount of iodine contrast agent should be kept as low as possible and depends mainly on the haemodynamic status and the size of the selected vessel. Despite lower contrast agent requirements with digital subtraction angiography, this technique is not routinely recommended, because most patients with massive PE cannot hold their breath. Nonselective angiography with large (>30 ml) amounts of contrast agent via power injector should be avoided due to the risk of worsening right ventricular failure.[40] To minimize the risk of pulmonary artery perforation, the main and lower lobe pulmonary arteries should be considered for treatment, and segmental branches with a diameter of <6 mm should not be approached.[57] Table 4 enlists the trials for catheter-directed therapy for pulmonary embolism.

Table 4: List of trials for catheter directed therapy for pulmonary embolism

Study	n	% receiving bilateral catheters	Alteplase dose	Catheter type	Heparin during thrombolytic infusion	Average change in mean pulmonary artery pressure (change in RV:LV ratio) (change in PA systolic pressure.)
ULTIMA	30	87%	Unilateral catheter: 10 mg Bilateral catheter: 20 mg	US-assisted CDT	Full dose (target Xa-1.0–0.7)	30 mm → 24 mm (1.28 → 0.99) (52 mm → 40 mm)

Contd...

Contd...

Study	n	% receiving bilateral catheters	Alteplase dose	Catheter type	Heparin during thrombolytic infusion	Average change in mean pulmonary artery pressure (change in RV:LV ratio) (change in PA systolic pressure.)
SEATTLE II	150	86%	24 mg	US-assisted CDT	Full dose (target PTT 60–80s)	? (1.55 → 1.13) (51 mm → 38 mm)
PERFECT	101	Not reported	76 patients: 28 +/- 11 mg 23 patients: urokinase	US-assisted CDT (36%) CDT without US (64%)	Low dose (300–500 units/h)	? (?) (51 mm → 37 mm)
Engelhardt 2011	24	79%	34 +/- 16 mg	US-assisted CDT	Full dose enoxaparine (1mg/kg bd)	? (1.33 → 1.00) (?)
Kennedy 2013	60	88%	35 +/- 11 mg	US-assisted CDT	Full dose (target PTT 60–80s)	27 mm → 20 mm (?) (47 mm → 38 mm)
Dumantepe 2014	22	28%	21 mg (range 16-33 mg)	US-assisted CDT	No heparin	33 mm → 20 mm (1.29 → 0.92) (67 mm → 34 mm)
McCabe 2015	53	Not reported	25 +/- 9 mg	US-assisted CDT	Intermediate dose (target PTT 40-60s)	34 mm → 27 mm (1.12 → 0.98) (51 mm → 41 mm)
Engelhardt 2015	52	83%	21 +/- 6 mg	US-assisted CDT	Full dose (target PTT 1.5-3x)	37 mm à 25 mm (1.42 → 1.06) (61 mm → 40 mm)
Bagla 2015	45	93%	24 mg	US-assisted CDT	Intermediate dose (target PTT 40-60s)	Not reported (1.59 → 0.93) (50 mm → 31 mm)

ROLE OF OPEN SURGERY IN ACUTE PULMONARY EMBOLISM

The role of open surgery in current scenario would be:
1. An absolute contraindication to thrombolysis
2. No facilities or expertise for catheter-based procedures.
3. Unstable patient despite thrombolysis/catheter-based procedure/s.

MANAGEMENT OF ACUTE PULMONARY EMBOLISM WITHOUT HYPOTENSION

If the patient presents without hypotension BP <90 mmHg) then it would be appropriate to stratify patients into low, intermediate or high probability cases for PE, based on either the modified Geneva scoring[58,59] or the Wells' scoring system[58,60] as shown in Tables 5 and 6.

Whichever is used, the proportion of patients with confirmed PE can be expected to be around 10% in the low-probability category, 30% in the moderate-probability category, and 65% in the high-clinical probability category, when using the three-level classification.[60] Depending on their scoring, patient should then be routed based on either a D-dimer assay or a CT Angiography as shown in Table 7.

Table 5: Geneva scoring system

Feature	Points (revised dichotomized score)	Points (simplified score)
Previous DVT or PE	3	1
Heart rate:		
75-94 bpm	3	1
≥95 bpm	5	2
Feature	Points (revised dichotomized score)	Points (simplified score)
Surgery or fracture < 1 month	2	1
Haemoptysis	2	1
Active malignancy	2	1
Unilateral lower limb pain	3	1
Pain on lower limb deep venous palpation or unilateral oedema	4	1\
Age > 65	1	1
Clinical probability		
PE unlikely	≤5	≤2
PE likely	>5	>2

Table 6: Wells' scoring system

Feature	Score
Previous DVT or PE	1.5
Heart rate >100 bpm	1.5
Surgery or bedridden <4 weeks	1.5
Haemoptysis	1
Active malignancy	1
Clinical symptoms of DVT	3
Alternative diagnosis less likely than PE	3
Clinical probability	
PE unlikely	<4
PE likely	>4

Table 7: Diagnostic yield of various D-dimer assays in excluding acute PE according to outcome studies

Study	D-dimer assay	Patients n	PE prevalence %	PE excluded by D-dimer and clinical probability n(%)	Three-months thrombolytic risk % (95% CI)
Carrier 2009 (meta-analysis)	Vidas Exclusion	56220	22	2246 (40)	0.1 (0.0-0.4)
Study	D-dimer assay	Patients n	PE prevalence %	PE excluded by D-dimer and clinical probability n(%)	Three-months thrombolytic risk % (95% CI)
Kearon, 2006 Wells, 2001	SimpliRed	2056	12	797 (39)	0.0 (0.0-0.5)
Leclercq, 2003; ten Wolde, 2004; van Belle, 2006	Tinaquant	3508	21	1123 (32)	0.4 (0.0-1.0)

Role of Lung Scintigraphy

Ventilation–perfusion scintigraphy (V/Q scan) is an established diagnostic test for suspected PE. It is safe and few allergic reactions have been described. The test is based on the intravenous injection of technetium (Tc)-99m-labelled macroaggregated albumin particles, which block a small fraction of the pulmonary capillaries and thereby enable scintigraphic assessment of lung perfusion. Perfusion scans are combined with ventilation studies, for which multiple tracers, such as xenon-133 gas, Tc-99m-labelled aerosols, or Tc-99m-labelled carbon microparticles can be used. The purpose of the ventilation scan is to increase specificity: in acute PE, ventilation is expected to be normal in hypoperfused segments (mismatch).[61,62]

According to the International Commission on Radiological Protection (ICRP), the radiation exposure from a lung scan with 100 MBq of Tc-99m macroaggregated albumin particles is 1.1 mSv for an average sized adult, and thus is significantly lower than that of CT angiography (2-6 mSv).[63,64] Being a radiation-and contrast medium-sparing procedure, the V/Q scan may preferentially be applied in young (particularly female) patients, in pregnancy, in patients with history of contrast medium-induced anaphylaxis and strong allergic history, in severe renal failure, and in patients with myeloma and paraproteinaemia.[65] The issues in most hospitals would be the availability of this facility in an emergency situation. In centres in which V/Q scintigraphy is readily available, it remains a valid option for patients with an elevated D-dimer and a contraindication to CT.[66]

Value of Lower Limb Compression Ultrasonography

Under certain circumstances, CUS can still be useful in the diagnostic work-up of suspected PE. CUS shows a DVT in 30-50% of patients with PE[67-69], and finding proximal DVT in a patient suspected of PE is sufficient to warrant anticoagulant treatment without further testing.[70] Hence, performing CUS before CT may be an option in patients with relative contraindications for CT such as in renal failure, allergy to contrast dye, or pregnancy.[71,72]

Markers of Right Ventricular Dysfunction

Right ventricular pressure overload is associated with increased myocardial stretch, which leads to the release of brain natriuretic peptide (BNP) or N-terminal (NT)-proBNP. The plasma levels of natriuretic peptides reflect the severity of haemodynamic compromise and (presumably) RV dysfunction in acute PE.[73] A meta-analysis found that 51% of 1,132 unselected patients with acute PE had elevated BNP or NT-proBNP concentrations on admission. These patients had a 10% risk of early death (95% CI 8.0-13) and a 23% (95% CI 20-26) risk of an adverse clinical outcome.[74] Importantly, persistently raised markers may be used as an indicator for catheter-based interventions in intermediate risk category of patients. RV dysfunction means the presence of at least one of the following.[75]

- RV dilation (apical 4-chamber RV diameter divided by LV diameter >0.9) or RV systolic dysfunction on echocardiography or CT
- Elevation of BNP (>90 pg/ml) or
- Elevation of N-terminal pro-BNP (>500 pg/ml) or
- ECG changes (new right bundle-branch block, antero-septal ST elevation or depression, or T-wave inversion)

Myocardial necrosis is defined as either Elevation of troponin I (>0.4 ng/ml)/troponin T (>0.1 ng/ml).[75]

Role of Echocardiography

Echocardiographic findings indicating RV dysfunction have been reported in ≥25% of patients with PE.[76] They have been identified as independent predictors of an adverse outcome[77] but are heterogeneous and have proven difficult to standardize.[78] Still, in haemodynamically stable, normotensive patients with PE, echocardiographic assessment of the morphology and function of the RV may help in prognostic stratification.

As already mentioned in the previous section on the diagnosis of PE, echocardiographic findings used to risk stratify patients with PE include RV dilation, an increased RV–LV diameter ratio, hypokinesia of the free RV wall, increased velocity of the jet of tricuspid regurgitation, decreased tricuspid annulus plane systolic excursion, or combinations of the above. Meta-analyses have shown that RV dysfunction detected by echocardiography is associated with an elevated risk of short-term mortality in patients without haemodynamic instability, but its overall positive predictive value is low.[79,80] In addition to RV dysfunction, echocardiography can also identify right-to-left shunt through a patent foramen ovale and the presence of right heart thrombi, both of which are associated with increased mortality in patients with acute PE.[6,37]

STRATEGY FOR NON-HIGH RISK PULMONARY EMBOLISM (FIG. 9)

1. **Intermediate risk**: This can be divided into **Intermediate high risk** (RV dysfunction by Echo &/or CTA and elevated cardiac enzymes) or **Intermediate low risk** (Either RV dysfunction by Echo &/or CTA or elevated enzymes or neither).
   - **Intermediate high risk:** Anticoagulation only, but rescue with reperfusion by systemic or Catheter directed procedure if situation deteriorates.
   - **Intermediate low risk:** Anticoagulation only but hospitalize.
2. **Low risk:** Anticoagulate but consider early discharge home.

Role of IVC Filters in Acute PE

Retrievable filters are indicated in the following settings only:[4]
1. Absolute contraindication to anticoagulants. This is on most occasions a temporary situation, either due to pre-existing coagulopathy, thrombocytopaenia or where there has been a transient deterioration in liver functions due to severe RV dysfunction.
2. Acute PE despite adequate anticoagulants indicating a high incidence of recurrent PE.
3. IVC filters are to be deployed in patients presenting with acute PE when a major surgery is in the offing in the immediate future, such as for abdominal malignancies.

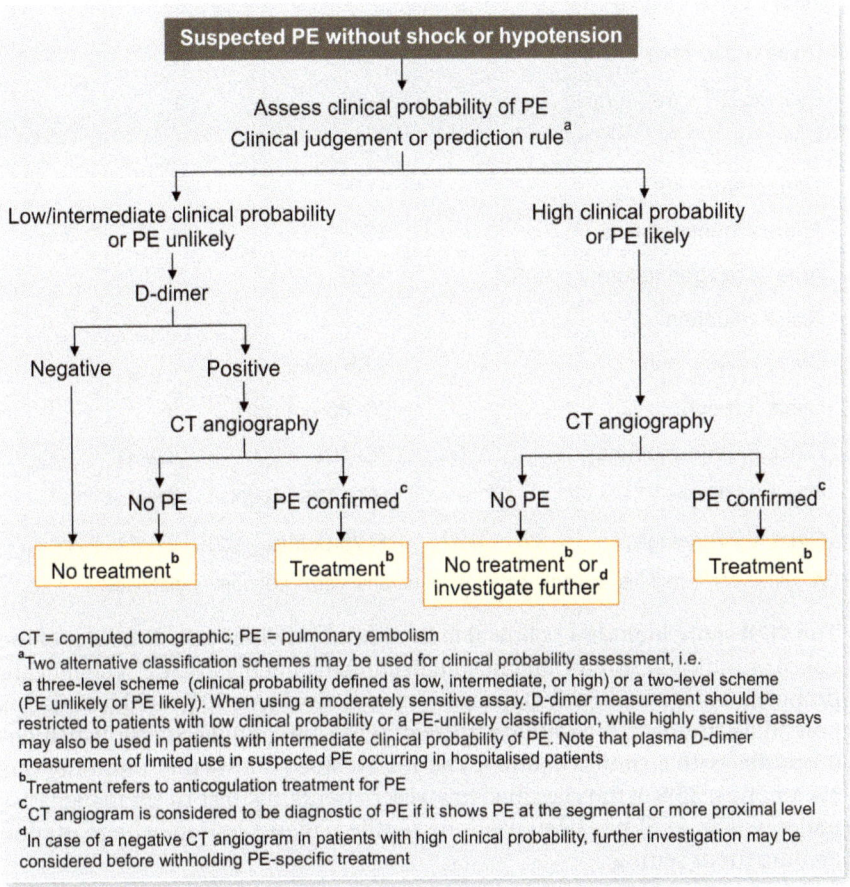

Figure 9: Proposed diagnostic algorithm for patients with suspected not high-risk pulmonary embolism[4]

PROGNOSTIC SCORING IN PULMONARY EMBOLISM (TABLE 8)

Table 8: PESI (the Pulmonary Embolism Severity Index)[81,82]		
Features	Points	
	Original version	Simplified version
Age	Years	>80 = 1
Male	+10	
History of cancer	+30	1
History of heart failure	+10	1[a]
History of chronic lung disease	+10	1[a]

Contd...

Contd...

Pulse > 110 bpm	+20	1
Systolic BP < 100 mmHg	+30	1
Respiratory rate > 30/min	+20	
Temperature <36 °C	+20	
Altered mental status	+60	
Arterial oxygen saturation <90%	+20	1
Risk evaluation		
Class I (Very low)	< 65 points	
Class II (Low)	66–85 points	
Class III (Intermediate)	86–105	Low: 0
Class IV (High)	106–125 points	High: >1
Class V (Very high)	>125 points	

*Variables combined into a single category of chronic cardiopulmonary disease

The PESI score include 11 clinical features and provides an estimation of the risk of mortality at 30 days after hospitalization in patients with PE. A significant proportion of low-risk patients (negative predictive value 99%) are identified as potential candidates for ambulatory treatment. The simplified version includes 6 features with a similar validity. The RIETE study shows that mortality was 1% amongst 36% of the classified low-risk patients, against 10.9% in high-risk patients. The PESI has been used to identify patients that may be treated in an outpatient setting.

GENEVA PROGNOSTIC SCORING (TABLE 9)[83]

Table 9: Geneva prognostic scoring

Feature	Points
History of cancer	2
History of heart failure	1
Previous DVT	1
DVT of ultrasound	1
PAS < 100 mmHg	2
PaO_2 < 8kPa	1
Clinical probability	
Low risk	<2
High risk	>2

Predictive risk value of low-mortality-risk patients, recurrent VET or increasing bleeding at 3 months. Patients with ≤ 2 points are considered low-level risk patients. This stratification might help identifying patients who could be treated in an outpatient setting.

ORAL ANTICOAGULATION SCHEDULE

1. **Provoked PE:** VTE is considered to be 'provoked' in the presence of a temporary or reversible risk factor (such as surgery, trauma, immobilisation, pregnancy, oral contraceptive use or hormone replacement therapy) within the last 6 weeks to 3 months before diagnosis. Major trauma, surgery, lower limb fractures and joint replacements, and spinal cord injury, are strong provoking factors for VTE. Here anticoagulation is recommended for atleast 3 months.[84]

2. **Unprovoked PE:** 'Unprovoked' refers to the absence there of. PE may also occur in the absence of any known risk factor. The presence of persistent—as opposed to major, temporary—risk factors may affect the decision on the duration of anticoagulation therapy after a first episode of PE. Here risk stratification is required prior to stopping/continuing with anticoagulation at 3 months.[84] In 2008, Rodger et al[85] proposed the HERDOO2 model, deriving data from a Canadian multicentre prospective cohort study that included 646 patients with a first unprovoked VTE event followed up for 18 months after discontinuing oral anticoagulation therapy In 2010, Eichinger et al. published the Vienna[86] prediction model that was validated on a prospective cohort study of 929 patients with a first unprovoked VTE. The third algorithm has been recently published by Tosetto et al. The proposed prediction model is named DASH[87] and includes the following factors (Table 10): D-dimer level measured 1 month after anticoagulation withdrawal, young Age, male Sex, and Hormonal therapy associated with the index VTE event. (Risk stratification for recurrence of VTE in PE can utilize the Vienna model for deciding duration of anticoagulation (Fig. 10).

Table 10: DASH prediction score derived from cox regression analysis[87]

DASH Predictors (N = 1,818 VTE cases)	b coefficient*	P-value	Recurrence score
1. D-dimer abnormal, after stopping AC	0.96	<0.0001	+2
2. Age <50 yr	0.43	0.002	+1
3. Sex—male	0.58	<0.0001	+1
4. Hormone use at VTE onset	-1.05	0.002	-2
DAST Prediction Rule			
DASH Score	≤1.0	2.0	≥3.0
Annualized VTE recurrence Rate	3.1%	6.4%	12.3%

* Cox regression coefficients after backward elimination and optimism correction
Source: Table adapted from Tosetto A, Iorio A, Marcucci M, et al. J Thromb Haemost. 2012; 366:1019-25.

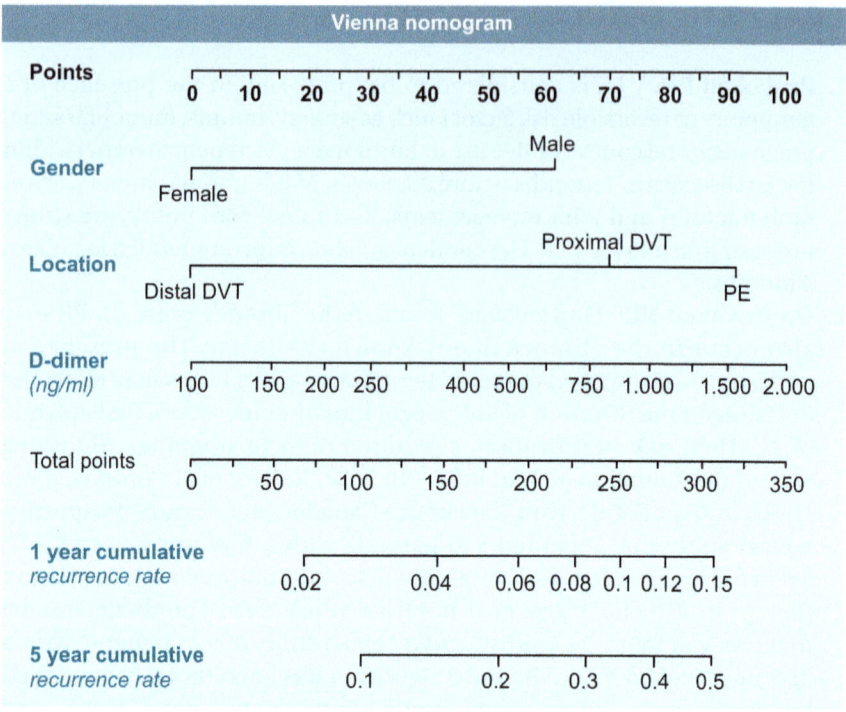

Figure 10: Vienna nomogram

Interpretation

The nomogram aims at estimating the recurrence risk following DVT or PE. Clinical (type of thrombosis and gender) and analytical (D-dimer measured at the time of suspension of anticoagulation) variables are taken into consideration. In practice, a line has to be drawn perpendicular to the top row (called *points*) that cuts the value of each of the three considered features (*gender, location* and *D-dimer*). The sum of the three responses is borne on a line *Total*, from which a perpendicular line is drawn to this value, which gives the cumulated risk at one year and, by drawing another perpendicular line, the cumulative risk at five years. For example: A man with a proximal DVT and a D-dimer of 400 µg/L will score 60 points for gender, 70 for proximal thrombosis and 46 points for D-dimer, totalizing 176 points, which corresponds to a probability of recurrence of 5.1% and 18.5%, at one and five years, respectively.

KEY POINTS FOR CLINICAL PRACTICE

1. The key to successful management of acute PE is early risk stratification
2. High risk case requires an early CT angiogram and reperfusion treatment.
3. Intermediate risk cases are managed by anticoagulation but a persistent or rising RV dysfunction may be an indicator for a reperfusion procedure.
4. Though systemic thrombolysis continues to be the most commonly employed reperfusion technique in treating acute PE, the lower incidence

of bleeding reported from catheter-based techniques makes it an exciting and potentially viable option.
5. In unprovoked VTE with PE, risk of recurrence makes it mandatory to have a strategy for stratification to decide period of anticoagulation to be prescribed.

REFERENCES

1. Kakkar N, Vasishta RK. Pulmonary embolism in medical patients: an autopsy-based study. Clinical and Applied Thrombosis/Hemostasis. 2007; Dec 26.
2. McIntyre KM, Sasahara AA. The hemodynamic response to pulmonary embolism in patients without prior cardiopulmonary disease. Am J Cardiol. 1971 Sep 30;28(3):288-94.
3. Lankeit M, Jiménez D, Kostrubiec M, Dellas C, Hasenfuss G, Pruszczyk P, et al. Predictive value of the high-sensitivity troponin T assay and the simplified pulmonary embolism severity index in hemodynamically stable patients with acute pulmonary embolism A Prospective Validation Study. Circulation. 2011 Dec 13;124(24):2716-24.
4. Konstantinides S, Torbicki A, Agnelli G, Danchin N, Fitzmaurice D, Galiè N, et al. 2014 ESC guidelines on the diagnosis and management of acute pulmonary embolism. Eur Heart J. 2014 Aug 28:ehu283.
5. Pollack CV, Schreiber D, Goldhaber SZ, Slattery D, Fanikos J, O'Neil BJ, et al. Clinical characteristics, management, and outcomes of patients diagnosed with acute pulmonary embolism in the emergency department: initial report of EMPEROR (Multicenter Emergency Medicine Pulmonary Embolism in the Real World Registry). J Am Coll Cardiol. 2011 Feb 8;57(6):700-6.
6. Torbicki A, Galié N, Covezzoli A, Rossi E, De Rosa M, Goldhaber SZ. Right heart thrombi in pulmonary embolism: results from the International Cooperative Pulmonary Embolism Registry. J Am Coll Cardiol. 2003 Jun 18;41(12):2245-51.
7. Ferrari E, Benhamou M, Berthier F, Baudouy M. Mobile thrombi of the right heart in pulmonary embolism: delayed disappearance after thrombolytic treatment. CHEST J. 2005 Mar 1;127(3):1051-3.
8. Pierre-Justin G, Pierard LA. Management of mobile right heart thrombi: a prospective series. Internat J Cardiol. 2005 Mar 30;99(3):381-8.
9. Krivec B, Voga G, Zuran I, Skale R, Pareznik R, Podbregar M, et al. Diagnosis and treatment of shock due to massive pulmonary embolism: approach with transesophageal echocardiography and intrapulmonary thrombolysis. CHEST J. 1997 Nov 1;112(5):1310-6.
10. Pruszczyk P, Torbicki A, Pacho R, Chlebus M, Kuch-Wocial A, Pruszynski B, et al. Noninvasive diagnosis of suspected severe pulmonary embolism: transesophageal echocardiography vs spiral CT. CHEST J. 1997 Sep 1;112(3):722-8.
11. Vieillard-Baron A, Qanadli SD, Antakly Y, Fourme T, Loubieres Y, Jardin F, et al. Transesophageal echocardiography for the diagnosis of pulmonary embolism with acute cor pulmonale: a comparison with radiological procedures. Intensive care medicine. 1998 May 1;24(5):429-33.
12. Stein PD, Fowler SE, Goodman LR, Gottschalk A, Hales CA, Hull RD, et al. Multidetector computed tomography for acute pulmonary embolism. N Engl J Medic. 2006 Jun 1;354(22):2317-27.

13. Goldhaber S, Heit J, Sharma GV, Nagel JS, Kim D, Parker JA, et al. Randomised controlled trial of recombinant tissue plasminogen activator versus urokinase in the treatment of acute pulmonary embolism. The Lancet. 1988 Aug 6;332(8606):293-8.
14. Meneveau N, Séronde MF, Blonde MC, Legalery P, Didier-Petit K, Briand F, et al. Management of unsuccessful thrombolysis in acute massive pulmonary embolism. CHEST J. 2006 Apr 1;129(4):1043-50.
15. Daniels LB, Parker JA, Patel SR, Grodstein F, Goldhaber SZ. Relation of duration of symptoms with response to thrombolytic therapy in pulmonary embolism. Am J Cardiol. 1997 Jul 15;80(2):184-8.
16. Wan S, Quinlan DJ, Agnelli G, Eikelboom JW. Thrombolysis compared with heparin for the initial treatment of pulmonary embolism a meta-analysis of the randomized controlled trials. Circulation. 2004 Aug 10;110(6):744-9.
17. Goldhaber SZ, Visani L, De Rosa M. Acute pulmonary embolism: clinical outcomes in the International Cooperative Pulmonary Embolism Registry (ICOPER). The Lancet. 1999 Apr 24;353(9162):1386-9.
18. Lobo JL, Zorrilla V, Aizpuru F, Uresandi F, Garcia-Bragado F, Conget F, et al. Clinical syndromes and clinical outcome in patients with pulmonary embolism: findings from the RIETE registry. CHEST J. 2006 Dec 1;130(6):1817-22.
19. Lin BW, Schreiber DH, Liu G, Briese B, Hiestand B, Slattery D, et al. Therapy and outcomes in massive pulmonary embolism from the Emergency Medicine Pulmonary Embolism in the Real World Registry. Am J Emerg Med. 2012 Nov 30;30(9):1774-81.
20. Jaff MR, McMurtry MS, Archer SL, Cushman M, Goldenberg N, Goldhaber SZ, et al. Management of massive and submassive pulmonary embolism, iliofemoral deep vein thrombosis, and chronic thromboembolic pulmonary hypertension a scientific statement from the American Heart Association. Circulation. 2011 Apr 26;123(16):1788-830.
21. Goldhaber SZ, Come PC, Lee RT, Braunwald E, Parker JA, Haire WD, et al. Alteplase versus heparin in acute pulmonary embolism: randomised trial assessing right-ventricular function and pulmonary perfusion. The Lancet. 1993 Feb 27;341(8844):507-11.
22. Sharifi M, Bay C, Skrocki L, Rahimi F, Mehdipour M. Moderate pulmonary embolism treated with thrombolysis (from the "MOPETT" Trial). Am J Cardiol. 2013 Jan 15;111(2):273-7.
23. Stein PD, Matta F. Thrombolytic therapy in unstable patients with acute pulmonary embolism: saves lives but underused. Am J Med. 2012 May 31;125(5):465-70.
24. Konstantinides S, Geibel A, Heusel G, Heinrich F, Kasper W. Heparin plus alteplase compared with heparin alone in patients with submassive pulmonary embolism. N Engl J Med. 2002 Oct 10;347(15):1143-50.
25. Meyer G, Vicaut E, Danays T, Agnelli G, Becattini C, Beyer-Westendorf J, et al. Fibrinolysis for patients with intermediate-risk pulmonary embolism. N Engl J Med. 2014 Apr 10;370(15):1402-11.
26. Kanter DS, Mikkola KM, Patel SR, Parker JA, Goldhaber SZ. Thrombolytic therapy for pulmonary embolism: frequency of intracranial hemorrhage and associated risk factors. CHEST Journal. 1997 May 1;111(5):1241-5.
27. Levine MN, Goldhaber SZ, Gore JM, Hirsh J, Califf RM. Hemorrhagic complications of thrombolytic therapy in the treatment of myocardial infarction and venous thromboembolism. CHEST Journal. 1995 Oct 1;108(4_Supplement):291S-301S.

28. Mikkola KM, Patel SR, Parker JA, Grodstein F, Goldhaber SZ. Increasing age is a major risk factor for hemorrhagic complications after pulmonary embolism thrombolysis. Am Heart J. 1997 Jul 31;134(1):69-72.
29. Wang C, Zhai Z, Yang Y, Wu Q, Cheng Z, Liang L, et al. Efficacy and safety of low dose recombinant tissue-type plasminogen activator for the treatment of acute pulmonary thromboembolism: a randomized, multicenter, controlled trial. CHEST Journal. 2010 Feb 1;137(2):254-62.
30. Chatterjee S, Chakraborty A, Weinberg I, Kadakia M, Wilensky RL, Sardar P, et al. Thrombolysis for pulmonary embolism and risk of all-cause mortality, major bleeding, and intracranial hemorrhage: a meta-analysis. JAMA. 2014 Jun 18;311(23):2414-21.
31. Ghignone M, Girling L, Prewitt RM. Volume expansion versus norepinephrine in treatment of a low cardiac output complicating an acute increase in right ventricular afterload in dogs. Anesthesiology. 1984 Feb;60(2):132-5.
32. Mercat A, Diehl JL, Meyer G, Teboul JL, Sors H. Hemodynamic effects of fluid loading in acute massive pulmonary embolism. Crit Care Med. 1999 Mar 1;27(3):540-4.
33. Manier G, Castaing Y. Influence of cardiac output on oxygen exchange in acute pulmonary embolism. Am Rev Resp Disease. 1992 Jan;145(1):130-6.
34. Capellier G, Jacques T, Balvay P, Blasco G, Belle E, Barale F. Inhaled nitric oxide in patients with pulmonary embolism. Intensive Care Med. 1997 Oct 1;23(10):1089-92.
35. Szold O, Khoury W, Biderman P, Klausner JM, Halpern P, Weinbroum AA. Inhaled nitric oxide improves pulmonary functions following massive pulmonary embolism: a report of four patients and review of the literature. Lung. 2006 Feb 1;184(1):1-5.
36. Kerbaul F, Gariboldi V, Giorgi R, Mekkaoui C, Guieu R, Fesler P, et al. Effects of levosimendan on acute pulmonary embolism-induced right ventricular failure*. Crit Care Med. 2007 Aug 1;35(8):1948-54.
37. Konstantinides S, Geibel A, Kasper W, Olschewski M, Blümel L, Just H. Patent foramen ovale is an important predictor of adverse outcome in patients with major pulmonary embolism. Circulation. 1998 May 19;97(19):1946-51.
38. Patocka C, Nemeth J. Pulmonary embolism in pediatrics. J Emerg Med. 2012 Jan 31;42(1):105-16.
39. Kuo WT, Banerjee A, Kim PS, DeMarco FJ, Levy JR, Facchini FR, et al. Pulmonary embolism response to fragmentation, embolectomy, and catheter thrombolysis (PERFECT): initial results from a prospective multicenter registry. CHEST Journal. 2015 Sep 1;148(3):667-73.
40. Engelberger RP, Kucher N. Catheter-based reperfusion treatment of pulmonary embolism. Circulation. 2011 Nov 8;124(19):2139-44.
41. Kuo WT, Gould MK, Louie JD, Rosenberg JK, Sze DY, Hofmann LV. Catheter-directed therapy for the treatment of massive pulmonary embolism: systematic review and meta-analysis of modern techniques. J Vasc Intervent Radiol. 2009 Jan 11;20(11):1431-40.
42. Konstantinides S, Tiede N, Geibel A, Olschewski M, Just H, Kasper W. Comparison of alteplase versus heparin for resolution of major pulmonary embolism. Am J Cardiol. 1998 Oct 15;82(8):966-70.
43. Becattini C, Agnelli G, Salvi A, Grifoni S, Pancaldi LG, Enea I et al. Bolus tenecteplase for right ventricle dysfunction in hemodynamically stable patients with pulmonary embolism. Thrombosis research. 2010 Mar 31;125(3):e82-6.

44. Engelberger RP, Kucher N. Ultrasound-assisted thrombolysis for acute pulmonary embolism: a systematic review. Eur H J. 2014 Mar 21;35(12):758-64.
45. Kucher N, Boekstegers P, Muller OJ, Kupatt C, Beyer-Westendorf J, Heitzer T, et al. Randomized, controlled trial of ultrasound-assisted catheter-directed thrombolysis for acute intermediate-risk pulmonary embolism. Circulation. 129 (4);2014:479-86.
46. Schmitz-Rode T, Janssens U, Duda SH, Erley CM, Günther RW. Massive pulmonary embolism: percutaneous emergency treatment by pigtail rotation catheter. J Am Col Cardiol. 2000 Aug 1;36(2):375-80.
47. Brady AJ, Crake T, Oakley CM. Percutaneous catheter fragmentation and distal dispersion of proximal pulmonary embolus. The Lancet. 1991 Nov 9;338(8776):1186-9.
48. Schmitz-Rode T, Janssens U, Hanrath P, Günther R. Fragmentation of massive pulmonary embolism by pigtail rotation catheter: possible complication. Eur Radiol. 2001 Oct 1;11(10):2047-9.
49. Eid-Lidt G, Gaspar J, Sandoval J, de los Santos FD, Pulido T, Pacheco HG, et al. Combined clot fragmentation and aspiration in patients with acute pulmonary embolism. CHEST Journal. 2008 Jul 1;134(1):54-60.
50. Kuo WT, van den Bosch MA, Hofmann LV, Louie JD, Kothary N, Sze DY. Catheter-directed embolectomy, fragmentation, and thrombolysis for the treatment of massive pulmonary embolism after failure of systemic thrombolysis. CHEST Journal. 2008 Aug 1;134(2):250-4.
51. Drasler WJ, Jenson ML, Wilson GJ, Thielen JM, Protonotarios EI, Dutcher RG, et al. Rheolytic catheter for percutaneous removal of thrombus. Radiology. 1992 Jan;182(1):263-7.
52. Zhu DW. The potential mechanisms of bradyarrhythmias associated with Angio Jet thrombectomy. J Invas Cardiol. 2008 Aug;20(8 Suppl A):2A-4A.
53. Engelberger RP, Kucher N. Catheter-based reperfusion treatment of pulmonary embolism. Circulation. 2011 Nov 8;124(19):2139-44.
54. Kucher N, Windecker S, Banz Y, Schmitz-Rode T, Mettler D, Meier B, et al. Percutaneous catheter thrombectomy device for acute pulmonary embolism: in vitro and in vivo testing 1. Radiology. 2005 Sep;236(3):852-8.
55. Owens CA. Ultrasound-enhanced thrombolysis: EKOS Endo Wave infusion catheter system. In Seminars in interventional radiology 2008 Mar (Vol. 25, No. 1, p. 37). Thieme Medical Publishers.
56. Skaf E, Beemath A, Siddiqui T, Janjua M, Patel NR, Stein PD. Catheter-tip embolectomy in the management of acute massive pulmonary embolism. Am J Cardiol. 2007 Feb 1;99(3):415-20.
57. Biederer J, Charalambous N, Paulsen F, Heller M, Müller-Hülsbeck S. Treatment of acute pulmonary embolism: local effects of three hydrodynamic thrombectomy devices in an ex vivo porcine model. J Endovas Therap. 2006 Aug 1;13(4):549-60.
58. Douma RA, Mos IC, Erkens PM, Nizet TA, Durian MF, Hovens MM, et al. Performance of 4 clinical decision rules in the diagnostic management of acute pulmonary embolism: a prospective cohort study. Annals Intern Medic. 2011 Jun 7;154(11):709-18.
59. Gibson NS, Sohne M, Kruip MJ, Tick LW, Gerdes VE, Bossuyt PM. Further validation and simplification of the Wells clinical decision rule in pulmonary embolism. Thrombosis & Haemostasis. 2008 Jan 1;99(1):229.
60. Ceriani E, Combescure C, Le Gal G, Nendaz M, Perneger T, Bounameaux H, et al. Clinical prediction rules for pulmonary embolism: a systematic review and meta-analysis. J Thromb Haemost. 2010 May 1;8(5):957-70.

61. Alderson PO, Martin EC. Pulmonary embolism: diagnosis with multiple imaging modalities. Radiology. 1987 Aug;164(2):297-312.
62. Miller RF, O'Doherty MJ. Pulmonary nuclear medicine. Eur J Nucl Med. 1992 May 1;19(5):355-68.
63. Roach PJ, Schembri GP, Bailey DL. V/q scanning using spect and spect/ct. J Nucl Med. 2013 Sep 1;54(9):1588-96.
64. Schembri GP, Miller AE, Smart R. Radiation dosimetry and safety issues in the investigation of pulmonary embolism. In Seminars in nuclear medicine. WB Saunders. 2010 Nov 30;40(6): pp. 442-54.
65. Reid JH, Coche EE, Inoue T, Kim EE, Dondi M, Watanabe N, et al. Is the lung scan alive and well? Facts and controversies in defining the role of lung scintigraphy for the diagnosis of pulmonary embolism in the era of MDCT. Eur J Nucl Medic Molec Imag. 2009 Mar 1;36(3):505-21.
66. Brenner DJ, Hall EJ. Computed tomography—an increasing source of radiation exposure. N Engl J Med. 2007 Nov 29;357(22):2277-84.
67. Righini M, Le Gal G, Aujesky D, Roy PM, Sanchez O, Verschuren F, et al. Diagnosis of pulmonary embolism by multidetector CT alone or combined with venous ultrasonography of the leg: a randomised non-inferiority trial. The Lancet. 2008 Apr 25;371(9621):1343-52.
68. Kearon C, Ginsberg JS, Hirsh J. The role of venous ultrasonography in the diagnosis of suspected deep venous thrombosis and pulmonary embolism. Annals Intern Medic. 1998 Dec 15;129(12):1044-9.
69. Turkstra F, Beek EJ, Büller HR. Ultrasonography of leg veins in patients suspected of having pulmonary embolism: letter. Annals of Intern Medic. 1998;128:244.
70. Le Gal G, Righini M, Sanchez O, Roy PM, Baba-Ahmed M, Perrier A, et al. A positive compression ultrasonography of the lower limb veins is highly predictive of pulmonary embolism on computed tomography in suspected patients. Thrombosis and haemostasis. 2006;95(6):963-6.
71. Elias A, Colombier D, Victor G, Elias M, Arnaud C, Juchet H, et al. Diagnostic performance of complete lower limb venous ultrasound in patients with clinically suspected acute pulmonary embolism. Thrombosis and haemostasis-stuttgart. 2004 Jan 1;91(1):187-95.
72. Righini M, Le Gal G, Aujesky D, Roy PM, Sanchez O, Verschuren F, et al. Complete venous ultrasound in outpatients with suspected pulmonary embolism. J Thrombosis and Haemost. 2009 Mar 1;7(3):406-12.
73. Henzler T, Roeger S, Meyer M, Schoepf UJ, Nance JW, Haghi D, et al. Pulmonary embolism: CT signs and cardiac biomarkers for predicting right ventricular dysfunction. Eur Respirat J. 2012 Apr 1;39(4):919-26.
74. Klok FA, Mos IC, Huisman MV. Brain-type natriuretic peptide levels in the prediction of adverse outcome in patients with pulmonary embolism: a systematic review and meta-analysis. Am J Respirat Critic Care Medic. 2008 Aug 15;178(4):425-30.
75. Dalal JJ, Amin P, Ansari AS, Bhave A, Bhagwat RG, Challani A, et al. Management of acute pulmonary embolism: Consensus statement for Indian Patients. J Assoc Physic India. 2015 Dec;63:41.
76. Kreit JW. The impact of right ventricular dysfunction on the prognosis and therapy of normotensive patients with pulmonary embolism. CHEST Journal. 2004 Apr 1;125(4):1539-45.
77. Kucher N, Rossi E, De Rosa M, Goldhaber SZ. Prognostic role of echocardiography among patients with acute pulmonary embolism and a systolic arterial pressure of 90 mm Hg or higher. Archives of Intern Med. 2005 Aug 8;165(15):1777-81.

78. ten Wolde M, Söhne M, Quak E, Mac Gillavry MR, Büller HR. Prognostic value of echocardiographically assessed right ventricular dysfunction in patients with pulmonary embolism. Archives of Intern Medic. 2004 Aug 9;164(15):1685-9.
79. Coutance G, Cauderlier E, Ehtisham J, Hamon M. The prognostic value of markers of right ventricular dysfunction in pulmonary embolism: a meta-analysis. Crit Care. 2011 Mar 28;15(2):R103.
80. Sanchez O, Trinquart L, Colombet I, Durieux P, Huisman MV, Chatellier G, et al. Prognostic value of right ventricular dysfunction in patients with haemodynamically stable pulmonary embolism: a systematic review. Eur H J. 2008 Jun 1;29(12):1569-77.
81. Aujesky D, Obrosky DS, Stone RA, Auble TE, Perrier A, Cornuz J, et al. Derivation and validation of a prognostic model for pulmonary embolism. Am J Resp Critic Care Medic. 2005 Oct 15;172(8):1041-6.
82. Jiménez D, Aujesky D, Moores L, Gómez V, Lobo JL, Uresandi F, et al. Simplification of the pulmonary embolism severity index for prognostication in patients with acute symptomatic pulmonary embolism. Archives of Intern Medic. 2010 Aug 9;170(15):1383-9.
83. Wicki J, Perrier A, Perneger TV, Bounameaux H, Junod AF. Predicting adverse outcome in patients with acute pulmonary embolism: a risk score. Thrombosis and haemostasis-stuttgart. 2000 Oct 1;84(4):548-52.
84. Baglin T, Luddington R, Brown K, Baglin C. Incidence of recurrent venous thromboembolism in relation to clinical and thrombophilic risk factors: prospective cohort study. The lancet. 2003 Aug 16;362(9383):523-6.
85. Rodger MA, Kahn SR, Wells PS, Anderson DA, Chagnon I, Le Gal G, et al. Identifying unprovoked thromboembolism patients at low risk for recurrence who can discontinue anticoagulant therapy. Canad Medic Associat J. 2008 Aug 26;179(5):417-26.
86. Eichinger S, Heinze G, Jandeck LM, Kyrle PA. Risk assessment of recurrence in patients with unprovoked deep vein thrombosis or pulmonary embolism. The Vienna prediction model. Circulation. 2010 Apr 13;121(14):1630-6.
87. Tosetto A, Iorio A, Marcucci M, Baglin T, Cushman M, Eichinger S, et al. Predicting disease recurrence in patients with previous unprovoked venous thromboembolism: a proposed prediction score (DASH). J Thromb Haemost. 2012 Jun 1;10(6):1019-25.

CHAPTER

15

Contrast-induced Nephropathy

Niranjan Kulkarni, Harshal Vora

INTRODUCTION

The use of intravascular iodinated contrast agents has continued to increase over recent years. There are potential risks associated with the intravascular administration of iodinated contrast agents. It is, therefore, essential that the persons administering iodinated contrast media and those performing the imaging procedures have an understanding of the indications for the use of iodinated contrast media as well as the potential side effects and their management. Contrast-induced nephropathy (CIN) is the third most common cause of iatrogenic acute kidney injury all over the world.[1,2] In recent years, the understanding of pathogenesis of CIN has improved, yet there are controversies in many aspects. Most of the patients who have been studied till date have received intra-arterial contrast agents. Intravenous use of contrast agents is believed to have a lower incidence of CIN.[3,4]

Definition and Incidence of CIN

The International Kidney Disease Improving Global Outcomes (KDIGO)[5] *defines* Acute Kidney Injury (AKI) when one of the following criteria is met:
- Serum creatinine rises by ≥26 µmol/l within 48 hours or
- Serum creatinine rises ≥1.5 fold from the baseline value, which is known or presumed to have occurred within one week or
- Urine output is <0.5 ml/kg/h for >6 consecutive hours.

The widely used definition of Contrast Induced-Acute Kidney Injury (CI-AKI) is a rise in serum creatinine of more than 25% or 0.5 mg/dl from the baseline creatinine value within 48 hours of intravascular administration of contrast agents.[6] Serum creatinine peaks at 3–5 days and usually returns to normal at 10–14 days (KATZBERG 1997).

There is a significant variability in the incidence of CIN in various studies. On an average, the incidence of CIN/CIAKI was 13.2% following non-coronary angiography, 8.5% following coronary angiography and 6.5% following CT Scans.[7]

Clinical Features

Usually, patients who develop CIN are asymptomatic and nonoliguric. They have reversible reduction in kidney function which returns to baseline value within 10–14 days.

Any persistent rise in serum creatinine or development of oliguria/anuria raises the possibilities of other aetiologies (e.g. cholesterol embolic syndrome, other nephrotoxic agents or ATN secondary to other aetiologies). Urine examination may exhibit tubular epithelial cells, granular casts or mild proteinuria but none of the findings are sensitive or specific for CIN.

Fractional Excretion of Na (FENa) is usually <1 in patients of CIN in contrast to a FeNa of >1 seen in most other causes of ATN.[8]

Risk Factors for CIN

Risk factors for CIN are well-known. Scoring systems are available to guide surgeons or physicians to determine the risk of developing CIN in a particular patient.[9]

Risk Factors

Risks for patients developing CI-AKI include
- Chronic kidney disease (CKD) eGFR <60 ml/min/1.73 m^2
- Older age (>75 years old)
- Cardiac failure
- Nephrotoxic medication
- Aminoglycosides
- NSAIDs
- Amphotericin B
- Hypovolaemia
- Sepsis
- Volume (dose) of contrast
- Intra-arterial administration.

It should be appreciated that often a number of these risk factors will be present together in a patient, and that there is currently no validated CI-AKI risk assessment available to recommend. The use of the estimated glomerular filtration rate (eGFR) to quantify kidney function should only be applied to patients with stable kidney function and should not be used in patients with AKI. Patients identified as at high risk of CI-AKI may be discussed with a renal physician to assess the individual risk/benefit associated with a specific contrast procedure. In some patients the risk of CI-AKI is outweighed by the potential benefit from the contrast study. It is recommended that these risks are explained to the patient in the context of the potential benefit of proceeding with the study. Imaging should not be delayed where the benefit of early imaging clearly outweighs the risk of waiting.

Contrast Agents

Many different forms of contrast agents have been developed over the last 50 years. They are ionic or non-ionic in nature. Contrast agents are divided into High osmolar contrast media (HOCM), Low osmolar contrast media (LOCM) and Isotonic contrast media (IOCM). Most HOCM are ionic in nature, while most LOCM are non-ionic in nature. HOCM are of very high osmolalities ranging approximately from 1500 to 2000 mosm/kg. LOCM varies from 600 to 1000 mosm/kg, which is still much higher than serum osmolality. IOCM can be ionic or non-ionic in nature with lower osmolalities. However, studies have not convincingly proven the superiority of IOCM over LOCM.[10-17] Some of the studies have shown less incidence of CIN with iodixanol (iso-osmolar agent) than with LOCM compound (iohexol),[18] but meta-analysis of all the data showed that lesser incidence of CIN with IOCM is not seen with entire spectrum of LOCM.[19-23] The European Society of Urogenital Radiology has recommended both IOCM and LOCM as contrast agents.[24] Superiority of IOCM or LOCM in comparison to HOCM is well known.[25,26] Use of HOCM as contrast agents has declined in the recent years.

Pathogenesis of CIN

Multiple pathophysiologic mechanisms have been suggested that contribute collectively in the development of CIN. The mechanisms include vasoconstriction and medullary hypoxia, direct toxic effects of contrast on tubular cells, free radical mediated injury. Volume depletion or drugs like ACE inhibitors or NSAIDs will potentiate the toxic effects of contrast agents. Many studies have demonstrated vasoconstriction as a mechanism of CIN.[27,28] Vasoconstriction is seen more in the medulla as oxygen delivery is lower. Liss et al, have demonstrated fall in oxygen tension from 30 to 15 mmHg after administration of low and iso-osmolar contrast agents.[29] A second important mechanism for development of CIN is direct cytotoxicity of contrast agents. Evidences supporting this theory come from renal biopsy specimens showing vacuolization and tubular cell necrosis from patients receiving intravascular contrast agents.[30] Increased viscosity of tubular fluid due to contrast increases direct tubular toxicity.

Outcomes of Contrast-induced Nephropathy

Multiple studies have shown that both short- and long-term mortality and progression of CKD is increased with CIN; however, its causal association is yet to be determined. Tables 1 and 2[31-37] demonstrates association of short-term and long-term mortality and CIN, respectively. Risk factors associated with an increase in the risk for CIN, e.g. heart failure are also independently associated.

Table 1: Association of contrast-induced nephropathy with short-term risk of mortality

Study authors	Number of patients	ODDS ratio of death	95% confidence interval
Levy et al.	357	5.5	2.9–13.2
Gruberg et al.	439	3.9	2.0–7.6
Shema et al.	1111	3.9	2–7.6
McCullough et al.	1826	6.6	3.3–12.9
From et al.	3236	3.4	2.6–4.4
Bartholomew et al.	20,479	22	16–31
Weisbord et al.	27,608	1.8	1.4–2.5

Table 2: Association of contrast-induced nephropathy with long-term risk of mortality[38-42]

Study authors	Patient numbers	Adjusted HR	95% CI
Goldenberg et al.	78	2.7	1.7–4.5
Solomon et al.	294	3.2	1.1–8.7
Harjai et al	985	2.6	1.5–4.4
Roghi et al.	2860	1.8	1–3.4
Brown et al.	7856	3.1	2.4–4.0

Preventing AKI

CIN is largely preventable provided patients who are at high risks are identified. Prevention of CIN can be divided into following steps.
1. Use of less nephrotoxic contrast agents.
2. Use of alternative diagnostic procedure when possible (e.g. MRI or ultrasonography).
3. Use of pharmacologic agents e.g. N-Acetyl cysteine.
4. Administration of IV fluids, e.g. normal saline.
5. Avoidance of other nephrotoxic agents or drugs like diuretics.

Choice of Contrast Agent

There are three types of contrast agents available at present. HOCM, LOCM and IOCM. Multiple studies have shown that LOCM/IOCM are better than HOCM to reduce the incidence of AKI.[43] Use of HOCM as a contrast agent is declining now. There are no significant differences found between IOCM and LOCM in most of the studies. The European Society of Urogenital Radiology and American College of Cardiology have recommended use of either IOCM or LOCM to reduce the incidence of CIN.[24]

Pharmacological Agents

Many pharmacological agents have been used to prevent CIN in the last few years. It includes periprocedural administration of isotonic saline, bicarbonate, dopamine, mannitol, diuretics, fenoldopam, theophylline and N-Acetylcysteine. Only intravenous fluids have shown definite evidences of effectiveness in prevention of CIN.[44] N-Acetylcysteine has an indeterminate role.

The rationale for use of N Acetylcysteine for the prevention of CIN relates to its capacity to prevent free radical mediated injury, as it has been thought to be an ROS scavenger. It thus stimulates the production of vasodilatory agents such as nitric oxide. Multiple trials have shown either positive or negative results for N-Acetylcysteine in the prevention of contrast-induced nephropathy (Tables 3 and 4).

Thus, it is not definite whether NAC will help to prevent CIN, however considering its low cost and minimal risk associated with oral NAC, the Kidney Disease Improving Global Outcomes (KIDIGO)[55] suggested its use in conjunction with isotonic crystalloid solution in patients who are undergoing contrast-associated procedures.

Role of IV Fluids in Prevention of CIN

Many of the clinical trials over the past 15 years have proven a definitive role of intravenous fluids in prevention of CIN. Solomon et al.[56] in 1994 published a clinical trial on the prophylactic effects of IV fluids alone or in combination with mannitol or furosemide. Among 28 patients who received intravenous fluids alone, three (11%) developed CIN, compared with 7 (28%) of 25 in the mannitol group and 10 (40%) in the furosemide group. In Table 5[56-61] randomised control trials have been elaborated on intravenous fluids.

Table 3: Positive studies[45-48]

Study authors	Patients	%CIN NAC	% CIN control
Drager et al	200	4%	12%
Miner et al.	171	9.6%	22%
Marenzi et al.	352	11.6%	33%
Baker et al.	80	5%	21%

Table 4: Negative studies[49-54]

Studies	Patients	% CIN NAC	%CIN control
Berwanger et al.	2308	12.7%	12.7%
Azmus et al.	399	7.1%	8.4%
Webb et al	487	23.3%	20.7%
Carbonnel et al.	216	10.3%	10.1%
Gomes et al	156	10.4%	10.1%
Fung et al.	91	13.3%	17.4%

Table 5: Randomised control trials prove a definitive role of IV fluid in prevention of CIN

Study	Nos. of patients	Type of IV fluids	Rates of CIN	P value
Solomon et al.	78	0.45% Nacl	11 vs 25 vs 40%	<0.05
Bader et al.	39	0.9% Nacl both groups (300 ml once vs. 2000 ml over 24 hours.)	15% vs 5.3%	0.605
Krauski et al.	63	0.45% NaCl vs 0.9% NaCl	10.8 vs 0.0%	0.136
Merten et al.	119	$NaHCO_3$ vs NaCl	1.6% vs 13.7%	0.02
Briguori et al.	336	$NaHCO_3$ vs NaCl	1.9 vs 9.9%	0.019
Recio-Mayoral et al.	111	$NaHCO_3$ vs NaCl	1.8 vs 21.8%	0.001

The last 3 studies were done to guide the ideal fluid composition for prevention of CIN. In the trials by Merten and Briguori,[59,60] positive results towards using bicarbonate as intravenous fluid of choice have been demonstrated. However, both the studies take significant statistical power to establish conclusively the superiority of bicarbonate infusion over normal saline. Adequately powered studies are needed to establish the importance of bicarbonate solution over normal saline. Recently Recio-Mayoral et al.[61] have done a study in 111 patients who were undergoing emergent coronary procedures compared normal saline with bicarbonate solutions. However, the major limitation of the study is that they did not use pre-procedural fluids in normal saline group.

Regarding the concentration of the solution, 0.9% normal saline was found to be better than 0.45% saline in study by Krauski et al.[58] However the study sample size is very small. In 2002, Mueller et al.[62] performed similar type of study comparing different concentration. The rate of CIN among group who have received 0.45% NaCl vs. 0.9% NaCl is 2.0% vs. 0.7%. Thus, both studies have at least shown that isotonic saline is more protective than hypotonic saline.

SUMMARY OF RECOMMENDATIONS FOR PREVENTION OF CIN

Prevention is important as there is no specific treatment and involves identification of patients at increased risk of CI-AKI. Wherever possible, alternative imaging modalities should be considered to reduce exposure to radio-iodine contrast media. Magnetic resonance angiography (MRA) may be considered as an alternative, but the use of gadolinium (Gd) in MRA is associated with the risk of developing Nephrogenic Systemic Fibrosis (NSF). Nephrogenic Systemic Fibrosis is a severe fibrosis of the skin resulting in extensive limitation in mobility. The condition has been reported mostly in patients with dialysis requiring CKD or AKI who have received Gd-containing contrast agents. The European Society of Urogenital Radiology has produced NSF guidelines with further advice issued from the European Medicines Agency.

Potentially nephrotoxic medications such as non-steroidal anti-inflammatory drugs and aminoglycosides should be withheld or avoided. Currently, there is insufficient evidence to support the routine discontinuation of angiotensin-converting enzyme inhibitors (ACE-I) or angiotensin receptor blockers (ARBs) in stable outpatients. However in acutely ill patients at an increased risk of developing AKI, it is suggested that withholding ACE-I and ARBs should be considered on an individual patient basis.

Metformin is not nephrotoxic but is exclusively excreted via the kidneys. Therefore patients on metformin who develop AKI following contrast are at risk of developing lactic acidosis due to the accumulation of the drug. The Royal College of Radiologists recommends that there is no need to stop metformin after receiving iodinated contrast if the serum creatinine is within the normal range and/or eGFR >60 ml/min/1.73 m². If serum creatinine is above the normal reference range or eGFR is <60 ml/min/1.73 m², any decision to stop it for 48 hours should be made in consultation with the referring clinician.

Acutely ill patients and patients who are identified at high risk of CI-AKI should have an assessment of their volume status and receive appropriate volume expansion prior to the procedure. Intravenous 0.9% sodium chloride at a rate of 1 ml/kg/h for 12 hours pre- and post-procedure has been shown to be more effective than 0.45% sodium chloride in reducing CI-AKI. It is currently recommended that either intravenous 0.9% sodium chloride or isotonic sodium bicarbonate should be used for volume expansion in patients at risk of CI-AKI. Oral volume expansion has not been shown to be as effective as intravenous volume expansion. It is generally accepted that high osmolar contrast media should be avoided in patients at risk of CI-AKI. The volume of contrast media should be minimised and further exposure to contrast media should be delayed until full recovery of renal function unless absolutely necessary. Renal function should be checked up to 48-72 hours following the procedure in a high-risk group to ensure stable renal function.

KEY POINTS FOR CLINICAL PRACTICE

- In the era of modern imaging techniques and interventions, CIN is a definite risk.
- Identification of risk groups and preventive efforts are mandated.
- Proper and accurate consenting of patients for CIN is mandatory, and cannot be overemphasised in an era where litigation is the buzz word in a modern patient doctor relationship.
- Use of isotonic bicarbonate solutions have provided greater benefits than normal saline but more powerful studies are required to establish its importance.
- In the current scenario, our recommendation is to administer either isotonic saline or isotonic bicarbonate solution at a rate of 1 ml/kg/h for 12 hours before or 12 hours after the procedure.
- In case of fluid overload status or in emergency 3 ml/kg/h of isotonic fluid for 1 hour before and then 1 ml/kg/h for 6 hours post-procedure is also recommended.

REFERENCES

1. Gupta R, Binbaum Y, Uretsky BF. The renal patient with coronary artery disease. Current concepts and dilemmas. J Am Coll Cardiol. 2004;44:1343-53.
2. Nash K, Hafeez A, Hou S. Hospital-acquired renal insufficiency. Am J Kidney Dis 2002;39:930-6.
3. Dong M, Jiao Z, Liu T, Guo F, Li G. Effect of administration route on the renal safety of contrast agents: a meta-analysis of randomized controlled trials. Journal of Nephrology.2012;25:290-301.
4. Karlsberg RP, Dohad SY, Sheng R. Contrast medium-induced acute kidney injury: comparison of intravenous and intraarterial administration of iodinated contrast medium. Journal of Vascular and Interventional Radiology. 2011;22(8):1159-65.
5. Lewington A, MacTier R, Hoefield R, Sutton A, Smith D, Downes M. Prevention of Contrast Induced Acute Kidney Injury (CI-AKI) In Adult Patients on behalf of The Renal Association, British Cardiovascular Intervention Society and the Royal college of Radiologists. Available from: http://www.renal.org/docs/defalt-source/guidelines-resources/joint-guidelines/Prevention_of_Contrast_Induced_Acute_Kidney_Injury_CI-AKI_In_Adult_Patients.pdf.
6. Barrett BJ, Parfrey PS. Preventing nephropathy induced by contrast medium. New England Journal of Medicine. 2006;354(4):379-86.
7. Weisbord SD, Mor MK, Resnick AL, Hartwig KC, Sonel AF, Fine MJ, Palevsky PM. Prevention, incidence, and outcomes of contrast-induced acute kidney injury. Archives of Internal Medicine. 2008;168(12):1325-32.
8. Fang LS, Sirota RA, Ebert TH, Lichtenstein NS. Low fractional excretion of sodium with contrast media-induced acute renal failure. Archives of internal medicine. 1980;140(4):531-3.
9. Lameire NH. Contrast-induced nephropathy—prevention and risk reduction. Nephrology Dialysis Transplantation. 2006;21(suppl 1):i11-23.
10. Aspelin P, Aubry P, Fransson SG, Strasser R, Willenbrock R, Berg KJ. Nephrotoxic effects in high-risk patients undergoing angiography. New England Journal of Medicine. 2003;348(6):491-9.
11. Solomon RJ, Natarajan MK, Doucet S, Sharma SK, Staniloae CS, Katholi RE, et al. Cardiac Angiography in Renally Impaired Patients (CARE) Study A randomized double-blind trial of contrast-induced nephropathy in patients with chronic kidney disease. Circulation. 2007;115(25):3189-96.
12. Chalmers N, Jackson RW. Comparison of iodixanol and iohexol in renal impairment. The British journal of radiology. 1999;72(859):701-3.
13. Jo SH, Youn TJ, Koo BK, Park JS, Kang HJ, Cho YS, et al. Renal toxicity evaluation and comparison between visipaque (iodixanol) and hexabrix (ioxaglate) in patients with renal insufficiency undergoing coronary angiography: the RECOVER study: a randomized controlled trial. Journal of the American College of Cardiology. 2006;48(5):924-30.
14. Carraro M, Malalan F, Antonione R, Stacul F, Cova M, Petz S, et al. Effects of a dimeric vs a monomeric nonionic contrast medium on renal function in patients with mild to moderate renal insufficiency: a double-blind, randomized clinical trial. European radiology. 1998;8(1):144-7.
15. Juergens CP, Winter JP, Nguyen-Do P, Lo S, French JK, Hallani H, et al. Nephrotoxic effects of iodixanol and iopromide in patients with abnormal renal function

receiving N-acetylcysteine and hydration before coronary angiography and intervention: a randomized trial. Internal medicine journal. 2009;39(1):25-31.
16. Laskey W, Aspelin P, Davidson C, Rudnick M, Aubry P, Kumar S, et al. DXV405 Study Group. Nephrotoxicity of iodixanol versus iopamidol in patients with chronic kidney disease and diabetes mellitus undergoing coronary angiographic procedures. American heart journal. 2009;158(5):822-8.
17. Nguyen SA, Suranyi P, Ravenel JG, Randall PK, Romano PB, Strom KA, et al. Iso-Osmolality versus Low-Osmolality Iodinated Contrast Medium at Intravenous Contrast-enhanced CT: Effect on Kidney Function 1. Radiology. 2008;248(1):97-105.
18. McCullough PA, Bertrand ME, Brinker JA, et al. A meta-analysis of the renal safety of isosmolar iodixanol compared with low-osmolar contrast media. Journal of the American College of Cardiology. 2006;48(4):692-9.
19. Clauss W, Dinger J, Meissner C. Renal tolerance of iotrolan 280—a meta-analysis of 14 double-blind studies. Eur Radiol. 1995;5:S79-S84.
20. Solomon R. The role of osmolality in the incidence of contrast-induced nephropathy: a systematic review of angiographic contrast media in high-risk patients. Kidney international. 2005;68(5):2256-63.
21. Sharma SK, Kini A. Effect of nonionic radiocontrast agents on the occurrence of contrast-induced nephropathy in patients with mild-moderate chronic renal insufficiency: Pooled analysis of the randomized trials. Catheterization and cardiovascular interventions. 2005;65(3):386-93.
22. Reed M, Meier P, Tamhane UU, Welch KB, Moscucci M, Gurm HS. The relative renal safety of iodixanol compared with low-osmolar contrast media: a meta-analysis of randomized controlled trials. JACC: Cardiovascular Interventions. 2009;2(7):645-54.
23. Heinrich MC, Häberle L, Müller V, Bautz W, Uder M. Nephrotoxicity of iso-osmolar iodixanol compared with nonionic low-osmolar contrast media: meta-analysis of randomized controlled trials 1. Radiology. 2009;250(1):68-86.
24. Thomsen HS. Guidelines for contrast media from the European Society of Urogenital Radiology. American Journal of Roentgenology. 2003;181(6):1463-71.
25. Rudnick MR, Goldfarb S, Wexler L, Ludbrook PA, Murphy MJ, Halpern EF, et al. Nephrotoxicity of ionic and nonionic contrast media in 1196 patients: a randomized trial. Kidney international. 1995;47(1):254-61.
26. Barrett BJ, Carlisle EJ. Meta-analysis of the relative nephrotoxicity of high- and low-osmolality iodinated contrast media. Radiology. 1993;188(1):171-8.
27. Caldicott WJ, Hollenberg NK, Abrams HL, Characteristics of response of renal vascular bed to contrast media. Evidence for vasoconstriction induced by renin angiotensin system. Invest Radiol. 1970;5(6):539-47.
28. Bakris GL, Burnett JC. A role for calcium in radiocontrast-induced reductions in renal hemodynamics. Kidney international. 1985;27(2):465-8.
29. Liss P, Nygren A, Erikson U, et al. Injection of low and iso-osmolar contrast medium decreases oxygen tension in the renal medulla. Kidney international. 1998;53(3):698-702.
30. Moreau JF, Droz D, Noel LH, Leibowitch J, Jungers P, Michel JR. Tubular nephrotoxicity of water-soluble iodinated contrast media. Investigative radiology. 1980;15:S54-60.
31. Levy EM, Viscoli CM, Horwitz RI. The effect of acute renal failure on mortality: a cohort analysis. Jama. 1996;275(19):1489-94.

32. Gruberg L, Mintz GS, Mehran R, Dangas G, Lansky AJ, Kent KM, et al. The prognostic implications of further renal function deterioration within 48 h of interventional coronary procedures in patients with pre-existent chronic renal insufficiency. Journal of the American College of Cardiology. 2000;36(5):1542-8.
33. Shema L, Ore L, Geron R, Kristal B. Contrast-induced nephropathy among Israeli hospitalized patients: incidence, risk factors, length of stay and mortality. The Israel Medical Association journal. 2009;11(8):460.
34. McCullough PA, Wolyn R, Rocher LL, Levin RN, O'Neill WW. Acute renal failure after coronary intervention: incidence, risk factors, and relationship to mortality. The American journal of medicine. 1997;103(5):368-75.
35. From AM, Bartholmai BJ, Williams AW, Cha SS, McDonald FS. Mortality associated with nephropathy after radiographic contrast exposure. In Mayo Clinic Proceedings. Elsevier. 2008;83(10)1095-100.
36. Bartholomew BA, Harjai KJ, Dukkipati S, Boura JA, Yerkey MW, Glazier S, et al. Impact of nephropathy after percutaneous coronary intervention and a method for risk stratification. The American journal of cardiology. 2004;93(12):1515-9.
37. Weisbord SD, Chen H, Stone RA, Kip KE, Fine MJ, Saul MI, et al. Associations of increases in serum creatinine with mortality and length of hospital stay after coronary angiography. Journal of the American Society of Nephrology. 2006;17(10):2871-7.
38. Goldenberg I, Chonchol M, Guetta V. Reversible acute kidney injury following contrast exposure and the risk of long-term mortality. American journal of nephrology. 2008;29(2):136-44.
39. Solomon RJ, Mehran R, Natarajan MK, Doucet S, Katholi RE, Staniloae CS, et al. Contrast-induced nephropathy and long-term adverse events: cause and effect?. Clinical Journal of the American Society of Nephrology. 2009;4(7):1162-9.
40. Harjai KJ, Raizada A, Shenoy C, Sattur S, Orshaw P, Yaeger K, et al. A comparison of contemporary definitions of contrast nephropathy in patients undergoing percutaneous coronary intervention and a proposal for a novel nephropathy grading system. The American journal of cardiology. 2008;101(6):812-9.
41. Roghi A, Savonitto S, Cavallini C, Arraiz G, Angoli L, Castriota F, et al. Impact of acute renal failure following percutaneous coronary intervention on long-term mortality. Journal of Cardiovascular Medicine. 2008;9(4):375-81.
42. Brown JR, Malenka DJ, DeVries JT, Robb JF, Jayne JE, Friedman BJ, et al. Transient and persistent renal dysfunction are predictors of survival after percutaneous coronary intervention: insights from the Dartmouth Dynamic Registry. Catheterization and Cardiovascular Interventions. 2008;72(3):347-54.
43. McClennan BL. Ionic versus nonionic contrast media: safety, tolerance, and rationale for use. Urologic radiology. 1989;11(1):200-2.
44. Stacul F, Adam A, Becker CR, Davidson C, Lameire N, McCullough PA, et al. Strategies to reduce the risk of contrast-induced nephropathy. The American journal of cardiology. 2006;98(6):59-77.
45. Drager LF, Andrade L, de Toledo JF, Laurindo FR, César LA, Seguro AC. Renal effects of N-acetylcysteine in patients at risk for contrast nephropathy: decrease in oxidant stress-mediated renal tubular injury. Nephrology Dialysis Transplantation. 2004;19(7):1803-7.
46. Miner SE, Dzavik V, Nguyen-Ho P, Richardson R, Mitchell J, Atchison D, et al.

N-acetylcysteine reduces contrast-associated nephropathy but not clinical events during long-term follow-up. American heart journal. 2004;148(4):690-5.
47. Marenzi G, Assanelli E, Marana I, Lauri G, Campodonico J, Grazi M, et al. N-acetylcysteine and contrast-induced nephropathy in primary angioplasty. New England Journal of Medicine. 2006;354(26):2773-82.
48. Baker CS, Baker LR. Prevention of contrast nephropathy after cardiac catheterisation. Heart. 2001;85(4):361-2.
49. Berwanger O, Cavalcanti AB, Sousa AM, Buehler A, Castello-Júnior HJ, Cantarelli MJ, et al. Acetylcysteine for the prevention of renal outcomes in patients with diabetes mellitus undergoing coronary and peripheral vascular angiography a substudy of the acetylcysteine for contrast-induced nephropathy trial. Circulation: Cardiovascular Interventions. 2013;6(2):139-45.
50. Azmus AD, Gottschall C, Manica A, Manica J, Duro K, Frey M, et al. Effectiveness of acetylcysteine in prevention of contrast nephropathy. The Journal of invasive cardiology. 2005;17(2):80-4.
51. Webb JG, Pate GE, Humphries KH, Buller CE, Shalansky S, Al Shamari A, et al. A randomized controlled trial of intravenous N-acetylcysteine for the prevention of contrast-induced nephropathy after cardiac catheterization: lack of effect. American heart journal. 2004;148(3):422-9.
52. Carbonell N, Blasco M, Sanjuán R, Pérez-Sancho E, Sanchis J, Insa L, et al. Intravenous N-acetylcysteine for preventing contrast-induced nephropathy: a randomised trial. International journal of cardiology. 2007;115(1):57-62.
53. Gomes VO, de Figueredo CP, Caramori P, Lasevitch R, Bodanese LC, Araujo A, et al. N-acetylcysteine does not prevent contrast-induced nephropathy after cardiac catheterisation with an ionic low osmolality contrast medium: a multicentre clinical trial. Heart. 2005;91(6):774-8.
54. Fung JW, Szeto CC, Chan WW, Kum LC, Chan AK, Wong JT, et al. Effect of N-acetylcysteine for prevention of contrast nephropathy in patients with moderate to severe renal insufficiency: a randomized trial. American Journal of Kidney Diseases. 2004;43(5):801-8.
55. Khwaja A. KDIGO clinical practice guidelines for acute kidney injury. Nephron Clinical Practice. 2012;120(4):c179-84.
56. Solomon R, Werner C, Mann D, D'Elia J, Silva P. Effects of saline, mannitol, and furosemide on acute decreases in renal function induced by radiocontrast agents. New England Journal of Medicine. 1994;331(21):1416-20.
57. Bader BD, Berger ED, Heede MB, Silberbaur I, Duda S, Risler T, et al. What is the best hydration regimen to prevent contrast media-induced nephrotoxicity?. Clinical nephrology. 2004;62(1):1-7.
58. Krasuski RA, Beard BM, Geoghagan JD, Thompson CM, Guidera SA. Optimal timing of hydration to erase contrast associated nephropathy: the OTHER CAN study. Journal of Invasive Cardiology. 2003;15(12):699-702.
59. Merten GJ, Burgess WP, Gray LV, Holleman JH, Roush TS, Kowalchuk GJ, et al. Prevention of contrast-induced nephropathy with sodium bicarbonate: a randomized controlled trial. Jama. 2004;291(19):2328-34.
60. Briguori C, Manganelli F, Scarpato P, Elia PP, Golia B, Riviezzo G, et al. Acetylcysteine

and contrast agent-associated nephrotoxicity. Journal of the American College of Cardiology. 2002;40(2):298-303.
61. Recio-Mayoral A, Chaparro M, Prado B, Cózar R, Méndez I, Banerjee D, et al. The reno-protective effect of hydration with sodium bicarbonate plus N-acetylcysteine in patients undergoing emergency percutaneous coronary intervention: the RENO Study. Journal of the American College of Cardiology. 2007;49(12):1283-8.
62. Mueller C, Buerkle G, Buettner HJ, Petersen J, Perruchoud AP, Eriksson U, et al. Prevention of contrast media-associated nephropathy: randomized comparison of 2 hydration regimens in 1620 patients undergoing coronary angioplasty. Archives of internal medicine. 2002;162(3):329-36.

CHAPTER

16

Carbon Dioxide Angiography and the Vascular Surgeon

Ashwini Naveen Gangadharan, Jessica Shah, R Sekhar

INTRODUCTION

The use of carbon dioxide (CO_2) as a contrast medium for angiography has not been widespread, despite its immense potential in clinical practice. Its usage was documented in the 1950s and 1960s as a venous contrast agent to evaluate for pericardial effusion and in 1969 Hipona[1] reported the safe use of CO_2 for the evaluation of the inferior vena cava (IVC). Following the safe, successful use in animals, Hawkins[2,3] applied the same principles to humans. Unfortunately, technology lagged behind and images obtained were suboptimal. During the 1980s, DSA evolved, as did tilting tables and a safe, reliable delivery system. As technology continued to improve, CO_2 evolved into a viable vascular imaging agent. Although used initially for renal failure and iodinated contrast allergy, the many unique properties of CO_2 and its multiple advantages in a multitude of scenarios alone or in combination with traditional contrast, makes it an exciting modality, especially in the Indian subcontinent, with the exponential rise in diabetics and CKD patients. In India, Madhusudhan and Sharma[4] in early 2009 reported good results with CO_2 in PAOD with a 'home made' delivery system. Much refinement has happened in delivery systems since then and CO_2 as a contrast medium for angiography is now routinely performed in high volume centres of vascular surgery in India.

This chapter will discuss the broad issues of this modality as applicable to the practicing vascular surgeon, rather than attempt to exhaustively elaborate on the various other applications of CO_2 angiography.

PRINCIPLES OF CO_2 ANGIOGRAPHY

CO_2 is a nontoxic, nonflammable, buoyant, compressible gas that has low viscosity and is produced endogenously at approximately 200–250 cc per minute. It is transported in the blood to the lungs by three mechanisms: dissolution directly in the blood (7%), bound to hemoglobin (10%), or predominantly carried as a bicarbonate ion (85%).

Because CO_2 is present endogenously there is no concern for allergy or renal toxicity, which has been confirmed by numerous animal and human studies. Its viscosity is 1/400 that of iodinated contrast and it is also highly soluble, roughly 20 times to 30 times greater than O_2. Therefore, it is less occlusive than other gases. When administered intravascularly, it tends to dissolve within a vessel in 30–60 seconds. CO_2 acts by displacement of blood and being lighter than blood, floats anterior to it. To render a representative image it must displace the blood in the vessel. As a result, the vessel is less dense and a negative image is obtained with digital subtraction angiography. The quality and accuracy of the image will depend on the amount of blood displaced by the CO_2 (Box 1).

Box 1: Properties of CO_2

Endogenous
Invisible
Nontoxic
High solubility (29 times that of O_2)
Low viscosity (/400 that of iodinated contrast)
Buoyant
Compressible
Nonallergenic
Non-nephrotoxic
Not diluted by blood lijke contrast
Dissolves rapidly in the blood and is removed by the lungs in one pass

---

TECHNICAL ASPECTS

CO_2 angiography technique is similar to conventional contrast DSA to start with, meaning that the same technique is employed for puncture and arterial access, using the same needles, wires and sheath (Box 2). However for proper delivery of the gas, Cho et al.[5] recommend an end-hole catheter. The delivery system for the gas could be the CO_2 manual syringe and connector (Optimed) shown (Figs 1 and 2) or the more recent but expensive automated CO_2 injector (Angiodroid). The patient must be counseled prior to the procedure for the discomfort that some might experience during

---

Box 2: Tips for improving images in CO_2 angiography

1. Elevate the feet 30 degrees (Trendelenburg)
2. Decrease patient motion
3. Selective injection
4. End-hole cateter
5. 1 ml (100–200 mg/ml) nitroglycerin intra-arterially prior to injection of CO_2
6. MA of 60 ms
7. Frame rate of 6 or more/sec
8. Stacking software to superimpose multiple frames for 1 composite image

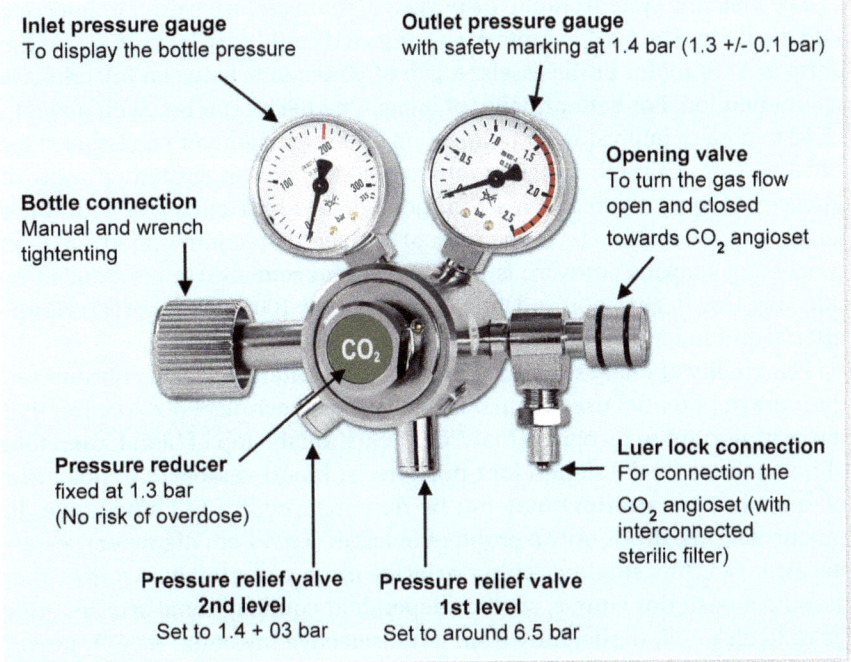

Figure 1: Gas adapter for injector (Optimed)

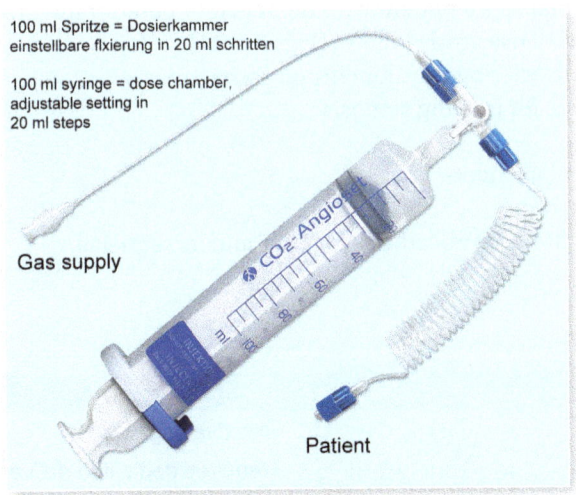

Figure 2: CO_2 manual syringe

injection, particularly because that might result in them moving the limb and reducing the clarity of pictures. Major cardiac issues like right to left shunts and pulmonary hypertension should be ruled out and no arterial injections are recommended above the diaphragm. Monitoring of BP, pulse and oxygen saturation is mandatory.

The injecting system should be purged of room air thrice prior to injecting into the body. The total volume of CO_2 injected could vary from 20 ml for the aorta to 5-10 ml for limb vessels. A gap of 30 seconds between injections is recommended. For better quality of images, catheters can be taken down to close to area of interest prior to injection and microcatheter can be used for tibial vessels. Titing the angiography table has been suggested to improve images but most centres, at least in India, do not have such a table in their facility in the cathlab. The frame rates of 6-7/sec are recommended and post processing stacking software is ideal. Bowel movement can be reduced by injecting 1mg IV glucagon and limb movements by 100-200 mcg of NTG intra-arterial and sedation (Table 1).

The quality of images that CO_2 presents, in centers in India, continues to discourage potential users. Funaki et al.[6] make a technical observation that it was important to recognise that CO_2 "floats" on the top of blood; therefore abnormalities in the dependent portions of blood vessels (e.g. posterior plaques in iliac arteries) may not be demonstrated to full advantage. In practical terms, this is only a problem in larger (i.e. >1 cm diameter) vessels because CO_2 fills smaller caliber arteries more completely. Arteries that assume a posterior course, such as dependent coursing renal arteries, may be difficult to fill, particularly from a nonselective injection. As CO_2 passes through bifurcations, the bolus dissipates into smaller bubbles that can create a "pseudostenosis".

In practice, the most common indication for use of CO_2 as a contrast for a vascular specialist is a patient with deranged or deteriorating renal function, and the areas of use are as follows (Figs 3 to 11):
1. Lower limb arteriograms for chronic ischaemias
2. Aortograms for treating stenosis
3. EVARs
4. IVC filter placements
5. AV fistulograms
6. Catheter directed procedures for DVT and its sequelae.

Table 1: Advantages and disadvantages	
Advantages	Disadvantages
Nonallergic	Requires dedicated delivery system
Non-nephrotoxic	Invisible to operator
Inexpensive	Patient motion artifacts
Unlimited volumes can be used	Labor intensive for operator
Low viscosity(<40 times that of contrast),so better accessibility	Cannot be used above diaphragm
Not diluted by blood like contrast	More radiation due to increase in frame rates.

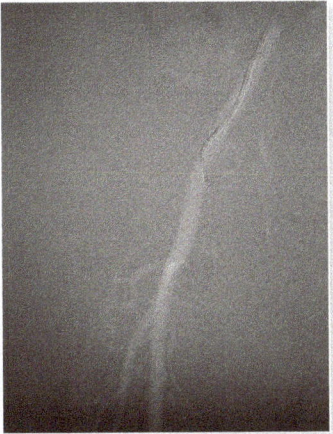

Figure 3: A normal CO_2 Angiogram showing CFA, Proximal SFA and profunda vessel

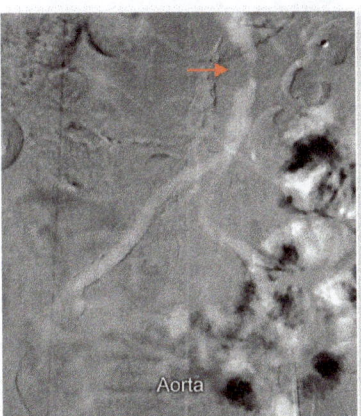

Figure 4: CO_2 angiogram showing aortic stenosis

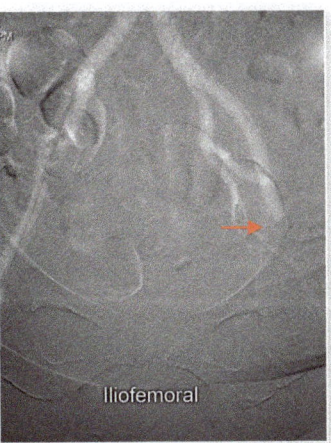

Figure 5: CO_2 angiogram of ileofemoral occlusion

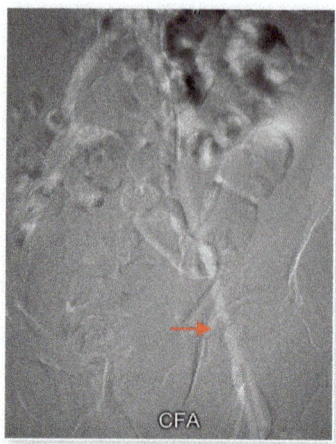

Figure 6: CO_2 angiogram of CFA occlusion

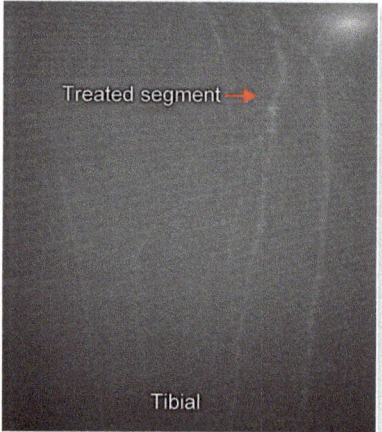

Figure 7: CO_2 angiogram of tibial vessels

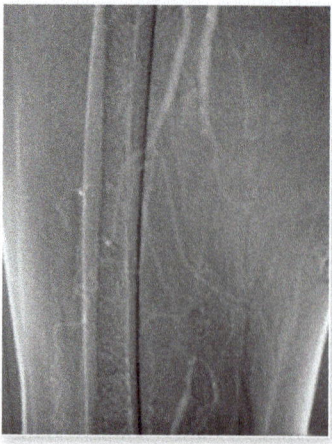

Figure 8: CO_2 angiogram showing SFA occlusion

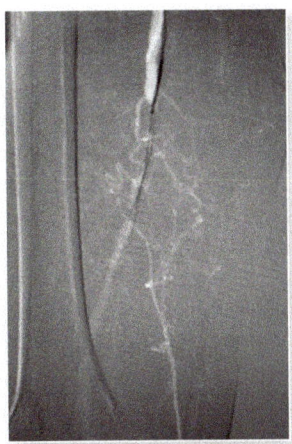

Figure 9: CO_2 angiogram after subintimal wire crossing

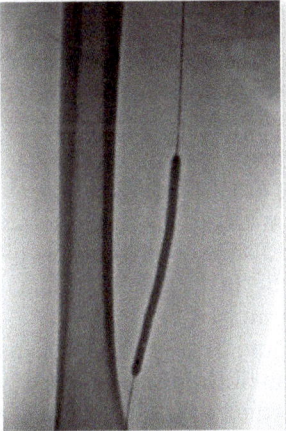

Figure 10: Balloon subintimal angioplasty of segment

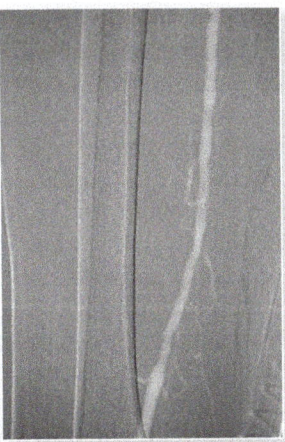

Figure 11: CO_2 angiogram on completion of SFA angioplasty

PRACTICAL EXPERIENCES WITH CO_2

Renal dysfunction after endovascular aortic aneurysm repair is an increasingly recognised problem. Carbon dioxide (CO_2) angiography has been used to limit the risk of contrast nephrotoxicity during endovascular procedures. A prospective study by Lee[7] evaluates the performance of CO_2 angiography during EVAR. Seventeen patients undergoing EVAR over a 12-month period were included. All were males with a median age of 74 (range 62–86) years. The median preoperative creatinine was 105 (range 77–165) μmol/L. CO_2 angiography was used routinely in all patients for graft positioning. Contrast was used for completion angiograms and whenever CO_2 did not satisfactorily demonstrate the anatomy. All patients had successful deployment of stent graft. The median contrast usage was 59 (range 20–250) ml. CO_2 angiography successfully demonstrated the aortic and iliac bifurcation in all 17 cases and the renal artery anatomy in 9.7 out of 17 patients had both CO_2 and contrast completion angiography. CO_2 correlated with contrast angiography in 6 of the 7 patients. There was no significant difference in pre- and postoperative creatinine values ($P > 0.9$; Wilcoxon test). They thus concluded that CO_2 angiography is a useful adjunct to contrast during the performance of EVAR and helps reduce contrast load and the risk of contrast nephrotoxicity.

Shaw and Kessel[8] however stated in a published review that it is important to be pragmatic and to use conventional contrast or alternative imaging rather than struggling with suboptimal CO_2 angiography. Also one must be aware of all reported complication with this procedure.

Johnston et al.[9] describe an episode of transient paralysis after CO_2 DSA most consistent with CO_2 embolus to the left iliolumbar artery following repair of a thoracoabdominal aneurysm.

DJ Spinosa, AH Matsumoto, et al.[10] describe transient mesenteric ischemia as a complication of carbon dioxide angiography.

Rundback et al.[11] described livedo reticularis, rhabdomyolysis, massive intestinal infarction, and death after carbon dioxide arteriography.

One question that comes to many a mind is whether a small supplement of iodinated contrast could be used just for the infragenicular or foot vessels. Spinosa et al.[12] tried to determine if the use of nonionic contrast material, as compared to the use of gadodiamide to supplement carbon dioxide angiography in patients with peripheral vascular disease (PVD) and chronic renal insufficiency (CRI), results in significant worsening of renal function. Lower extremity angiographic procedures (diagnostic and diagnostic/intervention) were performed in 40 patients with CRI (baseline serum creatinine [Cr] >1.5 mg/dl) using CO_2 alone or CO_2 supplemented with the use of either nonionic contrast material or gadodiamide (up to 0.4 mmol/kg). Serum creatinine levels were obtained before the procedure and at 48 hours after the procedure. The peak Cr level was also determined for patients with a significant (>0.5 mg/dl) Cr elevation. Forty-two lower extremity angiographic procedures (19 diagnostic and 23 diagnostic/interventions) were performed in 40 consecutive patients from August 1997 to October 1998, with a mean pre-procedure Cr of 2.2 mg/dl and a mean post-procedure Cr of 2.4 mg/dl. Twenty-five of the forty patients (63%) had diabetes mellitus. Fifteen procedures, including six interventions, were performed utilising CO_2 and nonionic contrast material in 15 patients. 6 of these 15 patients (40%) demonstrated a Cr increase >0.5 mg/dl at 48 hours. Seven procedures, including two interventions, were performed with CO_2 alone in seven patients. No patients in this group demonstrated an increase in serum creatinine of greater than 0.5 mg/dl at 48 hours. Twenty procedures, including 15 interventions, were performed with CO_2 and gadodiamide in 18 patients. In one of these 20 procedures (5%) there was an increase in Cr >0.5 mg/dl at 48 hours. The difference in worsening renal function for the nonionic contrast group (6 of 15) compared with the CO_2/gadodiamide group (1 of 20) was statistically significant ($P = .03$). When comparing the use of CO_2 and nonionic contrast material versus CO_2 alone and with gadodiamide (6 of 15 versus 1 of 27) the difference is also statistically significant ($P < 01$). The average volume of supplemental contrast material was similar in the nonionic contrast material and gadodiamide groups, as was the average volume of supplemental nonionic contrast material in the six patients with an increased Cr. They suggested that the use of small volumes of nonionic contrast material to supplement CO_2 angiography in patients with PVD and CRI can be associated with a significant increased risk of worsening renal function when compared to angiography performed with CO_2 alone or CO_2 and gadodiamide.

Successful correlation of CO_2 and iodinated contrast in PAOD was demonstrated by Seeger et al.[13] in the mid-1990s. They demonstrated a 92% correlation with an increase to 100% when a small amount of iodinated contrast was administered. It is well known that PAOD exists as part of a systemic process. Patients with intermittent claudication and rest pain undergoing angiography and intervention commonly have concomitant renal artery disease and insufficiency. In a review of 127 patients presenting with intermittent claudication or lower-limb ischaemia, approximately 45% had coexistent renal artery stenosis. 17% had mild, 16% had severe, and 12% had bilateral renal artery disease. In another review of 100 patients, greater than 50% had renal artery occlusion and unilateral or bilateral stenosis. More importantly than the actual stenosis is the occult renal impairment that accompanies PAOD even with a normal serum creatinine. In one series of 76 PAOD patients requiring angiography with normal serum creatinine, 86% had subnormal creatinine clearance with 65% below 60 mL/min. Authors have reported that serum creatinine is inaccurate in 33% of patients 40 years to 49 years of age and 90% of patients older than 70. This latter group is where most of the PAOD occurs. Considering these facts and the susceptibility of this group to CIN it would seem intuitive to use CO_2 as a contrast agent whenever possible. Again it can either eliminate or lower the total volume of iodinated contrast thereby lessening the potential for CIN.

From Asia, Jang Sang Park[14], Cheng Feng Ho[15] have published favourable results with CO_2 angiography for limb ischaemia.

With the availability of automated CO_2 injectors for angiography, several studies with CO_2 angiography using this technology have shown improved if not excellent results.

Corazza et al.[16] from Italy in their recent article state that the automated system permitted better results and less training than the original manual injector. Scalise et al.[17] compared the feasibility, safety, and diagnostic accuracy of automated CO_2 digital subtraction angiography (DSA) in comparison with ICM-DSA in the evaluation of critical limb ischaemic (CLI) patients. They performed DSA with both CO_2 and ICM on 40 consecutive CLI patients and directly compared the two techniques. 16 females and 24 males participated in the study (mean age, 71.7 years) and assessed the diagnostic accuracy of CO_2 in identifying arterial stenosis in the lower limb, with ICM-DSA used as the gold standard. The overall diagnostic accuracy of CO_2-DSA was 96.9% (sensitivity, 99.0%; specificity, 96.1%; positive predictive value, 91.1%; negative predictive value, 99.6%). Tolerable minor symptoms occurred in 3 patients. No allergic reactions or significant decline in renal function were observed in patients receiving the CO_2 injection. They concluded that carbon dioxide DSA is a valuable and safe alternative to traditional ICM-DSA for evaluating CLI patients. They suggested that this modality should be considered as the standard choice for CLI patients undergoing angiographic evaluation who are known to have renal insufficiency or contrast allergy. Similarly Palena et al.[18] studied the safety, efficacy, and diagnostic accuracy of automated carbon dioxide (CO_2) angiography (ACDA) for the evaluation of diabetic patients with critical limb ischaemia (CLI) and baseline renal insufficiency and compare ACDA with iodinated contrast medium (ICM) during endovascular treatment. From November 2014 to January 2015, 36 consecutive diabetic patients (mean age 74.8 ± 5.8 years; 27 men) with stage ≥3 chronic kidney disease (CKD ≥3) and CLI underwent lower limb angiography with both CO_2 and ICM followed by balloon angioplasty in a prospective single-center study. The primary outcome measure was the safety and efficacy of ACDA as the exclusive agent to guide angioplasty in this cohort. The secondary outcomes were the safety and diagnostic accuracy of ACDA injection as compared with ICM digital subtraction angiography (DSA) for invasive evaluation of these patients. ACDA safely and effectively guided angioplasty in all patients without complications. Transcutaneous oxygen pressure improved from 11.8 ± 6.3 to 58.4 ± 7.6 mmHg (p < 0.001). There were no complications related to ACDA during diagnostic imaging and no significant changes in the estimated glomerular filtration rate from baseline to 24 hours (44.7 ± 13.3 vs 47.0 ± 0.8 mL/min/1.73 m^2; nonsignificant). The diagnostic accuracy of CO_2 was 89.8% (sensitivity, 92.3%; specificity, 75%; positive predictive value 95.5%; negative predictive value 63.1%). There was no statistically significant difference in the qualitative diagnostic accuracy between the media (p = 0.197).They concluded that ACDA is an accurate, safe, and effective technique that can be utilized to guide endovascular interventions in diabetics with CLI and baseline CKD ≥3. Larger multicenter randomized studies are needed to validate these results. Sullivan et al.[19] studied the feasibility, safety, and potential role of carbon dioxide (CO_2) as a contrast agent for venography. Consecutive patients with contraindications to iodinated contrast agents or with unsatisfactory iodinated contrast studies underwent CO_2 digital subtraction venography. and complications were assessed. Over a 14-month period, 66 vein segments were studied in 21 patients. There was good correlation between experienced angiographers on CO_2 image quality (Ri = 0.80) and good agreement on diagnosis (k = 0.62). In 91% of the vein segments evaluated with CO_2 there was inter-observer agreement on the diagnosis. Upper extremity veins were adequately imaged with CO_2 alone in all (6/6) patients with contraindications to iodinated contrast. Following suboptimal iodinated contrast studies in six patients, CO_2 produced significantly better quality upper extremity central vein images ($p < 0.05$). Pain following injection into peripheral veins was the only CO_2-related complication. Inferior vena cava (IVC) filters were successfully deployed with CO_2 alone in 78% (7/9) of patients; two required iodinated contrast. Based upon initial experience, CO_2 venography can be recommended in patients with contraindications to iodinated contrast or unsatisfactory iodinated contrast studies. Sing et al.[20] studied the safety and accuracy of bedside carbon dioxide cavography for insertion of inferior vena cava filters in the intensive care unit. They concluded that carbon dioxide as a contrast agent is safe and provides accurate determination of vena caval diameter and anatomy. Carbon dioxide should be considered the contrast agent of choice in critically ill patients. Holtzman et al.[21] similarly compared results of carbon dioxide and iodinated contrast for cavography prior to inferior vena cava filter placement and concluded that CO_2 cavagrams accurately reflect the diameter of the IVC and the anatomy of the renal veins. Additionally, CO_2 cavagrams can be safely performed in the intensive care unit during bedside placement of IVC filters. Brown et al.[22] however mentioned in their study of gadolinium, carbon dioxide, and iodinated contrast material for planning inferior vena cava filter placement in a prospective trial, that CO_2 and gadolinium had limitations when compared with iodinated contrast material. Gadolinium provided superior consistency in identifying relevant landmarks for filter placement. CO_2 demonstrated significantly greater mean correlative error than gadolinium at initial and repeat readings. Heye et al.[23] studied preoperative mapping for haemodialysis access surgery with CO_2 venography of the upper limb. A total of 209 CO_2 venograms were obtained in 116 patients. In 89 patients (77%), 101 AVFs (21 forearm AVF (21%) and 80 elbow AVF (79%) were created. Surgical findings corresponded with CO_2 venography findings in 90% of patients. In 10 cases (10%), access was created at the elbow despite a patent forearm cephalic vein on CO2 venography ($n = 2$) or access was attempted with a vein which was thought to be unsuitable on CO2 venography ($n = 8$). Maturation rate of the latter was 50% (4/8) vs. 88% (80/91) for AVFs created with veins considered usable ($P = 0.004$). The overall maturation rate was 84% with 1-year primary, assisted primary and secondary patency rates of 63%, 70% and 71%, respectively. CO_2 venography is a useful tool for venous mapping prior to vascular access surgery, resulting in an overall maturation rate of 84% and good patency rates. Tumer et al.[24] studied CO_2 venography vs. conventional venography for AVF planning and AVF success. This included conventional ($n = 66$) and CO_2 venograms ($n = 44$). They concluded that the use of CO_2 venography prior to AVF creation is potentially equivocal and sufficient when compared to conventional venography, in AVF success. In our experience, CO_2 venography may be a suitable alternative for patients with renal insufficiency, not yet requiring HD, where prolonged preservation of renal function is desired.

In conclusion, it appears that with refinement in techniques, familiarity with the procedure and better technology, CO_2 angiography will gain wider acceptance in indicated cases.

KEY POINTS FOR CLINICAL PRACTICE

1. CO_2 angiography, despite some limitations, is a viable alternative modality to iodinated contrast in certain situations.
2. Potential users of this modality should familiarise themselves with not only the principles of the technique but also the properties of the gas.
3. Practice makes perfect, CO_2 angiography perfectly fits this adage; it is only with repeated usage that one can produce optimal images and results.
4. Better software for post processing and availability of CO_2 automated injectors will play a large role in acceptance of this modality amongst Interventionalist.

REFERENCES

1. Hipona FA, Ferris EJ, Pick R. Capnocavaography: a new technique for examination of the inferior vena cava. Radiology. 1969:92:606-9.
2. Hawkins IF. Carbon dioxide digital subtraction arteriography. AJR Am J Roentgenol. 1982;139(1):19-24.
3. Hawkins IF, Caridi JG. Carbon dioxide (CO_2) digital subtraction angiography: 26-year experience at the University of Florida. European radiology. 1998; 8(3):391-402.
4. Madhusudhan KS, Sharma S, Srivastava DN, Thulkar J, Metha SN, Prajad G, et al. Comparison of intra-arterial digital subtraction angiography using carbon dioxide by "home made" delivery system and conventional iodinated contrast media in evaluation of peripheral arterial occlusive disease of the lower limbs. J Med Imaging Radiat Oncol. 2009;53:40-49.
5. Cho KJ. CO_2 as a venous contrast agent: safety and tolerance. In: KJ Cho, IF Hawkins, eds. Carbon Dioxide Angiography: Principles, Techniques and Practices. New York: Informa Healthcare; 2007:37-44.
6. Funaki B. Carbon dioxide angiography. Semin Intervent Radiol. 2008;25(1): 65-70.
7. Lee AD, Hall RG. An evaluation of the use of carbon dioxide angiography in endovascular aortic aneurysm repair. Vasc Endovascular Surg. 2010;44(5):341-4.
8. Shaw D R, Kessel D O. The current status of the use of carbon dioxide in diagnostic and interventional angiographic procedures. Cardiovasc Intervent Radiol. 2006; 29:323-31.
9. Johnston WF, Zamora AJ, Upchurch Jr GR. Transient paralysis from carbon dioxide angiography in a patient after four-vessel endovascular thoraco-abdominal aortic aneurysm repair. Journal of vascular surgery. 2012;56(6):1717.
10. Spinosa, DJ, Matsumoto, AH, Angle, JF et al. Gadolinium-based contrast and carbon dioxide angiography to evaluate renal transplants for vascular causes of renal insufficiency and accelerated hypertension. JVIR. 1998;9:909-16.
11. Rundback JH, Shah PM, Wong J, Babu SC, Rozenblit G, Poplausky MR. Livedo reticularis, rhabdomyolysis, massive intestinal infarction, and death after carbon dioxide arteriography. Journal of vascular surgery. 1997;26(2):337-40.
12. Spinosa DJ, Angle JF, Hagspiel KD, Kern JA, Hartwell GD, Matsumoto AH. Lower extremity arteriography with use of iodinated contrast material or gadodiamide to supplement CO 2 angiography in patients with renal insufficiency. Journal of Vascular and Interventional Radiology. 2000;11(1):35-43.
13. Seeger JM, Self S, Harward TR, Flynn TC, Hawkins Jr IF. Carbon dioxide gas as an arterial contrast agent. Annals of surgery. 1993;217(6):688.

14. Park JS. CO2 angiography-1. Korean Journal of Vascular and Endovascular Surgery. 2011;27(2):52-60.
15. Ho CF, Chern MS, Wu MH, Wu HM, Lin WC, Chang CY, et al. Carbon dioxide angiography in lower limbs: a prospective comparative study with selective iodinated contrast angiography. The Kaohsiung Journal of Medical Sciences. 2003; 19(12):599-606.
16. Corazza I, Rossi PL, Feliciani G, Pisani L, Zannoli S, Zannoli R. Mechanical aspects of CO 2 angiography. Physica Medica. 2013;29(1):33-8.
17. Scalise F, Novelli E, Auguadro C, Casali V, Manfredi M, Zannoli R. Automated carbon dioxide digital angiography for lower-limb arterial disease evaluation: safety assessment and comparison with standard iodinated contrast media angiography. J Invasive Cardiol. 2015;27(1):20-6.
18. Palena LM, Diaz-Sandoval LJ, Candeo A, Brigato C, Sultato E, Manzi M. Automated Carbon Dioxide Angiography for the Evaluation and Endovascular Treatment of Diabetic Patients With Critical Limb Ischemia. Journal of Endovascular Therapy. 2015:1526602815616924.
19. Sullivan KL, Bonn J, Shapiro MJ, Gardiner GA. Venography with carbon dioxide as a contrast agent. Cardiovascular and interventional radiology. 1995;18(3):141-5.
20. Sing RF, Cicci CK, LeQuire MH, Stackhouse DJ. Bedside carbon dioxide cavagrams for inferior vena cava filters: preliminary results. Journal of vascular surgery. 2000; 32(1):144-7.
21. Holtzman RB, Lottenberg L, Bass T, Saridakis A, Bennett VJ, Carrillo EH. Comparison of carbon dioxide and iodinated contrast for cavography prior to inferior vena cava filter placement. The American journal of surgery. 2003;185(4):364-8.
22. Brown DB, Pappas JA, Vedantham S, Pilgram TK, Olsen RV, Duncan JR. Gadolinium, carbon dioxide, and iodinated contrast material for planning inferior vena cava filter placement: a prospective trial. Journal of vascular and interventional radiology. 2003;14(8):1017-22.
23. Heye S, Maleux G, Marchal GJ. Upper-Extremity Venography: CO2 versus Iodinated Contrast Material 1. Radiology. 2006;241(1):291-7.
24. Tumer Y, Resnick SA, Sato KT. CO_2 venography vs. conventional venography for AVF planning and AVF success. Journal of Vascular and Interventional Radiology. 2015;26(2):S48-9.

CHAPTER

17

Radiation Safety in Clinical Practice

Dayananda Shamurailatpam, R Sekhar

INTRODUCTION

Fluoroscopically guided interventional procedures are performed in large numbers world over. The number of procedures performed annually throughout the world has increased over the past 20 years.[1] The benefits of interventional procedures to patients are both extensive and beyond dispute, but many of these procedures also have the potential to produce patient radiation doses high enough to cause radiation effects and occupational doses to Interventionalist, be it a radiologist, a cardiologist or a vascular surgeon, high enough to cause concern.[1-4] One often forgets that Madame Marie Curie died due to excess exposure to her discovery, radium. Thomas Edison invented the fluoroscope, but he too stopped his work in this area when his assistant died of an x-ray overdose. Many years later, we have a better understanding of the dangers of radiation, and yet, we often fail to address safety issues adequately. This chapter is guided by recommendations by experts of Cardiovascular and Interventional Society of Europe (CIRSE) and the Society of Interventional Radiology (SIR) Safety and Health Committee.[5]

One of the root causes of excessive radiation exposure arises from the fact that many in the healthcare field who work with radiation have received only rudimentary limited or no radiation training. Whereas interventional radiologists are trained in the safe use of radiation, interventional cardiologists and vascular surgeons, for instance, typically receive minimal radiation training. Because they are unfamiliar with all of the sources of radiation exposure, they may know little about risk-reduction and safety strategies. Compounding the problem is that, while a radiologist's key team member is a radiologic technologist (who also has received radiation safety training), an interventional cardiologist or vascular surgeon's key team member may be a nurse, who likely has received little to no radiation safety training. That's not to say that all radiologists employ best radiation safety practices, either. Additionally, we often use far more radiation than necessary. In the United

States, there is an increased emphasis on ensuring the highest quality images, which means more radiation. That is not the case in Europe and Japan, where safety is more highly valued. The ideal dose is the least amount of radiation possible to produce an acceptable image. A good operator knows how to produce good images without excess radiation. In most hospitals, radiation safety is the joint responsibility of the facility's radiation safety officer and the technologists who work in the department. The safety officer keeps track of healthcare workers' radiation exposure via the dosimetry badges that should be worn at all times and turned in periodically for exposure assessment by an outside body, the BARC for instance in India. It is mandatory that hospitals provide protective devices, such as lead aprons and shields. They also require records be maintained regarding individual worker exposure, as recorded by dosimetry badges. But when no one's watching, it's easy to fall back into bad habits and complacency. Hospitals get busy and when a dosimetry badge value comes back high, some clinicians choose not to wear a badge, rather than take the time to determine the cause. What is particularly unfortunate is that the reason for the high dosimetry numbers often is easily resolved, and typically increases the safety of the worker and everyone around him or her (Figs 1 to 3).

UNDERSTANDING THE HAZARDS

Significant radiation exposure has the potential to impact the health of physicians performing interventions in the following ways:
- **Brain tumors:** A case report of brain tumors in 2 Canadian interventional cardiologists[6] first raised this concern. There were three additional cases

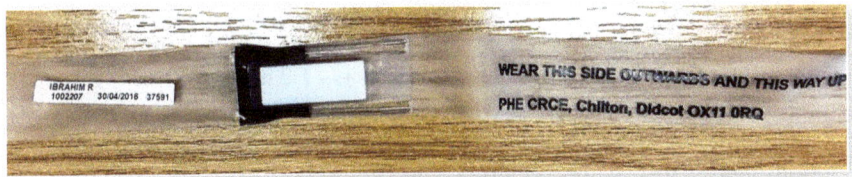

Figure 1: Dosimeter for head

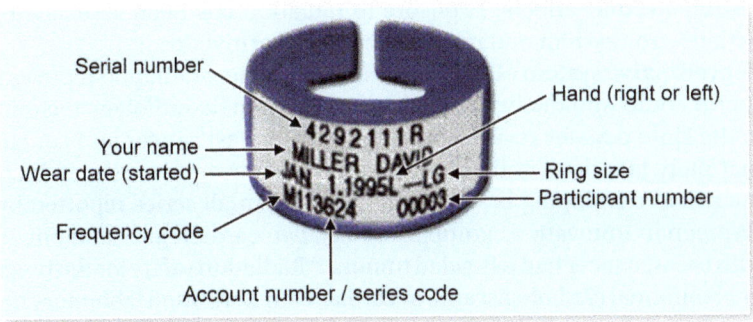

Figure 2: Ring dosimeter

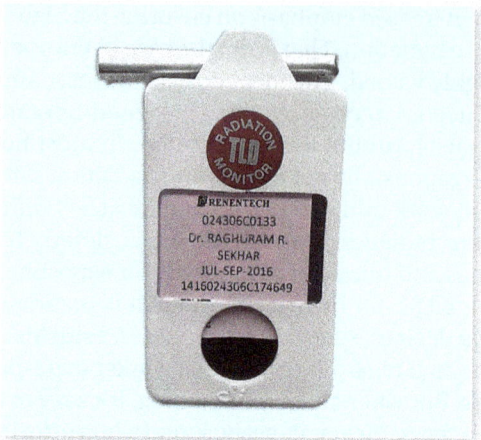

Figure 3: TLD badge: Body dosimeter

identified in a study from Sweden in physicians who had worked with fluoroscopy.[7] The left-sided predisposition of these tumors raised further concern when four additional cases were reported from France and Israel.[8] Active case findings from this group highlighted this concern further when they identified that 22 of 26 cases (85%) had a left-sided distribution of brain tumors, which is a phenomenon that is not noted in the general population.[9] In a study of 11 cardiologists performing invasive (diagnostic and interventional) procedures, radiation exposure to the outside left side and outside center of the head was significantly greater than the outside right side of the head (106.1 +/− 33.6 and 83.1 +/− 18.9 vs. 50.2 +/− 16.2 mrad, $p < 0.001$). This was significantly attenuated by the usage of a radiation protection cap (42.3 +/− 3.5 and 42.0 +/− 3.0 vs. 41.8 +/− 2.9 mrad) and only slightly higher than ambient control (38.3 +/− 1.2 mrad, $p = 0.046$).[10]

- **Cataracts:** Higher incidence of cataracts (specifically posterior subcapsular) has been reported in interventional cardiologists in a large French multicenter observational study.[11] Fortunately, this risk appeared to be mitigated in those who wore lead-lined glasses.[12]
- **Thyroid disease:** Structural as also functional changes as a result of radiation exposure have been reported in the thyroid gland.
- **Cardiovascular effects:** Exposure to radiation has been associated with both macro vascular and micro vascular abnormalities.
- **Reproductive system effects:** Exposure to ionizing radiation reduces both sperm count and quality. A study of 56,436 female radiology technicians in the United States revealed 1,050 cases of breast cancer and concluded that daily low-dose radiation exposure over several years may increase the risk of developing breast cancer.[13] In the small series reported by the "Women in Innovation" group for safety, two cardiologists and one nurse with breast cancer had left-sided tumors.[14] Radiation safety for the pregnant interventional cardiologist and/or cardiac catheterization laboratory nurse/technician is a pressing issue.

The adverse risks of radiation exposure may be described in terms of **stochastic** and **deterministic** effects. The **stochastic** effect is the non-threshold biologic effect of radiation that occurs by chance to a population of persons whose probability is proportional to the dose and whose severity is independent of the dose. Developing malignancy due to radiation exposure is a stochastic risk.

The deterministic effect is a dose-dependent direct health effect of radiation for which a threshold is believed to exist. Developing a skin burn as a result of a prolonged case is a deterministic effect.

Dose exposure is usually described in terms of the following parameters:

1. **Fluoroscopic time (min):** This is the time during a procedure that fluoroscopy is used but does not include cine acquisition imaging. Therefore, considered alone, it tends to underestimate the total radiation dose received.
2. **Cumulative air kerma (Gy):** The cumulative air kerma is a measure of X-ray energy delivered to air at the interventional reference point (15 cm from the isocenter in the direction of the focal spot). This measurement has been closely associated with deterministic skin effects.
3. **Dose-area product (Gy.cm^2):** This is the cumulative sum of the instantaneous air kerma and the X-ray field area. This monitors the patient dose burden and is a good indicator of stochastic effects.

In 2016, Kumar et al. helped us understand the above practical approach to the important issues related to ionizing radiation and its implications on physicians through a very elegant article,[15] excepts of which are shared in this chapter.

The radiation dose received by those performing interventions can vary for the same type of procedure and for similar patient dose.[4] There has been particular concern regarding occupational dose to the lens of the eye.[2] Data from exposed human populations suggest that lens opacities (cataracts) occur at doses far lower than those previously believed to cause cataracts.[16, 17] Statistical analysis of the available data suggests absence of a threshold dose, although if one does exist, it is possible that it is less than 0.1 Gy.[18, 19] Additionally, it appears that the latency period for radiation cataract formation is inversely related to radiation dose.[16] Occupational radiation protection requires both appropriate education and training for the performer and the availability of appropriate protection tools and equipment. Occupational radiation protection measures are necessary for all individuals who work in the interventional fluoroscopy suite. This includes not only technologists and nurses, who spend a substantial amount of time in a radiation environment, but also individuals such as anesthesiologists who may be in a radiation environment only occasionally. All of these individuals may be considered radiation workers, depending on their level of exposure and on national regulations. All workers require appropriate monitoring, as well as protection tools and equipment. They must also receive education and training appropriate to their jobs.[20] The level of training should be based on the level of risk.

RADIATION PROTECTION EQUIPMENT

The greatest source of radiation exposure to the operator and staff is scatter from the patient. Generally, controlling patient dose also reduces scatter and limits operator dose. However, chronic radiation exposure in the workplace mandates the use of protective tools in order to limit occupational radiation dose to an acceptable level. The purpose of radiation protection tools is to improve operator and staff safety without impeding the procedure or jeopardizing the patient's safety.

Shielding

There are three types of shielding:
- Architectural shielding
- Equipment mounted shields
- Personal protective devices.

Architectural shielding is built into the walls of the procedure room. In addition, rolling and stationary shields, which rest on the floor, are constructed of transparent leaded plastic and are available and useful for providing additional shielding for both operators and staff. They are particularly well suited for use by nurses and anesthesia personnel.[21]

Equipment-mounted shielding includes protective drapes suspended from the table and from the ceiling. Table-suspended drapes hang from the side of the patient table, between the under-table X-ray tube and the operator. These should always be employed, as they have been shown to substantially reduce operator dose.[22] Ceiling-suspended shields, generally constructed of a transparent leaded plastic, can also be used during cases of any significant length. Properly placed shields have been shown to dramatically reduce operator eye dose.[23,24] It now appears that the threshold dose for cataract formation can be reached within several years for a busy interventionalist, so suspended shields or some other form of eye protection should be used by anyone performing interventional procedures on a regular basis.[2] Disposable protective patient drapes are now available. These contain metallic elements (bismuth or tungsten–antimony) and are placed on the patient after the operative site has been prepared and draped.[25,26] They have been shown to reduce operator dose substantially, with reported reductions of 12-fold for the eyes, 26-fold for the thyroid, and 29-fold for the hands.[26] Although their use adds some cost to the procedure, disposable protective drapes should be considered for complex procedures and procedures in which the operator's hands must be near the radiation field.

Personal Protective Devices

Personal protective devices include aprons, thyroid shields, eyewear, and gloves. Protective aprons with thyroid shields are the principal radiation protection tool for interventional workers. They should be employed at all times. The vest/skirt configuration is preferred by many operators in order to reduce the risk of musculoskeletal/back injury.[27] This wrap-around style is typically 0.25 mm lead-equivalent so that, when worn, the double thickness anteriorly provides 0.5 mm lead equivalence.

Operators and staff who work in the interventional laboratory on a regular basis should be provided with properly fitted aprons, both to reduce ergonomic hazards and to provide optimal radiation protection.[28] Aprons should be inspected fluoroscopically on an annual basis to detect deterioration and defects in the protective material.[29] Because of the ergonomic hazards of personal protective devices (particularly leaded aprons), attempts to reduce the fatigue and injury associated with wearing heavy protective apparel have been made.[27] An early version of a "weightless apron" involved a rolling device from which the apron was hung. This was positioned behind the operator and rolled as the interventional radiologist moved.[30] A recently introduced innovation, travels on a set of ceiling-mounted rails and is easily donned within seconds.[31] This newer device extends from the head to the distal portions of the lower extremities and provides substantial protection to the wearer. Devices, such as these hold promise for improved ergonomics and safety. As new protective devices become available, they will be evaluated critically and adopted if shown to improve radiation protection and ergonomics.

Because the current ICRP occupational limit for eye exposure of 150 mSv/y may be too high, and because radiation cataract formation may be a stochastic effect, operators are strongly advised to use eye protection at all times.[2, 32] Leaded eyeglasses are an alternative to ceiling suspended shields for this purpose. Leaded eyeglasses with large lenses and protective side shields provide more protection than eyeglasses without these features. They help minimize scatter that approaches the operator from the side and scatter from the operator's own head.[33] The principal disadvantage of leaded eyeglasses is their weight and discomfort. In general, the operator's hands should be kept out of the primary radiation beam. The best way to protect the operator's hands is to keep them out of the radiation field. Leaded gloves are of benefit if the operator's hands will be near, but not in, the primary radiation beam (Figs 4 to 7).

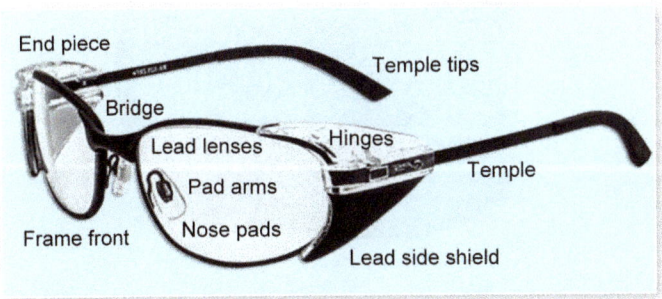

Figure 4: Safety lead glasses

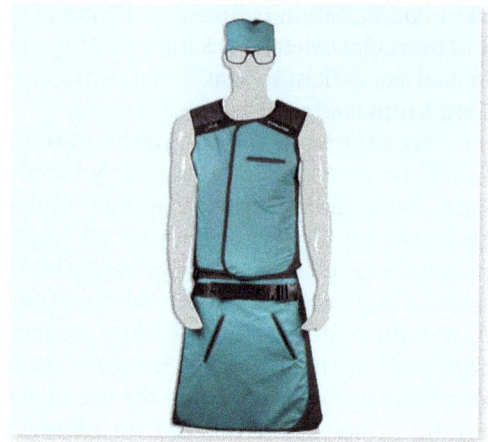

Figure 5: Lead apron

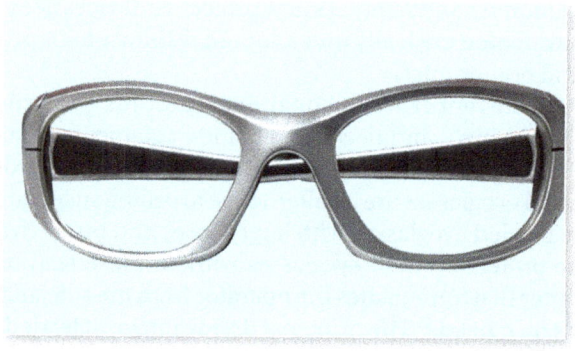

Figure 6: Radiation safety glasses

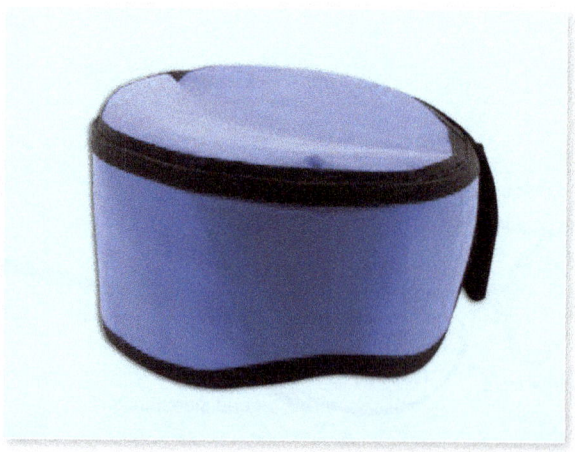

Figure 7: Radiation safety caps

Effectiveness of Shielding

The shielding material for protective aprons has evolved from heavy, lead impregnated vinyl or rubber with a shielding equivalent of 1 mm of lead, to lighter, composite (lead plus other high-atomic numbered elements) or entirely lead-free materials. These lighter materials have largely replaced the all-lead aprons of the past, and typically are designed to provide 0.5 mm lead-equivalent protection anteriorly.[34] Transmission of 70–100 kVp X- rays through 0.5 mm lead is approximately 0.5–5%.[35,29] The protection provided by 0.5 mm lead-equivalent composite and lead-free aprons has been found to vary, and ranges from 0.6% to 6.8% transmission.[29] Leaded glasses reduce the dose to the operator's eye from frontal exposure by a factor of approximately 8–10.[24,36] When side exposure is included (the typical situation in clinical practice), the protection factor is decreased to between two and three.[37] Combining various (Figs 8 and 9)

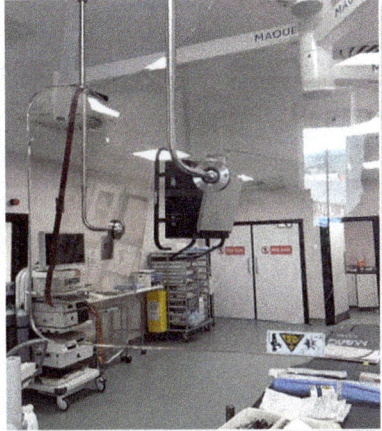

Figure 8: Ceiling-suspended screens

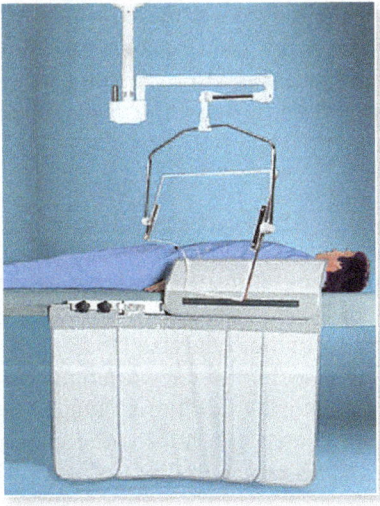

Figure 9: Table-suspended mobile lead skirts

types of shielding (i.e. table-suspended drapes, ceiling-suspended screens, aprons, leaded glasses, mobile shields, and disposable drapes) results in dramatic dose reduction for the operator.[21, 24]

Scatter

The magnitude and distribution of scattered radiation is affected by many factors, including patient size, gantry angulation, patient position, filtration, fluoroscopic settings, and the use of shielding. Overall, in an unshielded environment, and for a posteroanterior projection, the exposure is greatest below the table, less at the operator's waist level, and least at the eye level. However, substantial operator eye doses can be reached in unfavourable circumstances (e.g. large patient, high-dose fluoroscopy/ fluorography, gantry angulation), underscoring the importance of proper protection, particularly for the eyes.[38, 39]

PRACTICAL ADVICE TO REDUCE OR MINIMISE OCCUPATIONAL RADIATION DOSE

Decreasing patient dose will result in a proportional decrease in scatter dose to the operator. Therefore, techniques that reduce patient dose will generally also reduce occupational dose. This benefits both, the operator and patient. Notwithstanding the fact that the greatest reduction occurs when imaging is performed without ionizing radiation, such as with ultrasound, additional techniques can be used with fluoroscopically guided procedures to reduce occupational dose.

Minimise Fluoroscopy Time

Fluoroscopy should be used only to observe objects or structures in motion. Review the last-image-hold image for study, consultation, or education instead of additional fluoroscopic exposure. Use short taps of fluoroscopy instead of continuous operation. Fluoroscopy to determine or adjust collimator blade positioning can be eliminated by using the virtual collimation feature when present.

Minimise the Number of Fluorographic Images

For digital subtraction angiography, use variable frame rates tailored to the examination (e.g. 1 image/sec for 6 seconds, then one image every other second for 24 sec for arteriography of the celiac axis) instead of a constant frame rate (e.g. 2 images/second for 30 sec).[39,40] For documentation, use stored last-image-hold images instead of acquiring additional images. When available, use a stored fluoroscopy loop instead of a fluorographic acquisition if the image quality is adequate to document the findings.

Use Available Patient Dose Reduction Technologies

Available patient dose reduction technologies include low fluoroscopy dose rate settings, low frame rate pulsed fluoroscopy, removal of the antiscatter grid, spectral beam filtration, and use of increased X-ray beam energy. Improved image processing within the fluoroscopic unit can compensate to a considerable degree for the reduced image quality caused by decreased exposure levels. Catheters with highly radio-opaque tips are easier to see.

Use Good Imaging-chain Geometry

Position the patient support so that the patient is as far as possible from the X-ray tube. Place the image receptor as close as possible to the patient.

Use Collimation

Adjust collimator blades tightly to the area of interest. Tight collimation reduces patient dose and improves image quality by reducing scatter. When beginning a case, position the C-arm over the area of interest, with the collimators almost closed. Open the collimators gradually until the desired field of view is obtained.

Use All Available Information to Plan the Interventional Procedure

When appropriate, use pre-procedure imaging (US, MRI, CT) to define the relevant anatomy and pathology and to plan the interventional procedure.

Position Yourself in a Low-scatter Area

Stay as far away from the x-ray beam as possible. Use tubing extensions or needle holders so that your hands are away from the exposed field. Never place your hands in the X-ray beam. Use power injectors for contrast material injections when feasible, and step out of the procedure room during fluorographic acquisitions (digital subtraction angiography) when not personally washed up. When using angulated or lateral projections, keep in mind that the highest intensity of scattered radiation is located on the X-ray beam entrance side of the patient. When using these projections, the X-ray tube should be on the side opposite the operator whenever possible.

Use Protective Shielding

When you perform fluoroscopically guided interventions, you should wear a personal protective apron and a thyroid shield. Ceiling-suspended shields can provide significant additional dose reduction, especially to unprotected areas of your head and neck. Leaded eyewear is recommended if ceiling suspended shields cannot be used continuously during the entire procedure.

Under-table lead drapes reduce lower extremity dose substantially, and should be used whenever possible.

Use Appropriate Fluoroscopic Imaging Equipment

Imaging systems optimized for one type of procedure or body part may be suboptimal for others. Using fluoroscopy equipment under suboptimal conditions frequently results in increased radiation dose. Furthermore, high radiation dose procedures should be performed with fluoroscopic systems that incorporate recommended dose-reduction technology and comply with the most current International Electrotechnical Commission standards.[41] Encourage your institution to purchase this kind of equipment for interventional laboratories.

Obtain Appropriate Training

The International Atomic Energy Agency has produced a free training program, which can be downloaded at http://rpop.iaea.org/RPOP/RPoP/Content/AdditionalResources/Training/1_TrainingMaterial/Radiology.htm. The Multimedia and Audiovisual Radiation Protection Training in Interventional Radiology (MARTIR) project also produced a free training program, originally distributed on CD-ROM, that is now available on the Internet (Windows only) at http://ec.europa.eu/energy/wcm/nuclear/cd_rom_martir_project.zip. Oneself and all staff involved in the procedure should have a general knowledge of safe operating practices in a radiation environment. One should be thoroughly familiar with the operation of the particular fluoroscopy equipment one is using. If appropriate medical simulators are available, one should consider using them to learn and practice new skills before one applies them to patients.

Wear Your Dosimeters and Know Your Own Dose

One needs to know ones occupational dose in order to ensure that one is working safely. ones dose data will not be accurate unless one always wear ones dosimeters, and wears them correctly.

OCCUPATIONAL DOSIMETRY IN THE INTERVENTIONAL LABORATORY

Dosimeter Use

Radiation workers are monitored to determine their level of exposure. In order to allow adequate time for identification of practices leading to high personal dose and implementation of work habit changes, monthly monitor replacement is recommended for operators conducting interventional procedures. In some jurisdictions, monthly monitor replacement is mandatory. Several international and national organizations have published recommendations on occupational dosimetry that are applicable to workers in interventional laboratories. The relatively high occupational exposures in interventional radiology require the use of robust monitoring arrangements for staff. The International Commission on Radiological Protection (ICRP) recommends that interventional radiology departments develop a policy that staff wears two dosimeters, one under the apron and one at collar level above the lead apron.[42] Hand doses may also be monitored using an additional dosimeter.[43] For pregnant workers, fetal dose is usually estimated using a dosimeter placed on the mother's abdomen, under her radiation protective garments. This dosimeter overestimates actual fetal dose because radiation attenuation by the mother's tissues is not considered.

Dose Limits

Dose limits for occupational exposures are expressed in equivalent doses for deterministic effects in specific tissues, and as E for stochastic effects throughout the body. The occupational dose limits recommended by the ICRP have been adopted by most of the countries in the world, including the European Union and the United States.[32] The limits are described slightly differently in the European Union and the United States. In the European Union, the limit for E is 20 mSv per year, averaged over defined periods of 5 years. The E may not exceed 50 mSv in any one year. Individual members of the European Union may set stricter limits. Germany, for example, has established a 400-mSv lifetime dose limit. In the United States, individual state governments set occupational dose limits, but in most cases the recommendations developed by the NCRP are used.[44] These recommendations include an occupational limit of 50 mSv in any one year and a lifetime limit of 10 mSv multiplied by the individual's age in years. While the European Union and United States recommendations are not identical, they result in very similar outcomes. Additional restrictions apply to the occupational exposure of pregnant women. For women who may be pregnant, the ICRP recommends that the standard of protection for the conceptus should be broadly comparable to that provided for members of the general public.[32] After a worker has declared her pregnancy, her working conditions should ensure that the additional dose to the embryo/fetus does not exceed approximately 1 mSv during the remainder of the pregnancy. In the United States, the NCRP recommends a 0.5-mSv equivalent dose monthly limit for the embryo/fetus (excluding medical and natural background radiation) once the pregnancy is declared.[44] The dosimeter must be evaluated monthly. Electronic dosimeters can be used to provide rapid access to data.[45] In those centers where two-dosimeter worker monitoring systems are used, workers who may become pregnant should wear their "inside" monitor at waist level. Data from these inside monitors provide an estimate of fetal dose from conception to declaration. Workers whose inside badges show an average dose lower than 0.1 mSv/month are automatically in compliance with ICRP and NCRP recommendations. The current limit for the annual equivalent dose to the lens of the eye is 150 mSv. This limit is under review by an ICRP Task Group, as there is evidence that it is too high.[3,17,18] The annual limit for the hands and feet is 500 mSv. The dose received by specific tissues, such as the lens of the eye can be estimated by placing a dosimeter on or near the tissue of interest.

The "collar" badge is commonly used to estimate eye dose in interventional laboratories. This method is usually acceptable if the X-ray tube is mounted below the patient. It is not possible to accurately estimate an operator's hand dose using a body or wrist dosimeter because of the proximity of the hands to the x-ray beam. A ring badge is recommended to estimate hand dose.[43]

Risk Estimates

E is intended to be proportional to the risk of radiation-induced cancer. The ICRP and NCRP occupational limits and limits for the general public are stated in terms of E. (The ICRP refers to these values as dose limits; the NCRP refers to them as maximum permissible dose). Regulatory authorities require that a radiation worker receive a radiation dose no greater than the dose limit or maximum permissible dose. Interventional radiologists are unavoidably irradiated in the performance of their duties. However, a busy interventional radiologist who takes all appropriate radiation safety precautions is unlikely to have an E exceeding 10 mSv/y, and is more likely to have an E of 2–4 mSv/y.[35,46-48] These values are well below the European dose limits and United States maximum permissible doses. The risk to specific organs, such as the fingers or the lens of the eye is related to the physical dose delivered to these tissues.

EVALUATION OF PERSONAL DOSIMETRY DATA

Personal Dose Records

The information in a personal dose record will vary depending on the number, type, and location of personal dosimeters used. This record will contain information, assessed from the readings of one or two dosimeters worn on the chest or abdomen under and/or over the lead apron, and may contain information on the equivalent dose to the lens of the eye from the dosimeter worn at the collar level over the apron or thyroid collar, and the equivalent dose to the hand from a ring or bracelet dosimeter.

Copies of these dose reports should be sent to each department and individual at least once every year. The relevant information contained in the dosimetry report to an individual includes the doses for the current period and the current year.

Surveillance of Occupational Dose

The hospital's Radiation Safety section or Medical Physics Service should review the personal dose records of individual workers regularly. This review ensures that dose limits are not exceeded. It also evaluates whether the dose received is at the level expected for that worker's particular duties. Workers' recorded dose levels should be compared versus their own past dose levels and the average dose levels of others doing similar work at the same facility or at other facilities. Typical staff dose readings for different types of procedures have been published in the literature.[43,49-60] Depending on the type of procedure and the technique used, the operator dose, per procedure, ranges from 3 to 450 mSv at the neck over protective garments, from less than 0.1–32 mSv at the waist or chest under protective garments, and from 48 to 1,280 mSv at the hand. Unfortunately, most of the published data are stated in terms of dose per procedure, and most of the data are for physicians rather than assistants, nurses, technologists, or other staff. Translating these data into monthly or annual worker doses is difficult.

Investigation of High Occupational Dose

The World Health Organization recommends investigation when monthly exposure reaches 0.5 mSv for E, 5 mSv for dose to the lens of the eye, or 15 mSv to the hands or extremities.[61] The Radiation Safety Officer or a qualified medical physicist should contact the worker directly to determine the cause of the unusual dose and to make suggestions about how to keep the worker's dose as low as reasonably achievable. Badge readings for workers in interventional laboratories can be expected to be higher than for most other hospital workers. Most other hospital workers are expected to have minimal occupational radiation exposure.

WHAT IS THE ROLE OF THE INSTITUTION

The institution should provide an appropriate level of resources, such as staff, facilities, and equipment, to insure that radiation dose is adequately controlled. Facilities and equipment include, but are not limited to, shielding, radiation monitoring instruments, and protective clothing. Quality assurance is an essential component of any monitoring program.[62] Occupational doses should be analyzed by each department; high doses and outliers should be investigated. Protective aprons should be examined fluoroscopically every year and inspected visually on a daily or weekly basis for damage and defects.[29] Standardized methods for acceptance testing of protective aprons are needed because of the wide variation in actual attenuation values of aprons,[29,34] Adequate and relevant training programs should be provided for all levels of staff within the organization, including management, to develop a commitment to radiologic protection and in order that all concerned can contribute to the reduction and control of exposures.[62]

KEY POINTS FOR SAFE PRACTICE

- Minimise fluoroscopy time, the number of fluorographic images, use available patient dose reduction technologies
- Use collimation
- Use all available information to plan the interventional procedure (Fig. 10)
- Position yourself in a low-scatter area
- Use appropriate and recommended protective shielding
- Use appropriate fluoroscopic imaging equipment
- Obtain appropriate training
- Wear your dosimeters and know your own dose.

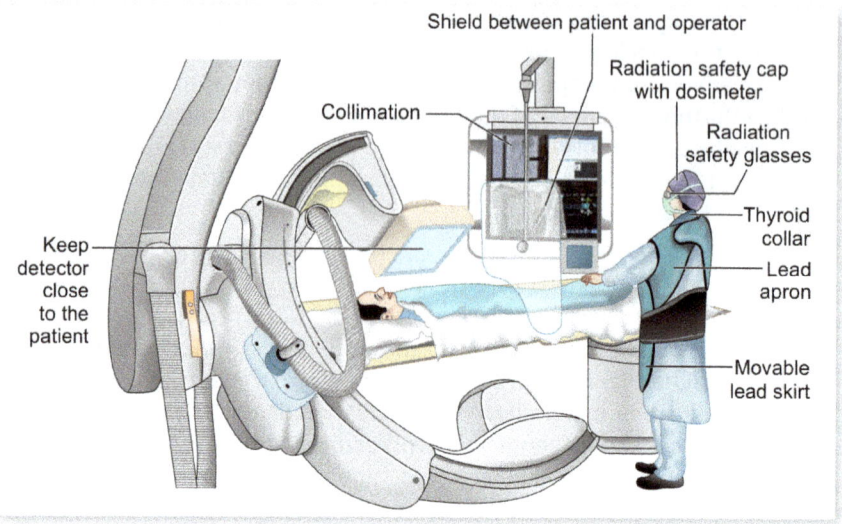

Figure 10: Perfect interventionalist

REFERENCES

1. Miller DL. Overview of contemporary interventional fluoroscopy procedures. Health Phys. 2008;95:638-44.
2. Vano E, Gonzalez L, Fernández JM, Haskal ZJ. Eye lens exposure to radiation in interventional suites:caution is warranted. Radiology. 2008;248:945-53.
3. Stecker MS, Balter S, Towbin RB, et al. Guidelines for patient radiation dose management. J Vasc Interv Radiol. 2009;20(Suppl):S263-73.
4. Kim KP, Miller DL, Balter S, et al. Occupational radiation doses to operators performing cardiac catheterization procedures. Health Phys. 2008;94:211-27.
5. Miller, Donald L. et al. Occupational Radiation Protection in Interventional Radiology: A Joint Guideline of the Cardiovascular and Interventional Radiology Society of Europe and the Society of Interventional Radiology. Journal of Vascular and Interventional Radiology. 2010;21:607-15.
6. Finkelstein MM. Is brain cancer an occupational disease of cardiologists? Can J Cardiol. 1998;14:1385-8.
7. Hardell L, Mild KH, Påhlson A, et al. Ionizing radiation, cellular telephones and the risk for brain tumours. Eur J Cancer Prev. 2001;10:523-9.
8. Roguin A, Goldstein J, Bar O. Brain tumours among interventional cardiologists: a cause for alarm? Report of four new cases from two cities and a review of the literature. EuroIntervention. 2012;7:1081-6.
9. Roguin A, Goldstein J, Bar O, et al. Brain and neck tumors among physicians performing interventional procedures. Am J Cardiol. 2013;111:1368-72.
10. Reeves RR, Ang L, Bahadorani J, et al. Invasive cardiologists are exposed to greater left sided cranial radiation:The BRAIN study (Brain Radiation Exposure and Attenuation during Invasive Cardiology Procedures). JACC Cardiovasc Interv. 2015;8:1197-206.

11. Jacob S, Boveda S, Bar O, et al. Interventional cardiologists and risk of radiation-induced cataract: results of a French multicenter observational study. Int J Cardiol. 2013;167:1843-7.
12. Vano E, Kleiman NJ, Duran A, et al. Radiation-associated lens opacities in catheterization personnel: results of a survey and direct assessments. J Vasc Interv Radiol. 2013;24:197-204.
13. Doody MM, Freedman DM, Alexander BH, et al. Breast cancer incidence in US radiologic technologists. Cancer. 2006;106:2707-15.
14. Buchanan GL, Chieffo A, Mehilli J, et al. The occupational effects of interventional cardiology: results from the WIN for Safety survey. Euro Intervention. 2012;8:658-63.
15. Gautam Kumar, MD, FACC; Syed Tanveer Rab, MBBS, FACC; American College of Cardiology. 2016.
16. Kleiman NJ. Radiation cataract. In: Working Party on Research Implications on Health and Safety Standards of the Article 31 Group of Experts, ed. Radiation Protection 145. EU Scientific Seminar 2006. New insights in radiation risk and basic safety standards. Brussels: European Commission, 2007;81-95.
17. Worgul BV, Kundiyev YI, Sergiyenko NM, et al. Cataracts among Chernobyl clean-up workers: implications regarding permissible eye exposures. Radiat Res. 2007; 167:233-43.
18. Nakashima E, Neriishi K, Minamoto A. A reanalysis of atomic-bomb cataract data, 2000-2002: a threshold analysis. Health Phys. 2006;90:154-60.
19. Neriishi K, Nakashima E, Minamoto A, et al. Postoperative cataract cases among atomic bomb survivors: radiation dose response and threshold. Radiat Res. 2007; 168:404-8.
20. European Commission. Radiation protection 116. Guidelines on education and training in radiation protection for medical exposures. Luxembourg: European Commission. Directorate-General for the Environment, 2000. Available at: http://ec.europa.eu/energy/nuclear/radiation_protection/doc/publication/116.pdf. AccessedAugust 16, 2009.
21. Luchs JS, Rosioreanu A, Gregorius D, Venkataramanan N, Koehler V, Ortiz AO. Radiation safety during spine interventions. J Vasc Interv Radiol. 2005;16:107-111.
22. Shortt CP, Al-Hashimi H, Malone L, Lee MJ. Staff radiation doses to the lower extremities in interventional radiology. Cardiovasc Intervent Radiol. 2007;30:1206-9.
23. Maeder M, Brunner-La Rocca HP, Wolber T, et al. Impact of a lead glass screen on scatter radiation to eyes and hands in interventional cardiologists. Catheter Cardiovasc Interv. 2006;67:18-23.
24. Thornton RH, Altamirano J, Dauer L. Comparing strategies for IR eye protection [abstract]. J Vasc Interv Radiol. 2009;20:S52-S53.
25. Dromi S, Wood BJ, Oberoi J, Neeman Z. Heavy metal pad shielding during fluoroscopic interventions. J Vasc Interv Radiol. 2006;17:1201-6.
26. King JN, Champlin AM, Kelsey CA, Tripp DA. Using a sterile disposable protective surgical drape for reduction of radiation exposure to interventionalists. Am J Roentgenol. 2002;178:153-7.
27. Klein LW, Miller DL, Balter S, et al. Occupational health hazards in the interventional laboratory: time for a safer environment. J Vasc Interv Radiol. 2009;20:147-52; quiz 153.
28. Detorie N, Mahesh M, Schueler BA. Reducing occupational exposure from fluoroscopy. J Am Coll Radiol. 2007;4:335-7.

29. Christodoulou EG, Goodsitt MM, Larson SC, Darner KL, Satti J, Chan HP. Evaluation of the transmitted exposure through lead equivalent aprons used in a radiology department, including the contribution from backscatter. Med Phys. 2003;30:1033-8.
30. Pelz DM. Low back pain, lead aprons, and the angiographer. AJNR Am J Neuroradiol 2000;21:1364.
31. Savage C, Carlson L, Clements J, Rees C. Comparison of the Zero Gravity system to conventional lead apron for radiation protection of the interventionalist. J Vasc Interv Radiol. 2009;20(Suppl):S53.
32. International Commission on Radiological Protection. The 2007 Recommendations of the International Commission on Radiological Protection. ICRP publication 103. Ann ICRP. 2007;37:1-332.
33. Cousin AJ, Lawdahl RB, Chakraborty DP, Koehler RE. The case for radio-protective eyewear/facewear. Practical implications and suggestions. Invest Radiol. 1987;22:688-92.
34. Finnerty M, Brennan PC. Protective aprons in imaging departments: manufacturer stated lead equivalence values require validation. Eur Radiol. 2005;15:1477-84.
35. Marx MV, Niklason L, Mauger EA. Occupational radiation exposure to interventional radiologists: a prospective study. J Vasc Interv Radiol. 1992;3:597-606.
36. Marshall NW, Faulkner K, Clarke P. An investigation into the effect of protective devices on the dose to radiosensitive organs in the head and neck. Br J Radiol 1992;65:799-802.
37. Moore WE, Ferguson G, Rohrmann C. Physical factors determining the utility of radiation safety glasses. Med Phys. 1980;7:8-12.
38. Balter S. Radiation safety in the cardiac catheterization laboratory: basic principles. Catheter Cardiovasc Interv. 1999;47:229-36.
39. Kandarpa K, Aruny JE. Handbook of interventional radiologic procedures, 3rd ed. Philadelphia: Lippincott Williams & Wilkins; 2002.
40. Bakal CW. Vascular and interventional radiology: principles and practice. New York: Thieme; 2002.
41. International Electrotechnical Commission. Report 60601 Medical electrical equipment-Part 2-43: Particular requirements for the safety of x-ray equipment for interventional procedures. Geneva: International Elelctrotechnical Commission, 2000.
42. International Commission on Radiological Protection. Avoidance of radiation injuries from medical interventional procedures. ICRP Publication 85. Ann ICRP. 2000;30:7-67.
43. Whitby M, Martin CJ. A study of the distribution of dose across the hands of interventional radiologists and cardiologists. Br J Radiol. 2005;78:219-29.
44. National Council on Radiation Protection and Measurements. Limitation of Exposure to Ionizing Radiation. NCRP Report No. 116. Bethesda, MD: National Council on Radiation Protection and Measurements, 1993.
45. Balter S, Lamont J. Radiation and the pregnant nurse. Cath Lab Digest 2002;10:e1. Available at: http://www.cathlabdigest.com/article/357. Accessed August 16, 2009.
46. Tsapaki V, Kottou S, Vano E, et al. Occupational dose constraints in interventional cardiology procedures: the DIMOND approach. Phys Med Biol. 2004;49:997-1005.

47. Delichas M, Psarrakos K, Molyvda-Athanassopoulou E, et al. Radiation exposure to cardiologists performing interventional cardiology procedures. Eur J Radiol. 2003;48:268-73.
48. Dendy PP. Radiation risks in interventional radiology. Br J Radiol. 2008;81:1-7.
49. Vañó E, González L, Guibelalde E, Fernández JM, Ten JI. Radiation exposure to medical staff in interventional and cardiac radiology. Br J Radiol. 1998;71:954-60.
50. Stratakis J, Damilakis J, Hatzidakis A, Theocharopoulos N, Gourtsoyiannis N. Occupational radiation exposure from fluoroscopically guided percutaneous transhepatic biliary procedures. J Vasc Interv Radiol. 2006;17:863-71.
51. Layton KF, Kallmes DF, Cloft HJ, Schueler BA, Sturchio GM. Radiation exposure to the primary operator during endovascular surgical neuroradiology procedures. AJNR Am J Neuroradiol. 2006;27:742-3.
52. Stavas JM, Smith TP, DeLong DM, Miller MJ, Suhocki PV, Newman GE. Radiation hand exposure during restoration of flow to the thrombosed dialysis access graft. J Vasc Interv Radiol. 2006;17:1611-7.
53. Lipsitz EC, Veith FJ, Ohki T, et al. Does the endovascular repair of aortoiliac aneurysms pose a radiation safety hazard to vascular surgeons? J Vasc Surg. 2000; 32:704-10.
54. Buls N, Pages J, Mana F, Osteaux M. Patient and staff exposure during endoscopic retrograde cholangiopancreatography. Br J Radiol. 2002;75:435-43.
55. Sulieman A, Theodorou K, Vlychou M, et al. Radiation dose optimisation and risk estimation to patients and staff during hysterosalpingography. Radiat Prot Dosimetry. 2008;128:217-26.
56. Hellawell GO, Mutch SJ, Thevendran G, et al. Radiation exposure and the urologist: what are the risks? J Urol. 2005;174:948-52.
57. Botwin KP, Thomas S, Gruber RD, et al. Radiation exposure of the spinal interventionalist performing fluoroscopically guided lumbar transforaminal epidural steroid injections. Arch Phys Med Rehabil. 2002;83:697-701.
58. Harstall R, Heini PF, Mini RL, Orler R. Radiation exposure to the surgeon during fluoroscopically assisted percutaneous vertebroplasty: a prospective study. Spine 2005;30:1893-8.
59. Kallmes DF, O E, Roy SS, et al. Radiation dose to the operator during vertebroplasty: prospective comparison of the use of 1-cc syringes versus an injection device. AJNR Am J Neuroradiol. 2003;24:1257-260.
60. Synowitz M, Kiwit J. Surgeon's radiation exposure during percutaneous vertebroplasty. J Neurosurg Spine. 2006;4:106-9.
61. World Health Organization. Efficacy and radiation safety in interventional radiology. Geneva: World Health Organization; 2000.
62. International Commission on Radiological Protection. General principles for the radiation protection of workers. ICRP Publication 75. Ann ICRP. 1997;27:1-60.

CHAPTER
18

Current Management of Lymphoedema of Limbs

Rajesh Hydrabadi, Waldemar L. Olszewski, Marzanna T Zaleska

INTRODUCTION

Lymphatic fluid forms an important part of the circulatory system in our body.[1] Daily about 12 litres of extracellular fluid is formed in the human body and drained by lymphatic channels where it is named lymphatic fluid to the venous system. The production increases in myriad of conditions like inflammation infection or deep vein thrombosis. The lymphatic fluid is active immunologically as it forms a part of the defence mechanisms of the body. Plus it transports the bacteria as well as dead cells to be phagocytosed at the nearest lymph nodes. Lymphoedema of limbs affects around 300 million people worldwide as per WHO estimates (Fig. 1). It occurs due to partial or total obstructions of lymphatic channels following:
1. Skin and soft tissue infection
2. Trauma
3. Surgery for cancer and radiotherapy.

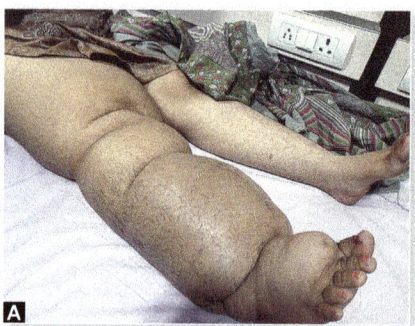
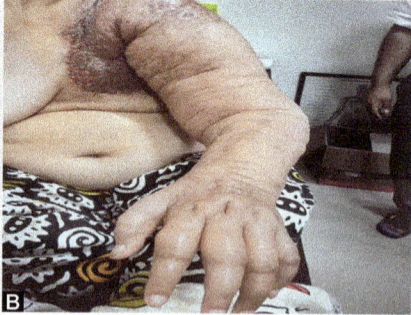

Figure 1: Typical pictures of lymphoedema of lower arm (postinflammatory) and upper arm (postmastectomy) lymphoedema

The age old belief that gross lymphoedema is caused by filariasis is a myth which needs to be put to rest once and for all. We have not seen any proof of filarial cause in spite of extensive search. Even in patients in areas endemic for filariasis, we believe it is the bacterial infection and cellulitis following mosquito bite which somehow causes lymphatic oedema. It is diagnosed as dermato-lymphangio-adenitis (DLA).[2] Presence of dead filarial larvae in these patients is mistakenly blamed for lymphatic oedema.

Why Treat?

The disease process is a chronic in nature with intermittent episodes of infection resulting in acute increase in the size of the oedema. By the time, the clinically evident signs are visible the process has been on for a long time gradually increasing in severity. Unfortunately in humans, the lymphatic channels that are destroyed are never regenerated. If the infection episode is of a virulent organism it can result in systemic involvement and may lead to septicaemia and even mortality. Over and above this, the cosmetic effects and resultant psychological effects on the patient are quiet devastating resulting in withdrawal from social activities and severe depression. It is further reinforced by medical community telling them that there is no treatment available. Hence, every possible attempt should be made to treat these patients as early as possible in their disease process

1. Stasis of lymphatic fluid in a limb brings about
2. Recurrent infections (Figs 2 and 3),
3. Increase in the size of limb (Fig. 4)
4. Fibrosis of skin and subcutaneous tissue (Fig. 5)
5. Reduced quality of life over an above the cosmetic disfigurement.

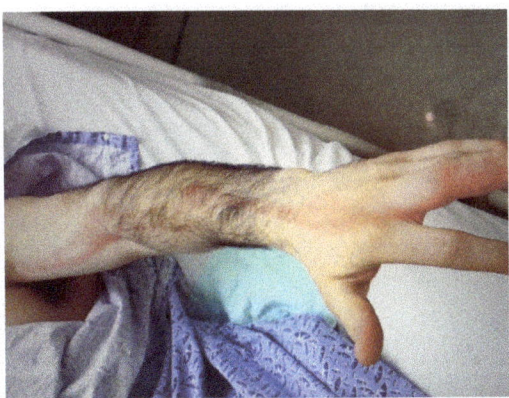

Figure 2: Picture of dermato-lymphangio-adenitis (DLA) (cellulitis, erysipelas) of upper limb. Red streaks along the lymphatic collectors. *From with Permission* New England Journal of Medicine.

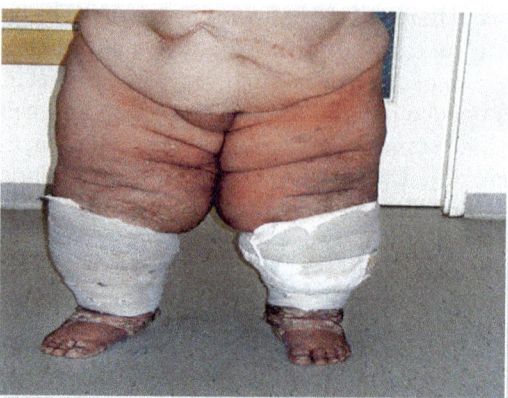

Figure 3: Acute dermato-lymphangio-adenitis (DLA) of both lower lymphedoematous limbs. Note erythema and lymph leakage from the whole surface. Lymphedema developed after inguinal lymphadenectomy because of penis cancer. Lymph cultures showed presence of *Staphylococcus epidermidis*

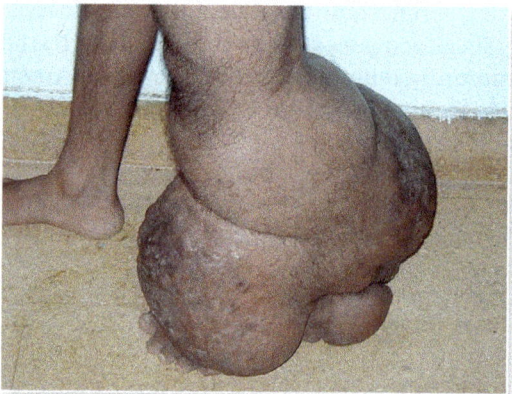

Figure 4: Typical picture of very advanced obstructive lymphoedema of lower limb for surgical treatment. Conservative therapy would be unsuccessful. This spectacular case is one of millions in the world and a challenge for prevention and early therapy of lymphedema

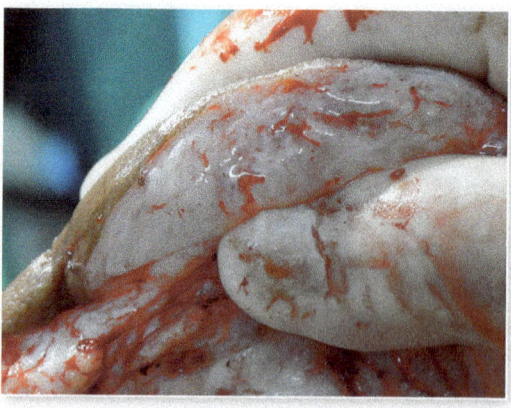

Figure 5: Fragment of skin and subcutis excised from the oedematous limb showing fibrosis and tissue fluid/lymph on the cut surface

HISTORY AND CLINICAL EXAMINATION

The first consultation usually tries to give us the cause of the disease.

Usually, patient needs to be proud to know the exact duration and the event that lead to it, plus it is important to find if it started groin downwards or foot upwards. The frequency of recurrent infections decides the urgency of treatment.

Recent rapid increase in size points to a threatened limb calling for early intervention. In a case of post-mastectomy or post-pelvic surgery for malignancy.

The incidence of lymphoedema increases as the survival increases and to identify this patients early in their course is easy as they are under care of oncologist. Only we need to educate the concerned oncologists to refer the patients early. The duration of oedema determines the amount of fibrous tissue in the subcutaneous plane and the elasticity of the skin determines the response to compression therapy. The amount of fluid in the tissues determines the response to any drainage procedure.

CLINICAL CLASSIFICATION

A. Congenital, as part of vascular malformation.
B. Acquired
   - Following infection and trauma
   - Following treatment of cancer.

The so called lipoedema (obese limbs and hips) should not be considered as lymphoedema, however, in course of time limb lymphatics become damaged by infections (Fig. 6).

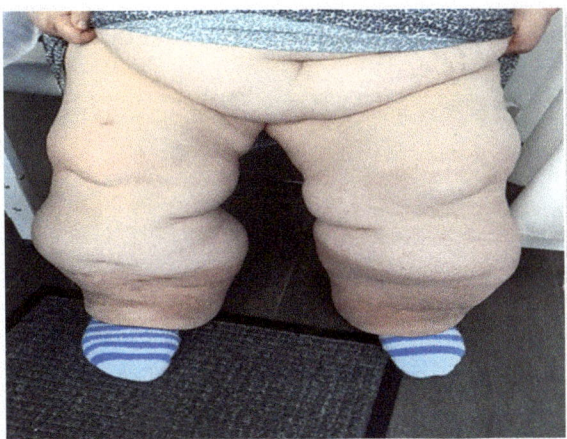

Figure 6: A case of the so called "lipoedema" of lower limbs, hips and abdomen. It is very frequently mistakenly considered to be lymphoedema. In majority of such cases, lymphoscintigraphy shows normal lymphatics, at least as long as there were no previous leg skin infections and inflammation. There is little of free interstitial fluid but most adipocytes forming fat globules. Compression of limbs and surgical methods used for treatment of lymphoedema are not applicable

INVESTIGATION

Lymphoscintigraphy technetium 99 labelled nanocoll particles are infected in the web space and the heel of the effected and the opposite limb.

The gamma camera traces the passage of the particles along the lymphatic drainage to the inguinal or axillary lymph nodes and beyond and the time taken (Figs 7 and 8). It gives a good sense of the disease being treated and is mandatory. Before any decision is made about definitive treatment.

Indocyanine green lymphography. Unlike lymphoscintigram. Here florescent dye is injected in the inter-digital space and the progress of the dye is followed by the camera. It gives information about the collection of oedema fluid under skin of the oedematous limb (Figs 9 and 10).

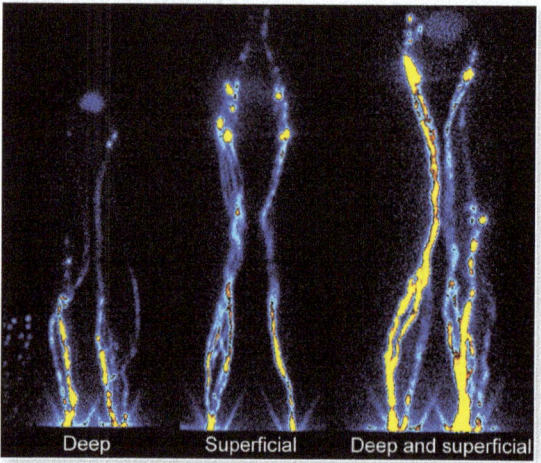

Figure 7: Normal lymphoscintigram of lower limbs. Lymphatic collectors of the superficial and deep system and inguinal nodes. Colors from blue to red show the level of radioactivity

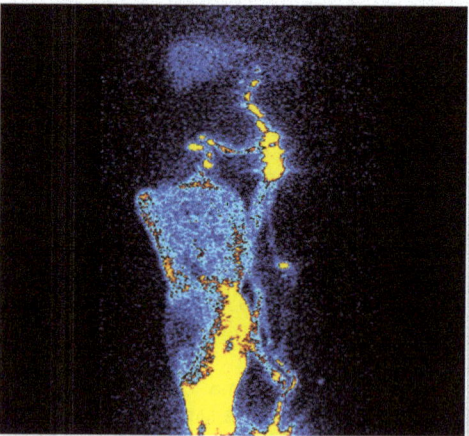

Figure 8: Lymphoscintigram of a lymphoedematous lower limb. Spread of isotope in the tissue spaces in the calf. In the thigh isotope in the subepidermal and dermal plexus finding its way to the hypogastrium bypassing the obstructed calf and thigh collectors

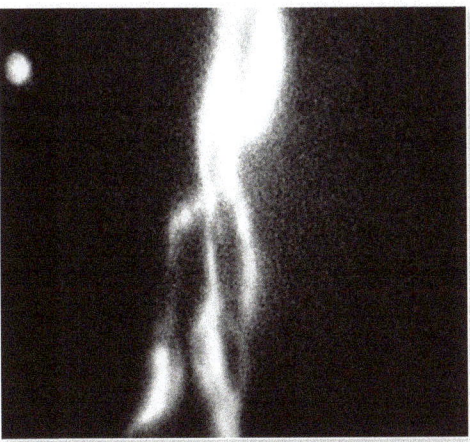

Figure 9: Indocyanine green lymphographic pictures of the foot and lower calf superficial lymphatics in a normal leg

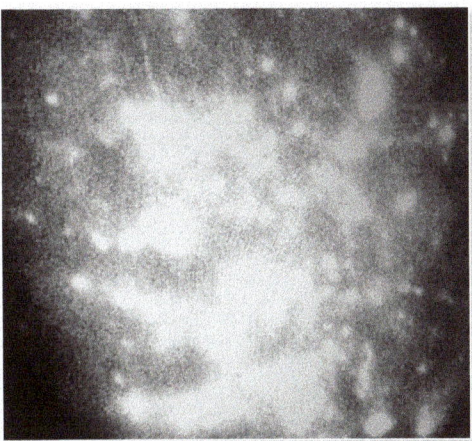

Figure 10: Indocyanine green lymphographic pictures of lymphoedematous tissues with obstructed collectors. Dye is spread in the tissue spaces and subepidermal lymphatic plexus. Analysis of isotope and indocyanine green lymphographies together give an insight of most lymphatics of the limb

Ultrasound gives information about the thickness of subcutaneous tissue and, to some extent, the proportion of fibrous tissue and fluid in a long standing case as well as tissue structure in inflammation. It is also done to check the arterial and venous circulation (Fig. 11).

Computed tomography enables to evaluate the volume of subcutaneous compartment vs muscular compartment in order to differentiate between lymphatic and venous obstruction. Deep venous thrombosis brings about expansion of the the muscular, whereas, lymph stasis the subcutaneous compartment. Moreover, scan of abdomen and pelvis shows information about pelvic lymph nodes and lymphatic bundle around the iliac vessels (Fig. 12).

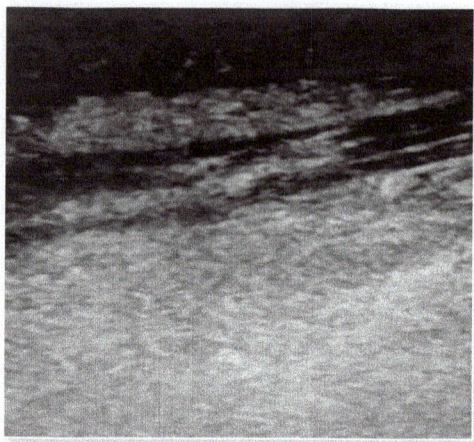

Figure 11: Ultrasound picture of skin and subcutaneous tissue of lower limb in a case with DLA. Inflamed tissues give a picture of homogenous fluid-rich structure. This methods also helps in evaluation of the thickness of skin usually overgrown in lymphoedema

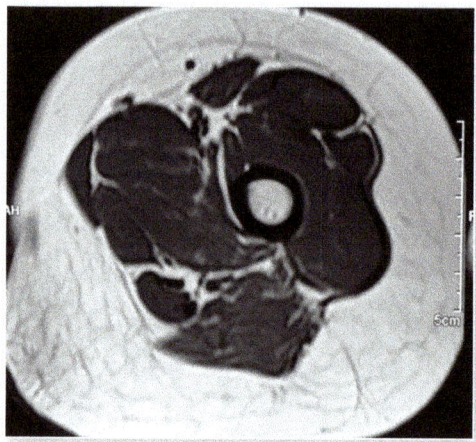

Figure 12: Computer tomography of a lymphoedematous limb shows enlarged subcutaneous compartment with normal muscles compartment. This helps to discriminate between lymphoedema and thrombosis in muscles

Magnetic resonance imaging will show the thickness of the lymphoedema compartment as well as any enlarged or fibrotic lymph nodes and any other anomalies the compartment (Fig. 13).

DERMATO-LYMPHANGIO-ADENITIS

Lymphatic oedema especially of lower limbs, is subclinical or clinical inflammation or infection due to presence of microbes in the fluid (Fig. 14). The number of bacterial population increases in the fluid it produces DLA.[3] Treatment by oral antibiotics for the initial two or three months to try and reduce the bacterial colony count is recommended. Long-acting penicillin

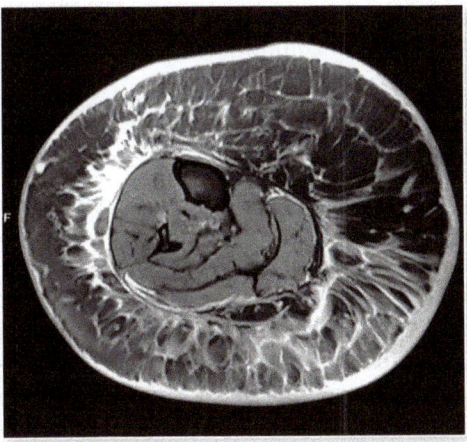

Figure 13: Magnetic resonance imaging is helpful in evaluation of mass of fibrous tissue, fat and free fluid between these structures

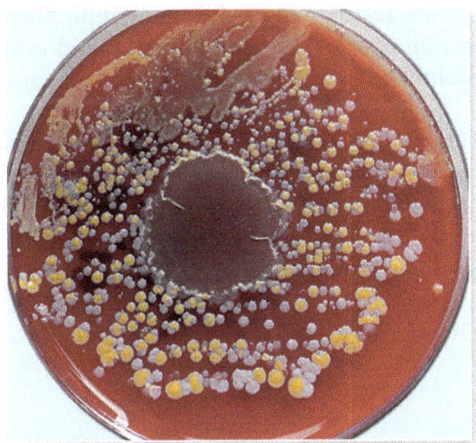

Figure 14: Bacteriological culture plate showing bacterial colonies grown from a drop of lymph from a patient with DLA. White and yellow colonies are of *S. epidermidis* and *aureus*. In the middle necrosis of confluent colonies

Penidur LA 12 prophylaxis for a long-term or in some cases for the life time of the patient becomes obligatory.[4] Acute cases of DLA are treated with wide-spectrum. The most common bacteria found in the lymphatic fluid are gram positive cocci methicillin sensitive. The dominant is *S. epidermidis* sensitive to amoxicillin. Linezolid and clindamycin are also found to be effective.

Compression Therapy

Bandaging

The main story of management of patient with lymphatic oedema has been conservative bandaging and compression therapy for many countries and are still the therapy of choice for patients. Short stretch or elastic stocking or penta hose of II or III degree compression or elastic bandaging (40 mmHg) are recommended.

Intermittent Pneumatic Compression

The manual lymphatic drainage requires trained personnel to treat the large number of patients. Intermittent pneumatic compression devices do the same task mechanically and are advices in all the patients (Fig. 15). It is expected the patient to buy the machine for daily use. The machine should have an inflation cycle which is equal to take the time to move the lymphatic fluid in the patient's limb.[5] Longer inflation time cycle works better in patients with long standing lymphoedema. Recommended is sequential intermittent pneumatic massage with sleeve pressure of 80–120 mmHg, 1 hour twice a day, for 10–30 days followed immediately by bandaging or stockings or sleeves.

Surgical Procedures

Surgical operations for restoration of stagnant lymph flow or bypassing the lymphatic obstruction sites to facilitate oedema fluid evacuation from the affected limb are complementary measures to intensive compression therapy. These are:
1. Microsurgical lymph node-vein or lymphatic-vein anastomoses.
2. Replacement of the obliterated lymphatic collectors by implantation of silicone tubings bypassing the site of lymphatic obstruction.
3. Debulking of redundant tissues including liposuction.
4. Surgical methods in the stage of clinical experiment: (i) transplantation of lymphatic trunks and (ii) lymph nodes with afferent lymphatics bridging the site of mechanical barriers for lymph flow.

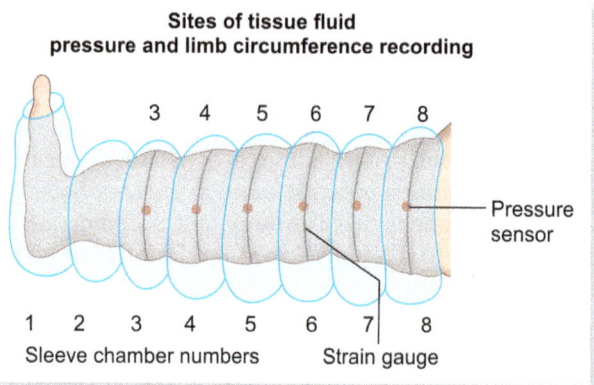

Figure 15: Scheme of • chamber sleeve for intermittent pneumatic compression (biocompression) and sites of tissue fluid pressure and limb circumference measurements. Measurements provide data on decrease of oedema fluid brought about by compression

Physiological Operations

Lymphonodo-vein or Lymphatico-venous Microsurgical Shunts

The operation of microsurgical lymphovenous was designed in 1966 by Olszewski et al.[6,7] for decompressing the lymphoedematous limb of the accumulated lymph and direct its flow to the venous system distally to the site of lymphatic obstruction. The physiological principles of the operation were based on the observations of natural anatomical lymphovenous communications in the retroperitoneal space in animals and in humans in cases of obstruction of the thoracic duct. The lymph node was cut transversely and lymph oozing started from the cortical sinuses (Fig. 16). Then, the node was implanted end-to-side into an excised wall window of the neighbouring

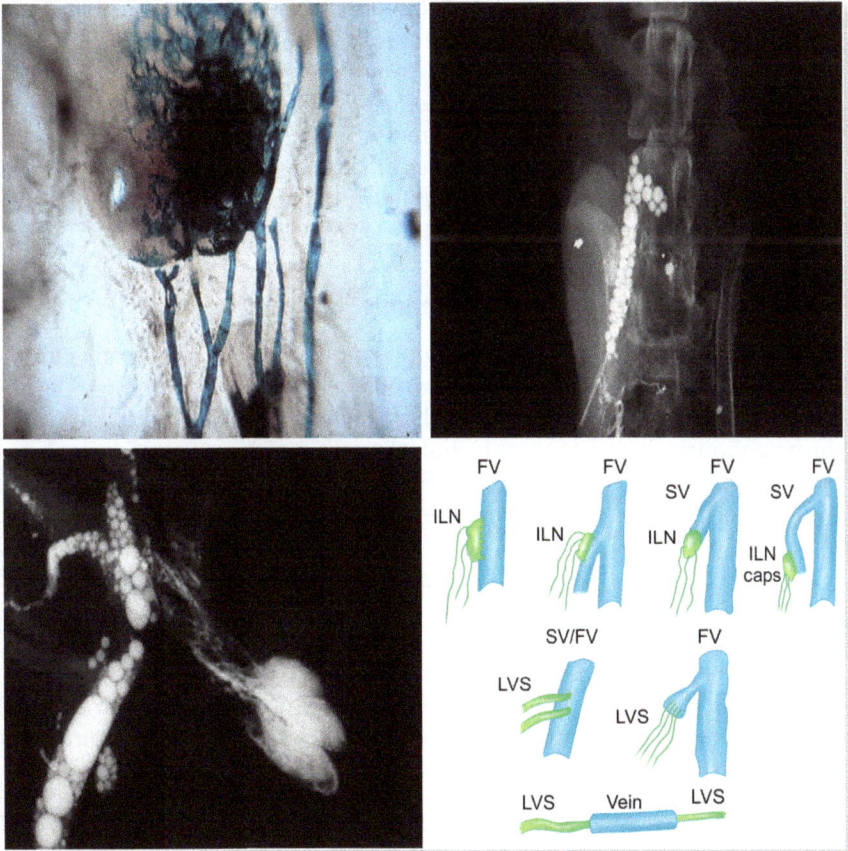

Figure 16: Historical pictures illustrating the first lymphovenous microsurgical shunts performed in dogs in 1966. Upper left-lymph node with afferent lymphatics and node sinuses. Lower left-transverse section of the node and implantation to the vein, contrast medium injected into the node flowed to the vein. Upper right-contrast medium injected into the vein implanted mesenteric node flows to the IVC. Lower right-human operations, various modifications of microsurgical lymph node and lymphatic-vein anastomoses. Over hundred thousand of these operations have now been performed allover the world
Abbreviations: FV-femoral vein, ILN-inguinal lymph node, SV-sapneous vein, LVS-lymphatic vessels, ILN caps-inguinal lymph node capsule (no parenchyma).

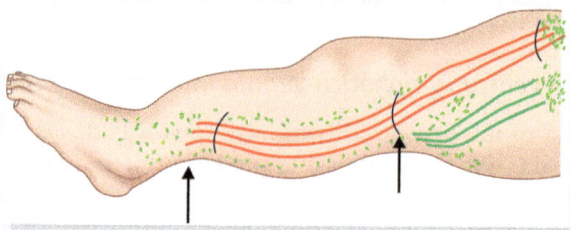

Figure 17: Schematic presentation of a lower limb with implanted silicone tubings bypassing the groin running subcutaneously above the inguinal ligament

vein. Over the course of time various modifications of the lymphovenous shunt operations have been introduced and tried by us and other authors. They included end-to-end, end-to-side anastomoses, interposition of vein fragments bridging the ends of severed lymphatics (Fig. 17). The number of operations around the world cannot at present be accurately estimated, however, more than 100 thousand should have been performed. The worldwide experience in indications, technique and results were described in abundant previous and recent literature.[8,9] At present two types of shunts are performed, the lymph node-saphenous vein (LNSV) and afferent lymphatics-saphenous vein (LVSV) or other peripheral superficial veins.

Super-microsurgical Lymphatico-venous Shunts

Development of high dissolving power optics and super-fine atraumatic sutures as well as infrared lymphography opened the way for performing multiple anastomoses between the small peripheral patent superficial lymphatics and the neighbouring veins. Various technical modifications of anastomoses have been proposed.[10,11] The early results seems to be satisfactory, however, only the long-term follow-up will prove their effectiveness.

Artificial Lymph (Oedema Fluid) Flow Pathways by Implantation of Hydrophobic Silicone Tubings

None of the so far applied conservative and surgical methods proved to restore the shape and function of limbs to normal conditions. In advanced cases of lymphoedema all main lymphatics are obstructed and tissue fluid accumulates in the interstitial spaces, spontaneously forming "blind channels" or "lakes". The only solution would be to drain these spaces by creating artificial pathways for oedema fluid flow away to the non-obstructed regions where absorption of fluid can take place. This can be achieved by formation of artificial pathways for oedema fluid flow by subcutaneous implantation of silicone tubings "lymphatics" placed along the limb from the most distal parts to its root and continue to more proximal regions with fluid absorption capacity (Figs 17 and 18). In lower limbs, this is an implant from foot to the hypogastrium or lumbar region, in upper limbs from hand dorsum to the scapular area.[12,13] This is a three-modality procedure: 1. Silicone tubing implantation, 2. Intermittent pneumatic compression and elastic support, 3. Prophylactic antibiotics to

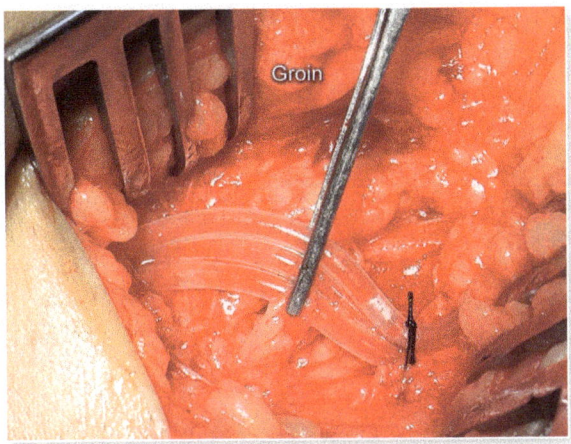

Figure 18: Subcutaneously implanted silicone tubings in the groin. Upper end in the lumbar region, lower above the internal ankle. See tissue fluid in their lumen

prevent bacterial colonisation. Postoperative lymphoscintigraphy and tubing angiography showed patency even at the five-year follow-up (Figs 19 to 22).

Debulking Procedures

This operation holds strong its established position in the lymphatic surgery in lymphoedema of lower limbs stage IV, previously known as elephantiasis. The number of patients in this advanced stage can be counted in millions, especially in the developing countries. It is still not uncommon in the Western Hemisphere.

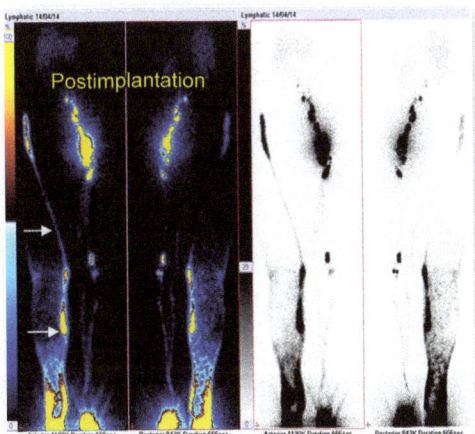

Figure 19: Lymphoscintigram 6 months after subcutaneous implantation in the lower lymphoedematous limb (arrows). Patent implant bypassing the site of obstruction at the inguinal level

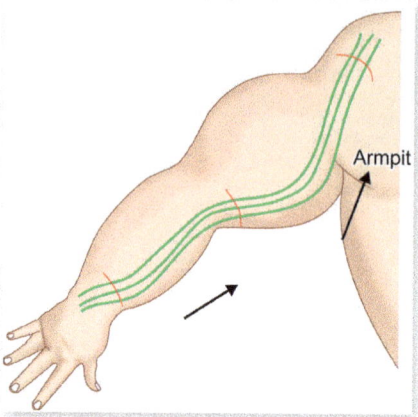

Figure 20: Schematic presentation of upper limb with implanted silicone tubings bypassing the axillary pit

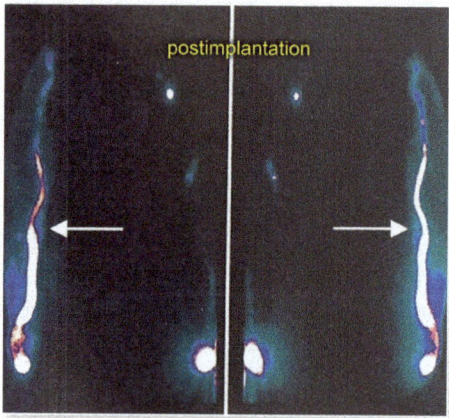

Figure 21: SPECT-CT lymphoscintigram of the upper limb after mastectomy with implanted patent silicone tubings (arrows)

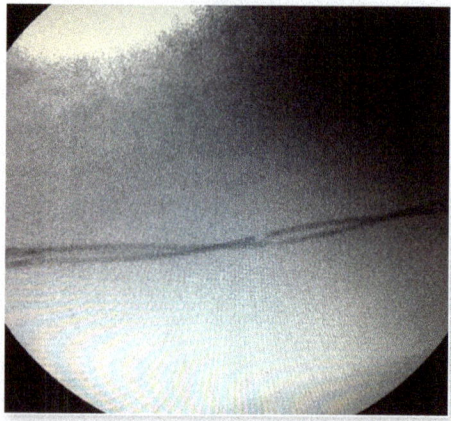

Figure 22: Contrasted silicone tubings injected with arterial nonionic medium one year after implantation. Contrast medium in and around tubings with visible lateral openings

Surgical Procedures

Olszewski et al. redesigned the surgical procedures by introducing new elements in debulking surgery, as: 1. Long-term systemic antibiotic preparation (1-3 months), 2. Resection of longitudinal strips of redundant skin and subcutaneous tissue (with fibrotic lymphatics) in the calf and thigh and covering the denuded surface with pedunculated flaps (Figs 23 and 24), and 3. Excision of the thickened fibrotic fascia.

Liposuction

The technique of liposuction of lymphoedematous tissues has been transferred from plastic surgery treating local fat deposits disfiguring the limbs, neck, breast, abdomen and other regions of the body. The technique has been adapted to therapy of lymphoedema by many authors.[14] According to the published literature satisfactory results are obtained in postmastectomy lymphoedema and some types of lipoedema of lower limbs in females. In these cases the dominant tissue in the subcutis is fat which can not be decreased in volume using the compression garments and intermittent pneumatic compression. The limitation of the method are difficulties in suction of fibrous tissue dominating in advanced stages of lower limb lymphoedema, large internal wound surface, formation of haematoma and redundancy of skin.

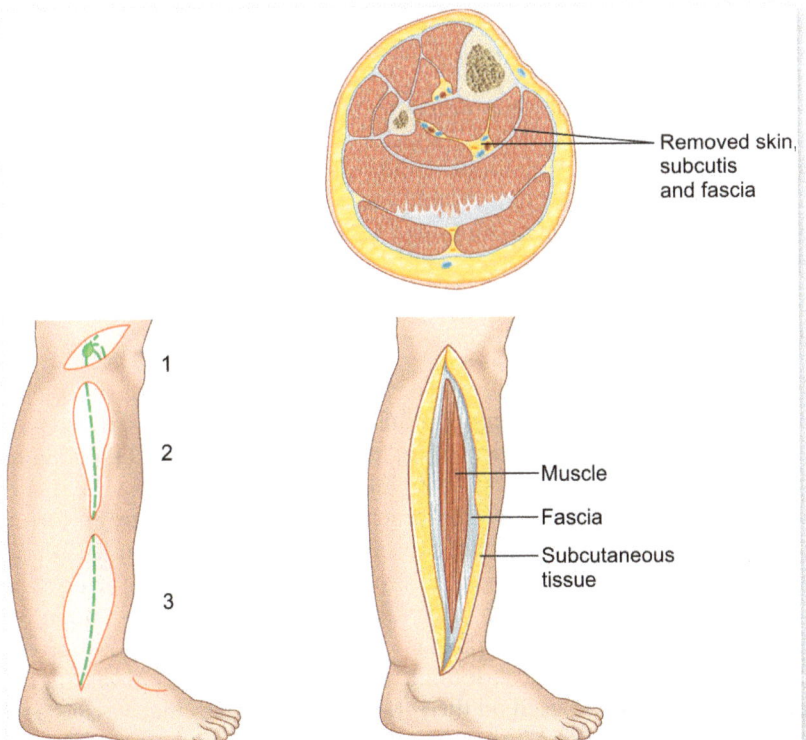

Figure 23: Schematic drawing of partial debulking operations in advanced stage IV of lymphoedema of lower limb (previously elephantiasis). Total denuding of the calf is no more practiced

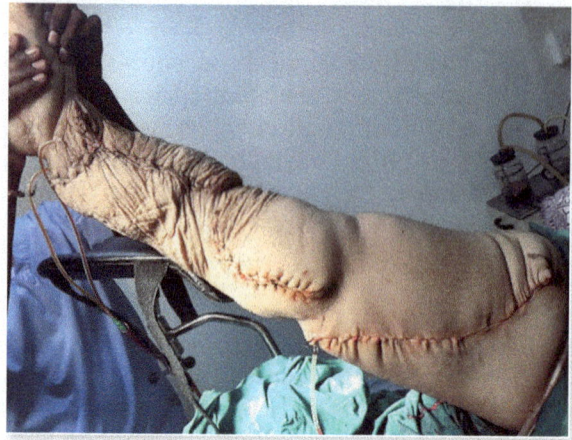

Figure 24: Postoperative picture of a lower limb after debulking according to the scheme as on Figure 23

Surgical Methods in the Stage of Clinical Experiment

These are: 1. Transplantation of lymphatic trunks, and 2. Lymph nodes with afferent lymphatics bridging the site of mechanical barriers for lymph flow.

Free Transplants of Lymphatics

They were developed by Baumeister and served mainly therapy of the postmastectomy lymphoedema.[15] The effectiveness of this methods has been proved in some cases on lymphoscintigrams. Again, as with other surgical methods of treatment of lymphoedema, with exception of debulking, the net results have been overshadowed by the parallel physiotherapy and administration of antibiotics.

Transplantation of Vascularised Lymph Nodes

The microvascular lymph node transfer (LNT) is the recent promising method for treatment of postmastectomy lymphoedema, especially in its early stage.[16,17] The recipient sites are the wrist, axilla, and forearm. A groin flap containing lymph nodes based on the superficial circumflex iliac vessels and the anastomoses to the superficial radial artery and cephalic vein were performed. Others used similar groin flaps but as recipient vessels the circumflex scapula vessels. The superficial branch of the superficial circumflex iliac artery as the dominant vessel responsible for the vascularisation of the lymph nodes was reported with the wrist and the anastomosis to the radial artery. Combined the breast reconstruction using abdominal flaps with the transfer of vascularised inguinal lymph nodes based on the superficial circumflex iliac vessels or the superficial inferior epigastric vessels, and the anastomoses performed from the deep inferior epigastric vessels end-to-end to the thoracodorsal vessels were reported. Different criteria for staging do not allow objective evaluation of results, especially the anatomical site with the maximum improvement. Altogether, authors claim 70% cases had satisfactory results in terms of decrease of circumference and relief of neuropathic pains.

GENERAL CONCLUSION

Taken together, an evident progress has been made since mid of the XXth century in therapy of lymphoedema. Elephantiasis has practically disappeared in the Western Hemisphere. This has been the effect of combined manual drainage, pneumatic compression, elastic garments and administration of long-term antibiotics for prevention of chronic and recurrent acute dermato-lymphangio-adenitis (DLA), as well as surgical procedures with first of all lymphovenous shunts, followed by novel types of debulking. The search for methods for restoration of lymphatic drainage by transplantation of lymphatics and lymph nodes is a promising effort in regenerative medicine. The indications for surgical treatment of lymphoedema should be diversified depending of the aetiology of this condition. The majority of lymphoedema cases around the world are of post-inflammatory (post-infective?) type with gradual obliteration of peripheral lymphatics. The inflammatory causative factor remains and adversely affects patency of the constructed anastomoses. The post-traumatic type of lymphoedema has at least two pathological components as prolonged healing of damaged tissues like bones and muscles and wound infection, that may gradually damage the draining lymphatics and nodes. The post-surgical oncological cases are the most favourable for early microsurgical shunts as the peripheral lymphatic trunks are healthy and retain their contractility for years. Lymphoscintigraphic and infrared lymphographic functional pictures decide upon the site and expected effectiveness of the microsurgical shunts. Most promising new approach of implantation of silicone tubings replacing the non-functioning (obliterated or excised) lymphatics, easy to perform in millions of patients, operation lasting for 30 minutes, valued at 300–500 USD only, should be widely applies to evaluate its effectiveness. Early surgical intervention has now become a must, taking in consideration that lymphoedema is an on-going process of fibrosis of subcutis and muscular fascia and in advanced stages fibrous and fat tissues dominate in volume over the excess of stagnant tissue fluid. All surgical procedures should be followed by external compression of limbs and administration of long-term low-dose penicillin controlling bacteria present in the stagnant tissue fluid.

REFERENCES

1. Olszewski WL (Ed). Lymph stasis-pathomechanism, diagnosis and treatment. CRC Press, USA, 1997.
2. Olszewski WL, Jamal S, Manokaran G, Pani S, Kumaraswami V, Kubicka U, et al. Bacteriologic studies of skin, tissue fluid, lymph, and lymph nodes in patients with filarial lymphedema. Am J Trop Med Hyg. 1997;57(1):7-15.

3. Olszewski WL, Jamal S, Manokaran G, Pani S, Kumaraswami V, Kubicka U, et al. Bacteriological studies of blood, tissue fluid, lymph and lymph nodes in patients with acute dermatolymphangioadenitis (DLA) in course of 'filarial' lymphedema. Acta Trop. 1999;15;73(3):217-24.
4. Olszewski WL. Episodic dermatolymphangioadenitis (DLA) in patients with lymphedema of the lower extremities before and after administration of benzathine penicillin: a preliminary study. Lymphology. 1996;29:126-31.
5. Zaleska M, Olszewski WL, Durlik M. The effectiveness of intermittent pneumatic compression in long-term therapy of lymphedema of lower limbs.Lymphat Res Biol. 2014;12(2):103-9.
6. Olszewski WL. Experimental lympho-venous anastomoses. Proceedings of the Congress, Polish Society of Surgeons 1966:62. Lodz.
7. Nielubowicz J, Olszewski WL. Surgical lymphatico-venous anostomosis. (Preliminary note.) Minerva Cardioangiol. 1967;15:254-6.
8. Degni M. New technique of lymphatic-venous anastomosis (buried type) for the treatment of lymphedema. VASA. 1974;3:479-83.
9. Olszewski WL. Lymphovenous microsurgical shunts in treatment of lymphedema of lower limbs: a 45-year experience of one surgeon/onecenter. Eur J Vasc Endovasc Surg. 2013;45:282-90.
10. Koshima I, Inagawa K, Urushibara K, et al. Supermicrosurgical lymphaticovenular anastomosis for the treatment of lymphedema in the upper extremities. J Reconstr Microsurg. 2000;16:437-42.
11. Maegawa J, Hosono M, Tomoeda H, et al. Net effect of lymphaticovenous anastomosis on volume reduction of peripherallymphoedema after complex decongestive physiotherapy. Eur J Vasc Endovasc Surg. 2012;43:602-8.
12. Olszewski WL, Zaleska M. A novel method of edema fluid drainage in obstructive lymphedema of limbs by implantation of hydrophobic silicone tubes. J Vasc Surg Venous Lymphatic. 2015;3:(4);401-8.
13. Olszewski WL, Zaleska M. Treatment of postmastectomy lymphedema by bypassing the armpit with implanted silicone tubings. Int Angiol. 2015 Nov 23. [Epub ahead of print]
14. Brorson H, Freccero C, Ohlin K, et al. Liposuction of postmastectomy arm lymphedema completely removes excess volume: a 15-year study. Lymphology. 2010;43(Suppl):108-10.
15. Baumeister RG, Siuda S, Bohmert H, et al. Reconstruction of interrupted lymphatic pathways: autologous lymph-vessel transplantation for treatment of lymphedemas. Scand J Plast Reconstr Surg. 1986;20:141-6.
16. Becker C, Assouad J, Riquet M, et al. Postmastectomy lymphedema: long-term results following microsurgical lymph node transplantation. Ann Surg. 2006;243:313-5.
17. Cheng MH, Huang JJ, Nguyen DH, et al. A novel approach to the treatment of lower extremity lymphedema by transferring a vascularized submental lymph node flap to the ankle. Gynecol Oncol. 2012;126:93-8.

CHAPTER

19

A Novel Noninvasive Tool for Interventions: Magnetic Resonance-guided Focussed Ultrasound Surgery

Shrinivas B Desai, Ritu K Kashikar

INTRODUCTION

Embolisation of the uterine arteries has been a standard treatment modality for fibroids and has been performed regularly by interventional physicians in India for some time now. It requires good angiographic equipment, material and trained personnel. Treatment time is about 1 hour in high volume centers. The procedure is frequently accompanied by pain. A novel new alternative to uterine artery embolization (UAE) for managing fibroids in women is MRgFUS. The method is noninvasive and is connected with short hospitalisation, as compared to other methods. Magnetic resonance-guided focussed ultrasound (MRgFUS) is a revolutionary, completely noninvasive treatment option for various solid tumours like uterine fibroids as well as non-tumorous conditions like adenomyosis. It was approved by FDA in October 2004 for treatment of uterine fibroids. This technology combines high-intensity focused ultrasound beam that heats and destroys targeted tissues noninvasively with MRI system that visualises patient anatomy and controls the treatment by monitoring tissue effect in real time.

MRgFUS allows the radiologist to localise, target, monitor, and control the energy delivered by the ultrasound machine to kill the lesion, without knife or needle.

PHYSICS PRINCIPLES OF MRGFUS

The goal of MRgFUS is to deliver focussed high-energy ultrasound wave into tissue to cause thermal coagulation of the targeted tissue. A piezoelectric plate within the ultrasound transducer generates the ultrasound wave. The ultrasound field that is generated by a transducer depends on the size, shape, and vibration frequency of the source. The ultrasound wave is then focussed by lenses or reflectors, or by making the transducer self-focussing. The sound waves pass through the skin and non-target tissue to focus on and deliver the energy to that target (Fig. 1).

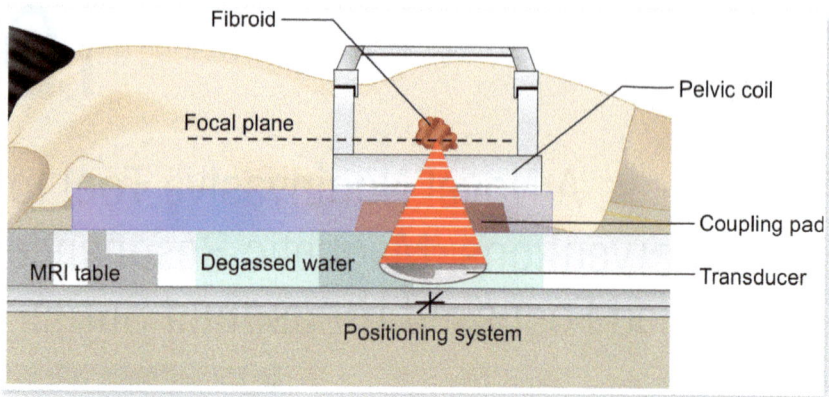

Figure 1: Physics of MRgFUS

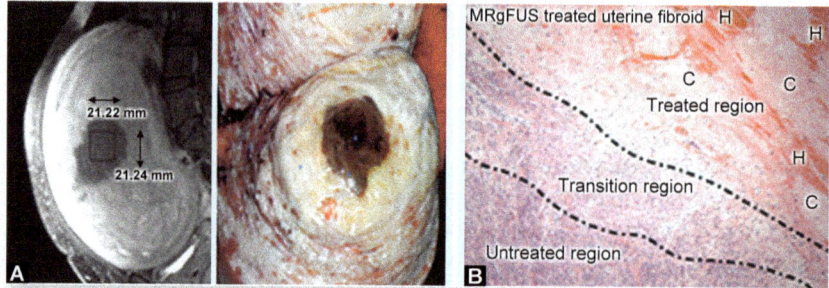

Figure 2: Physiology of thermal therapy. (A) MRgFUS treated fibroid: Coagulated regions seen in macropathology image; (B) Histology analysis shows a sharp demarcation between treated and nontreated regions (-------------- 0.1 mm)

In the ExAblate system, there is a phased-array transducer with 208 array elements that are individually controlled. There is a computer-controlled positioning system, a multichannel RF amplifier system, and a user interface. These components are integrated with a MR imaging system (standard is 1.5 T, but the system can also be used with a 3 T machine). The lateral position and angle of the transducer is mechanically controlled, and the focussing depth and size of the focal zone are controlled by the phased array with beam steering. This equipment allows the high-intensity ultrasound waves to be targeted within a small focal volume of tissue.

The high-intensity focussed ultrasound causes an increase in the temperature of the tissue in the focal area. When the temperature in the target is raised to an appropriate level, protein denaturation occurs, resulting in cell death and creation of a coagulation necrosis. However, the tissue in the path of the ultrasound beam, away from the focus, is warmed, but only to sublethal temperatures (Fig. 2).

MRI Temperature Measurement Principles (MR Thermometry)

MRI has excellent soft-tissue contrast and the ability to provide fast, quantitative temperature imaging in a variety of tissues. For the ExAblate equipment, real-time thermal mapping at the target site is achieved using phase imaging on the basis of the shift in PRF caused by temperature rise. Phase-difference fast-spoiled gradient-echo MR imaging or "phase map" imaging, is performed at the targeted region before, during, and immediately after sonication. These images are used to construct the temperature images acquired during the sonications. Those images are automatically compared with a reference image obtained immediately before the sonications to create a real-time thermal map. The benefit of combining MR with the focused ultrasound treatment is real-time monitoring of the localisation of the individual sonications, enabling the measurement of energy deposition and the temperature changes in the region being treated, and feedback on the effectiveness of the sonications (Figs 3 and 4).

EQUIPMENT CONFIGURATION

The system requires a GE MRI scanner. A special MRI table contains the focussed ultrasound device with a sealed water bath and the focussed array ultrasound transducer. The phased-array transducer has 208 elements, with frequency of 0.95–1.15 MHz. The electronic components that control the transducer allow the transducer to be moved in the water bath; the transducer

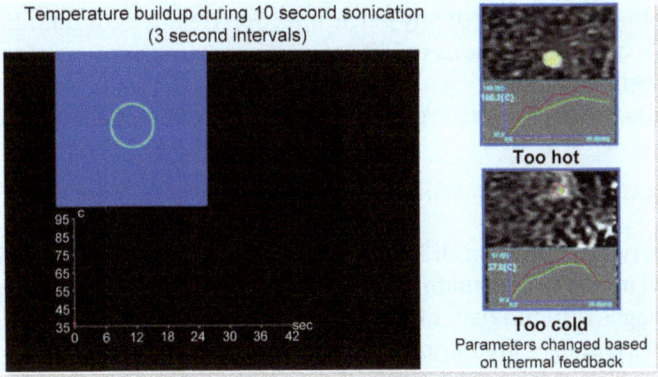

Figure 3: Real-time thermometry

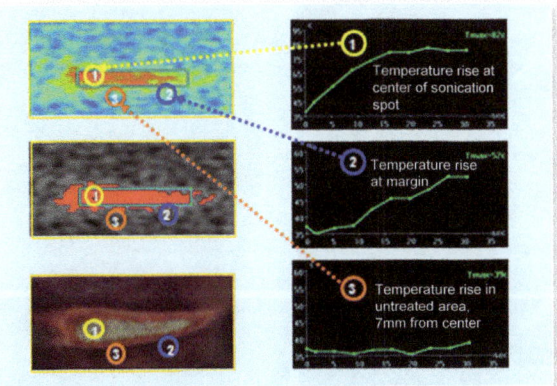

Figure 4: Real-time MR thermometry and tissue ablation: MR thermometry demonstrates clear correlation with tissue ablation and sharp edges of sonication

can also pitch and roll to achieve angulations up to 25°. The depth of focus can also be varied electronically. There is also a workstation in the control room at which the operator plans and performs the procedure.

UTERINE FIBROIDS

Inclusion Criteria

Patients who are diagnosed with uterine fibroids—Fibroids that are homogeneous and hypointense (dark) on T2 respond better than fibroids that are heterogeneous and hyperintense (bright) on T2. Fibroids should be enhancing because if they are degenerated/infarcted (lost their blood supply), there is no reason to treat them.

Exclusion Criteria

- MRI incompatible implants (pacemaker, cochlear implant)
- Pregnant patients
- Patients with cardiac, cerebrovascular, bleeding, haematological, neurological disorder or any pelvic infection (relative contraindication)
- Known adverse reactions to MR contrast agent (in case is used to evaluate treatment outcomes)
- Patients with intrauterine device that could interfere with the treatment.

Pre-treatment Screening

MRI pelvis with contrast in all 3 planes. T2W1 images provide information about the signal intensity and anatomy of fibroids. Fibroids that are hypointense on T2W1 images respond better to treatment than hyperintense fibroids (Fig. 5). Postcontrast images are important to know fibroid viability (Fig. 6). Gradient sequences show blood products/and or calcification within the fibroid.

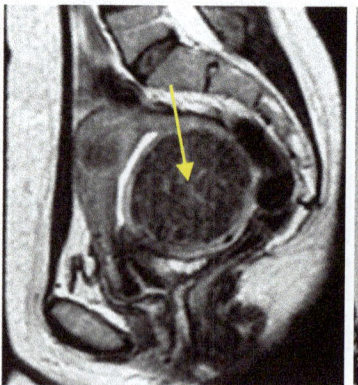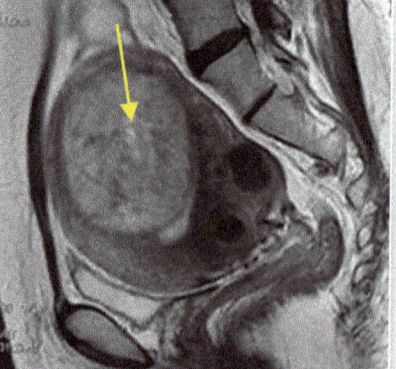

Figure 5: Texture: Bright fibroids T2w images (relative to the uterus wall) are less susceptible to the treatment

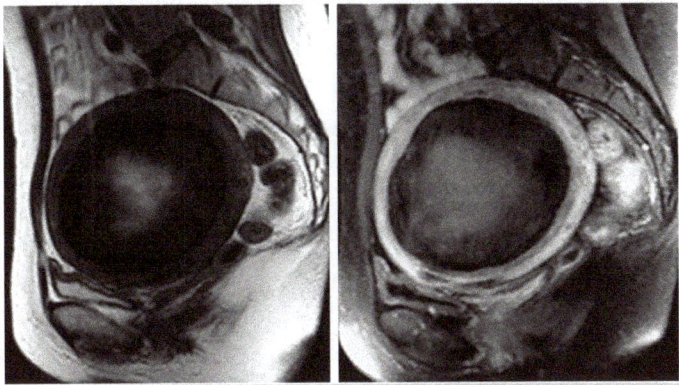

Figure 6: Viability: Non-enhancing fibroids cannot be treated as they are already non-viable

The purpose of MR screening is to acquire information about:
- Identification of the fibroids
- Number, size and location (Figs 7 to 9)
- Identification of possibly symptomatic fibroids
- Signal intensity (Fig. 5)
- Distance from transducer
- Position of organs (bladder, bowel, nerves) (Fig. 10)
- Presence of scars, surgical clips in the beam path (Fig. 11).

MR-GUIDED FOCUSSED ULTRASOUND PROCEDURE

Preparation of the Patient

1. The patient is asked to fast overnight
2. The skin on the lower abdominal wall from the umbilicus to the pubic symphysis is shaved to prevent any air bubbles being trapped in the hair,

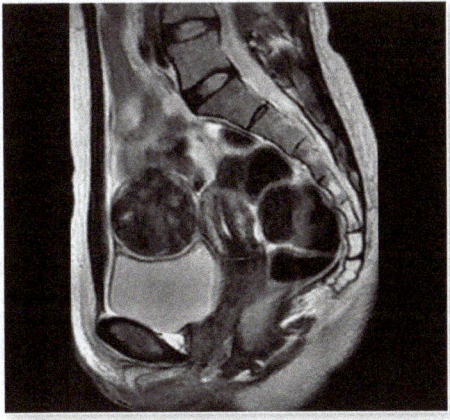

Figure 7: Pedunculated fibroid. If the thickness of the pedicle is <50% of that of the fibroid, the fibroid should not be treated, as there is a risk of the fibroid falling after treatment

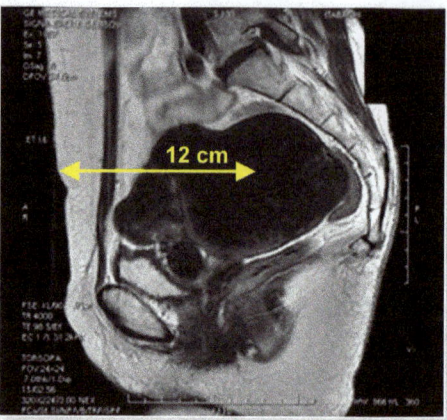

Figure 8: Location of disease: Arrow line shows maximum treatable depth. Exclude patient with a significant portion that is deeper than 14 cm from the skin line

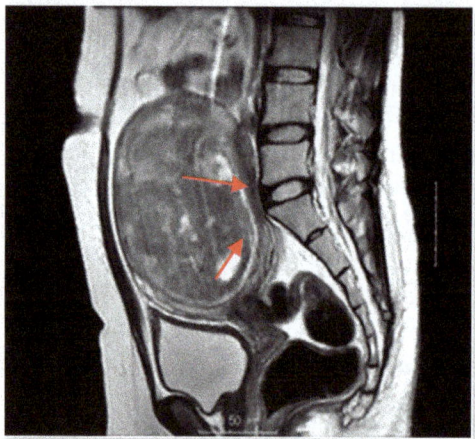

Figure 9: Location of disease: Minimum distance from bone. The center of the targeted fibroid volume must be at least 4 cm from a bone surface

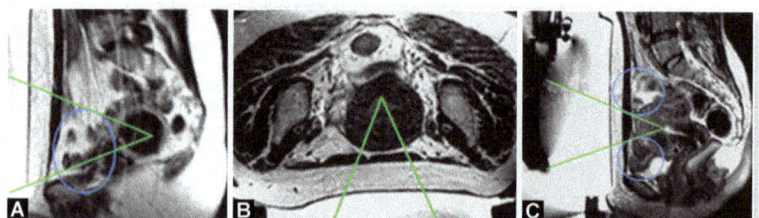

Figure 10: Accessibility: Bowels should not be present in the beam path, as it may contain of air or energy absorbing particles. (A) No access; (B) Full access; (C) Limited access

which would interfere with the ultrasound beam and potentially increase the risk of skin burns.
3. The skin is cleaned to remove any lotion, oils, or powder on the skin that might put the patient at risk for burn.

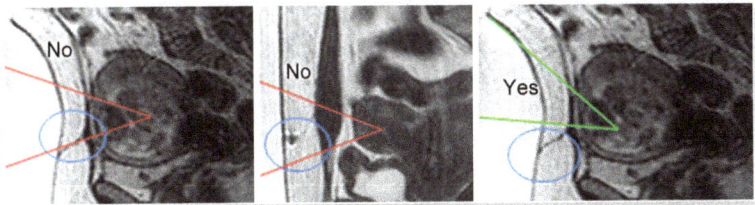

Figure 11: Accessibility: Refrain from other obstacles on the beam path as: IUD, surgical clip, surgical scars. These can be avoided by beam steering and scar patches

4. An intravenous catheter is placed.
5. A Foley catheter is placed because the patient will be undergoing the procedure for up to 4 hours and it is important to be able to keep the bladder empty.
6. Rectal gel is instilled to push the uterus anteriorly closer to the transducer and also to prevent damage to bowel wall which lies in the far beam.

The procedure is performed with the patient lying in a prone position on the treatment table with her pelvis positioned over the transducer. The abdomen is in a water bath, of degassed deionised water, in contact with an acoustic gel pad. The procedure is performed in conscious sedation.

Treatment Planning

Baseline T2-weighted MRI images in axial, coronal and sagittal planes are obtained. This insures that the patient is in the proper position and allows planning of the treatment parameters. These images are transferred to the ExAblate planning console. The treatment area is manually defined and drawn by the radiologist, and the target volume is analysed with superimposition of ultrasound beam paths in all three planes (Fig. 12). The beam pathway is evaluated to avoid any structures that would be in the path, such as bowel, pubic bone, bladder, or nerves. No sonication should be performed within 4 cm of a bony structure in the far field of the beam. The path is also examined

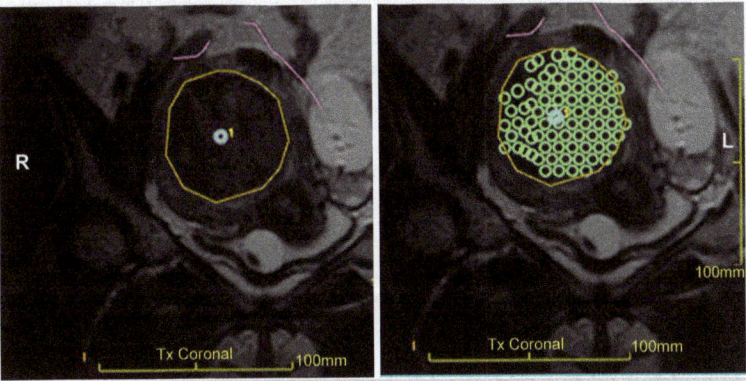

Figure 12: Treatment planning in coronal plane green circles represent individual ROTs

to make sure that there are no scars, surgical clips, or air bubbles that might cause ultrasound aberrations. The number and position of sonications are planned to encompass the entire target volume. Fiducial markers are placed on the uterus in all planes so that any patient motion that causes the uterus to shift in its position can be recognised.

If there is bowel anterior to the uterus, positioned between the abdominal wall and the uterus, the bladder can be filled using the Foley catheter, and this will elevate the uterus and may displace the bowel.

Once the treatment area is defined, preliminary low-energy, subtherapeutic sonications are performed to determine the accuracy of the system targeting and to make appropriate adjustments. A sonication with temperature imaging is first performed in the coronal plane, perpendicular to the direction of the ultrasound beam. Then the sonication is repeated in the sagittal plane parallel to the ultrasound beam. The images obtained are evaluated to ensure correct targeting of the focal coordinates. These verification sonications are low energy, sublethal sonications and generate a very low temperature rise at the focal point. Any discrepancy caused by the mechanical alignment of the system or movement in the location of the focal spot can be corrected at this point. Once verification of the system has been determined, then the treatment begins with a gradual ramping up of the ultrasound to full therapeutic power (Figs 13 and 14). It is desirable to try and reach 70–80°C, which ensures real tissue necrosis. Sonications last 20–40 seconds, there is a cooling period in between sonications lasting up to 90 seconds.

The patient is given a "panic button" to hold during the treatment that allows her to stop the equipment if she experiences severe pain or heating during the procedure. She is asked to be particularly aware of burning sensation on the abdominal wall, or of pain radiating down her legs. The patient is also made

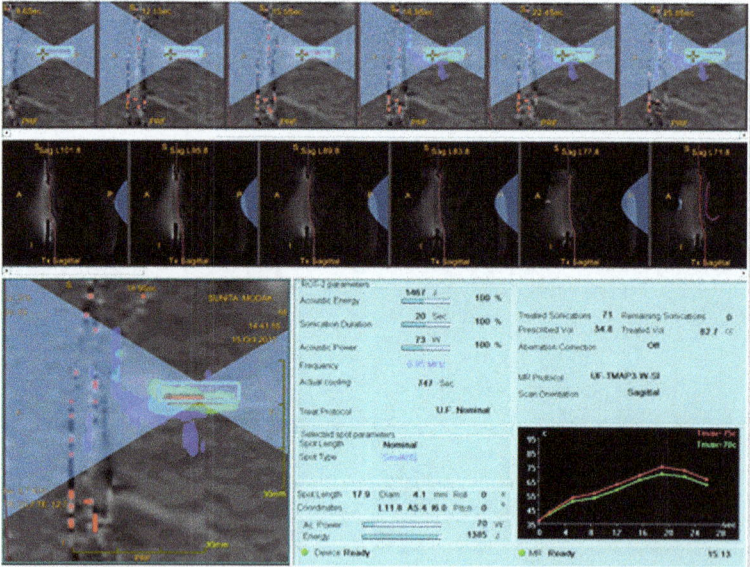

Figure 13: Individual sonication. Green box indicates ROT. The beam path is indicated in blue. MR-guided thermometry graph is seen on the right

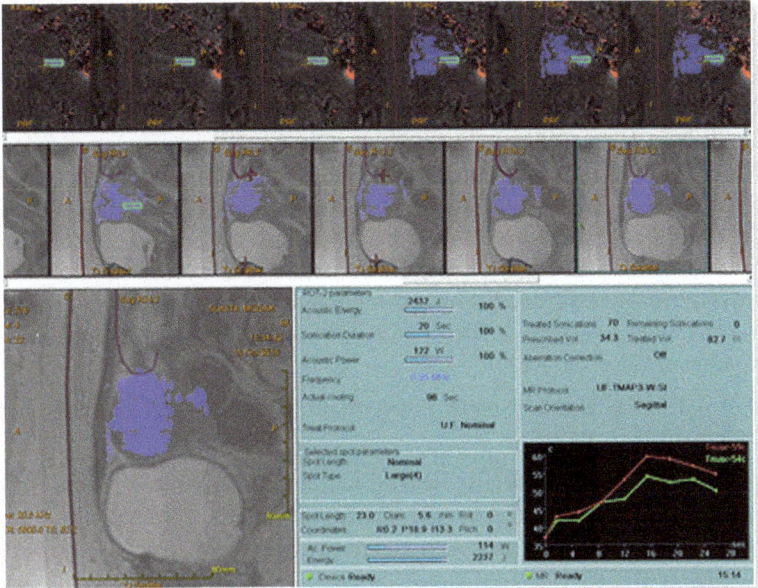

Figure 14: Accumulated dose—blue area represents treated tissue and accumulated dose

aware that the procedure is not painless. Most patients relate that they have a cramping sensation during each sonication.

Following the treatment, fat-saturated, T1-weighted contrast-enhanced images are obtained in the sagittal, coronal, and axial planes to evaluate the extent of the ablated area. The volume of ablated tissue can then be calculated, and a percentage of treated versus non-treated fibroid tissue can be determined

COMPLICATIONS

1. Skin burns—from air being trapped between the transducer and the patient's skin. Such burns are more likely to be small and superficial. Skin burns seem to be most common and most serious when there is an abdominal scar, usually from a prior caesarian section or laparotomy.
2. Bowel perforation—extremely important to evaluate the space between the abdominal wall and the uterus to make sure that no bowel is trapped in front of the uterus. During the procedure it is important to continuously evaluate the images for evidence of bowel moving into the field. Particularly patients who are fidgeting in the scanner, the bowel may shift
3. Sciatic nerve damage—heating of the bone close to the nerves and may take months to resolve

RESULTS

- At the end of the treatment, results are evaluated with post-contrast study.
- Simultaneously non-perfused volume (NPV) is calculated which correlates

to the volume of the uterine fibroid which has been ablated during the treatment.
- Aim of the treatment is to achieve minimum NPV of 70%.
- Symptom severity score (SSS) is evaluated from the day of treatment upto 1 year follow-up.

Pelvic pain and pressure symptoms seem to resolve most quickly, with women commenting that the fibroid feels softer and the pressure particularly on the bladder seems decreased. Improvement in menstrual bleeding seems to take longer, commonly taking three menstrual cycles before noticing improvement. Measurable fibroid shrinkage does not occur immediately and it may be at least 3-4 months before the patient notices any change in the size of the fibroid (Figs 15 to 17).

How does MRgFUS compare with other surgery and Uterine artery embolization?

MRgFUS treatment of uterine fibroid leads to clinical improvement with fewer significant clinical complications and adverse events compared to hysterectomy at 6 months' follow-up and are in the range of currently accepted criteria for cost-effectiveness (Table 1).

Table 1: Comparism of MRgFUS with hysterectomy and myomectomy

Features	Hysterectomy	Myomectomy	MRgFUS
Complication rate	10%–15%	11%–lap 35%–open	0–0.01%
Hospital stay	several days	5–7 days	1 day (depending on number of sessions)
Recovery period	about 6 weeks	2–4 weeks	Can return to work the next day

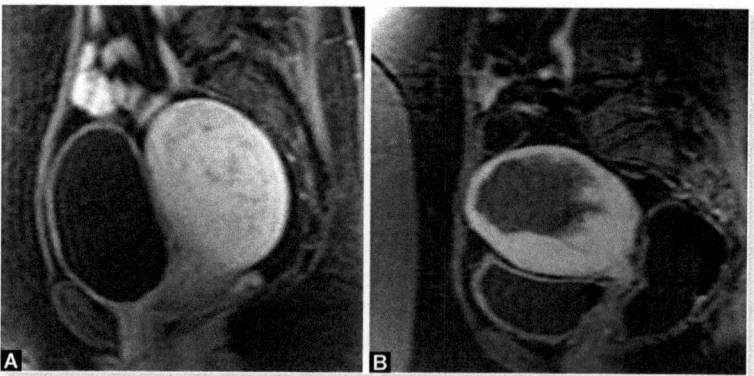

Figure 15: 37-year-old female patient: H/o urinary retention since 1 month; Symptom severity score (SSS) before treatment: 24; Number of fibroids: 1; Treatment duration: 3 hours; Number of sonications: 46; Nonperfused volume: 93%; Complications: None; Symptom severity score after treatment: 12; Follow up: Symptomatic reduction. (A) Pretreatment; (B) Post-treatment

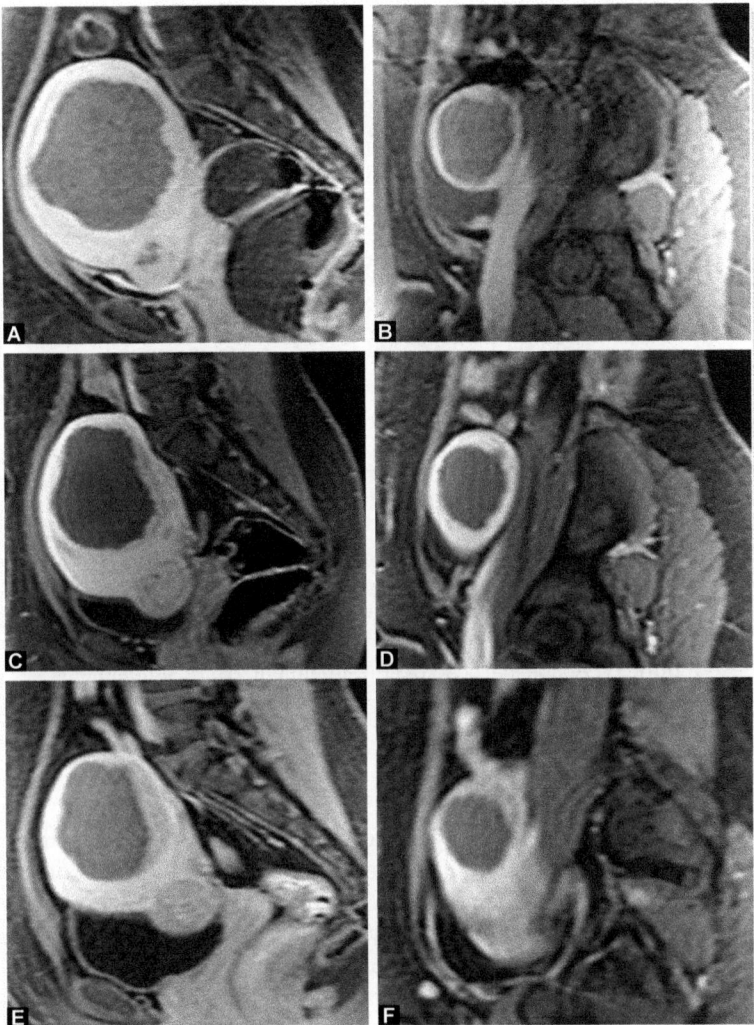

Figure 16: 30-year-old female patient: Heavy bleeding and severe abdominal pain during periods since 2 years; Symptom severity score (SSS) before treatment: 26; Number of fibroids: 2; Treatment duration: 5 hours; Number of sonications: 157; Nonperfused volume: 93%; Complicaions: None; Symptom severity score after treatment: 18. (A and B) Immediate post-treatment fibroid volume: 271 cc and 61.2 cc, respectively; (C and D) 6-month follow-up approx volume: 137 cc and 40 cc (40–45% reduction); (E and F) 1 year follow-up approx volume: 90 cc and 19 cc (60–70% reduction)

Recurrence rates are encouraging, in the range of 11 % at 24 month follow up, which is comparable to laparoscopic surgery and lower than uterine artery embolization .

Pregnancy experience after MRgFUS is encouraging, with a high rate of delivered and ongoing pregnancies suggesting good pregnancy outcomes.

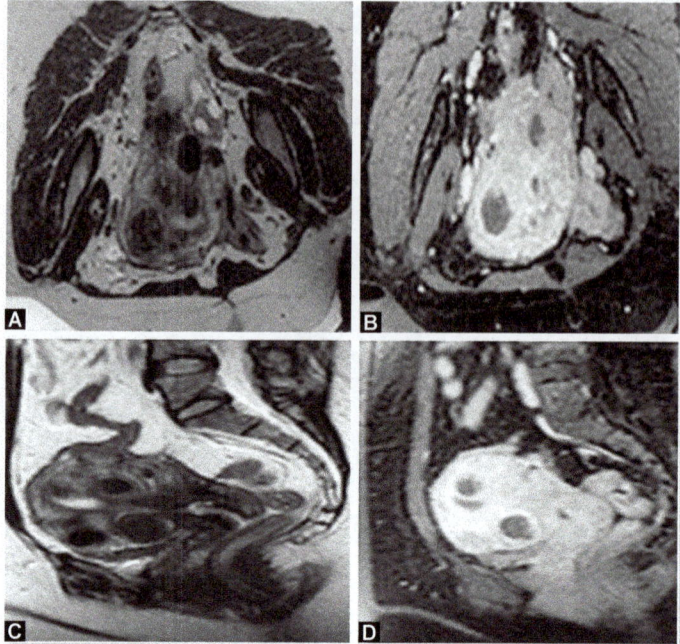

Figure 17: Abdominal scar: (A) Pre-treatment; (B) Post-treatment. Adherent bowel loop: (C) Pre-treatment; (B) Post-contrast

ADENOMYOSIS

- Adenomyosis is a benign gynaecologic growth characterised by the presence of ectopic endometrial glands and stroma in the myometrium and hyperplasia of adjacent smooth muscles.
- The major symptoms due to adenomyosis are dysmenorrhoea, menorrhagia, menometrorrhagia, chronic pelvic pain and subfertility.
- It can be either focal or diffuse and is often asymmetric, predominating in the posterior uterine corpus.
- Current treatment involves conservative management with NsAIDs and hormonal control, uterine artery embolisation, surgery, and endometrial ablation.
- MRgFUS can provide effective treatment of adenomyosis with good relief of symptoms
- Both focal and diffuse adenomyosis can be treated.

The pretreatment screening, procedure, post-treatment follow-up remain similar to fibroids.

Results

Adenomyosis-related dysmenorrhoea is often the first symptom to be relieved following treatment. Similar to fibroid treatment, improvement in menstrual bleeding may takes a few months to resolve. Encouraging results are seen in incidence of pregnancies and live births following MRgFUS (Figs 18 to 20).

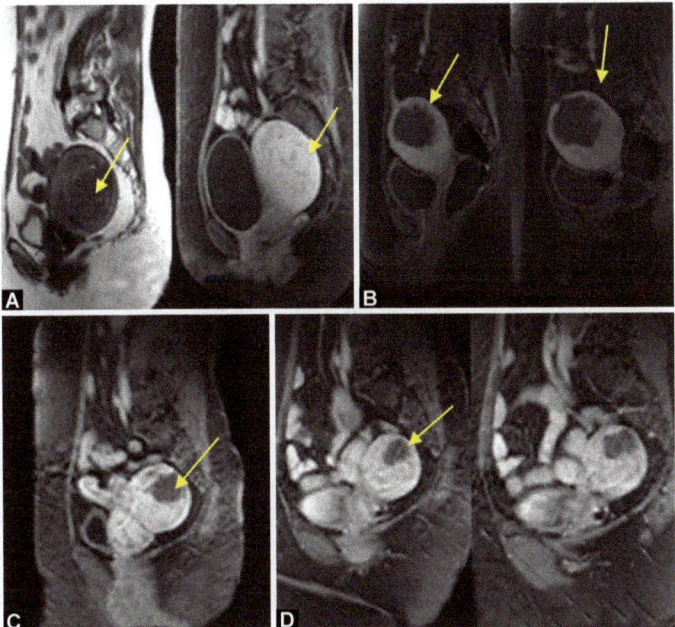

Figure 18: 40 years with menorrhagia and dysmennorrhea posterior wall adenomyosis. Immediate post-treatment scan shows good ablation of endometriotic tissue. Follow-up scans obtained at 3 and 6 months show shrinkage of ablated lesion. (A) Pre-treatment; (B) Immediate post-treatment; (C) 3-month follow-up; (D) 6-month follow-up

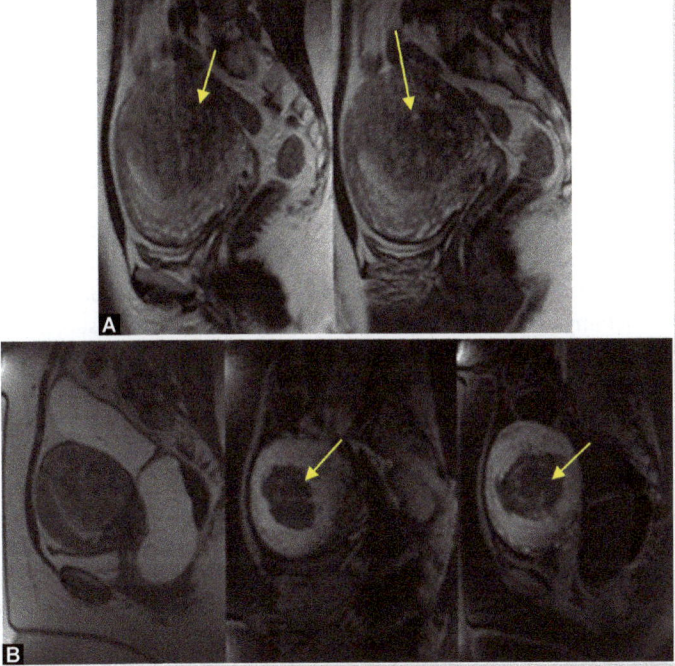

Figure 19: Posterior wall adenomyosis. Estimated adenomyosis: Volume 322 cc. Treated adenomyosis: Volume 195 cc; NPV 60; Adenoreduction 52%. (A) Pre-treatment; (B) Post-treatment

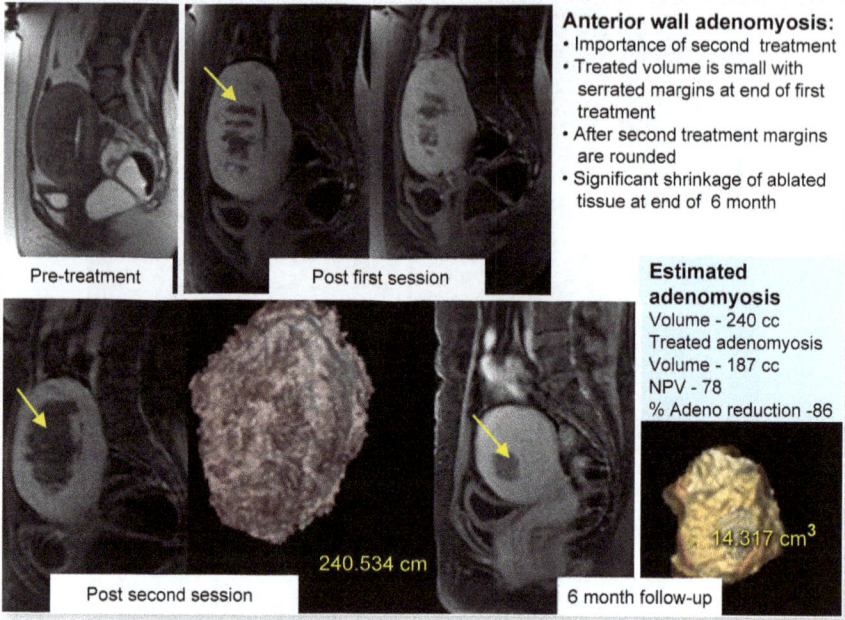

Figure 20: Anterior wall adenomyosis

Our experience with this modality has been excellent, and to date, we have successfully performed 950 procedures for uterine fibroids and 85 procedures for adenomyosis. We strongly recommend this modality as a part of the treatment armamentarium for the above conditions and as an alternative to the standard uterine artery embolisation.

FURTHER READING

1. Fennessy FM, Kong CY, Tempany CM, Swan JS. Quality-of-life assessment of fibroid treatment options and outcomes. Radiology. 2011;259(3):785-92.
2. Fennessy FM, Tempany CM, McDannold NJ, So MJ, Hesley G, Gostout B, et al. Uterine leiomyomas: MR imaging-guided focused ultrasound surgery - results of different treatment protocols. Radiology. 2007;243:885-93.
3. Funaki K, Fukunishi H, Funaki T, Sawada K, Kaji Y, Maruo T. Magnetic resonance-guided focused ultrasound surgery for uterine fibroids: Relationship between the therapeutic effects and signal intensity of preexisting T2-weighted magnetic resonance images. Am J Obstet Gynecol. 2007;196:184.
4. Hindley J, Gedroyc WM, Regan L, Stewart E, Tempany C, Hynyen K, et al. MRI guidance of focused ultrasound therapy of uterine fibroids: Early results. AJR Am J Roentgenol. 2004;183:1713-9.
5. Inbar Y, Eylon SC, Schiff E, Hananel A, Freundlich D. Pregnancy and live birth after focused ultrasound surgery for symptomatic focal adenomyosis: a case report. Hum

Reprod 2006;21(5):1 e Assessment of Fibroid Treatment Options and Outcomes. 2011;259(3).
6. Kim KA, Yoon SW, Lee C, Seong SJ, Yoon BS, Park. H. Short-term results of magnetic resonance imaging-guided focused ultrasound surgery for patients with adenomyosis: symptomatic relief and pain reduction. Fertil SteriL. 2011;95(3):1152-5. doi: 10.1016/j.fertnstert.2010.09.024.
7. Magnetic Resonance-guided Focused Ultrasound Treatment for Uterine Fibroids: First Study in Indian Women. Shrinivas B Desai, Abhijit A Patil, Rahul Nikam, Ajinkya S Desai, Vrushali Bachhav. Department of Imaging and Interventional Radiology, Jaslok Hospital and Research Center, Mumbai, J Clin Imaging Sci. 2012;2:74.
8. Rabinovici J, Inbar Y, Eylon SC, Schiff E, Hananel A, Freundlich D. Pregnancy and live birth after focused ultrasound surgery for symptomatic focal adenomyosis: a case report. Hum Reprod 2006;21(5):1255-9. Epub 2006 Jan 12.
9. Taran FA, Tempany CM, Regan L, Inbar Y, Revel A, Stewart EA. Ultrasound Obstet Gynecol. 2009;34(5):572-8.
10. Zowall H, Cairns JA, Brewer C, Lamping DL, Gedroyc WM, Regan L. Cost-effectiveness of magnetic resonance-guided focused ultrasound surgery for treatment of uterine fibroids. BJOG. 2008;115:653-62.

Index

Page numbers followed by *f* and *t* refer to figure and table, respectively.

A

Abdomen, lipoedema of 271*f*
Activated partial thromboplastin time 26, 202
Adductor canal level 98*f*
Adenomyosis 296, 297*f*
  anterior wall 298*f*
  posterior wall 297*f*
Adjunctive catheter-directed thrombolysis 188
Adjunctive venous angioplasty and stenting 191
Adult stem cells 4
American College of Cardiology 38
American Heart Association 38, 138, 172
American Stroke Association Guidelines for Primary Prevention of Stroke 138
Aminoglycosides 226
Amphotericin B 226
Aneurysmal disease 7
Angiogenesis 3
Angiogram 85f, 87*f*
Angiojet power pulse thrombectomy 189*f*
Angiojet system 188
Angioplasty 78, 81, 158
Angiotensin
  converting enzyme inhibitor 231
  receptor blocker 43, 231
Anglo-Scandinavian cardiac outcomes trial 42
Ankle brachial indexes 4, 40
Antegrade-retrograde intervention 122
Anticoagulants 204*t*
Antiplatelet therapy 89
Aortic
  aneurysms 39
    abdominal 49, 50, 52*t*
  catheterisation 63
  disease 63
  dissection 62, 64, 65*f*
    management of 62
  insufficiency, murmur of 63
  rupture 65, 65*f*
  stenosis 241*f*
  valve disease 63
Apixaban 17, 20, 25
Arterial disease, peripheral 38, 76, 96, 117
Arteriovenous malformation 140
Artery 103
  cerebral 141
  disease, coronary 39
  femoral 77*f*, 104
  peroneal 100*f*
  recanalisation of 105
Artificial lymph flow pathways 278
Aspiration devices 186
Atherectomy devices 89, 121
Atherosclerosis, regression of 1
Atherosclerotic carotid disease, asymptomatic 175
Atherothrombosis 40
Atrial fibrillation 23
Automated carbon dioxide angiography 246

B

Bacterial colonies grown 275*f*
Balloon
  angioplasty techniques 122
  subintimal angioplasty 243*f*
Biomimetic stents 90
Blood
  flow, cerebral 150, 151*f*
  peripheral 4
  pressure 43
Bone marrow 4
Bowel loop 296*f*
Brain tumors 251
Branch vessel malperfusion 65

C

Canakinumab Anti-inflammatory Thrombosis Outcome Study 3
Carbon dioxide 237
  angiography 237
Cardiac failure 226
Cardiovascular

and Interventional Society of Europe 250
disease, atherosclerotic 38
inflammation reduction trial 3
mortality 39
Carotid
    artery 140
        stenting 160f, 172, 174
    atherosclerosis study, asymptomatic 175
    disease 176t
        asymptomatic 175
    interventions 166
    revascularisation 175t
    stenting 166t
    subclavian bypass 66f
Cataracts 252
Catheter directed thrombolysis 183, 204
Cellulitis 269f
Cerebrovascular disease 39, 41
Chest pain, substernal 199
Cholesterol ester transfer protein 2
CO_2 angiogram 242f, 243f
Compression therapy 275
Concentric distal filter devices 159f
Contemporary catheter techniques 205
Contrast-induced nephropathy, association of 228t
Cough 199

D

Dabigatran 17, 19, 23
Dalteparin 204
Deep vein thrombosis 22, 180
Dermato-lymphangio-adenitis 269, 269f, 270f, 274
Digital subtraction angiography 246
Diluted thrombin time 26
Direct thrombin inhibitors 16, 17
Distal balloon
    inflation 162f
    occlusion 163f
Distal filter device 159f
    advantages of 158t
    disadvantages of 158t
Distal occlusion device 157, 161
    advantages of 161t
    disadvantages of 161t
Distal protection devices 157
Doppler ankle brachial indices 76
Drug
    coated angioplasty balloons 83, 86, 119
    eluting
        stents 83
        technology 83
Duplex ultrasound 174
Dyslipidaemia 1
Dysmenorrhoea 297f
Dyspnoea 199

E

Echocardiography, role of 213
Edoxaban 17, 21, 25
Ekosonic pulmonary embolism system 208f
Ekosonic system 190, 191f
Elastase inhibition 8
Elastic recoil 111
Embolectomy 204
Embolic protection devices 156, 157
Embolism 110
Embolus, fragmentation of 206f
Endometriotic tissue 297f
Endothelial cells 37
Endovascular
    aneurysm repair 49
    stent grafts 52t
        principles of 50
    stroke treatment 141, 146
    therapy 80
End-stage renal disease 43
Enoxaparin 204
Erysipelas 269f
Erythema 270f
Estimated glomerular filtration rate 226
European Carotid Surgery Trial 172
European Society for Vascular Surgery 172
Extensive infrapopliteal venous thrombosis 183f

F

Facial droop 138
Fatty streaks 37
Femoro-popliteal lesions, classification of 77f
Fever 199
Fibernet system 168f
Fibrinolysis, intra-arterial 141
Fibroblast growth factor 4
Fluoroscopic time 253
Fluoroscopically guided interventional procedures 250
Foot ulcers, chronic 5

G

Gastrointestinal bleeding 23
Geneva prognostic scoring 216
Geneva scoring system 211*t*
Glyceryl trinitrate 103
Graft
    failure 130
    types of 52
Granulocyte-colony stimulating factor 5
Great toe gangrene 123*f*
Green fluorescent protein 5

H

Haematoma
    intramural 68, 69*f*
    periaortic 67
    retroperitoneal 111
Haemoptysis 199
Haemorrhage, symptomatic
    intracerebral 141
Hallux gangrene 83*f*
Heart
    and renal protection, study of 44
    protection study 40
    valves 28
Heel ulceration 124*f*
Hepatocyte growth factor 4
Hips, lipoedema of 271*f*
Hybrid procedures 88
Hypertension 63
Hypotension 200, 211
Hypovolaemia 226
Hysterectomy 294*t*

I

Ileofemoral occlusion, CO_2 angiogram of 241*f*
Iliac vein 193
Indigo system 187*f*
Indocyanine green lymphographies 273*f*
Infarction, cerebral 141
Infections, recurrent 269
Inferior vena cava 237, 247
Infrapopliteal lesions, classification of 118*f*
Infusion catheter 184*f*
Injuries, cerebral 168
Intermittent pneumatic compression 276

International Commission on Radiological Protection 261
Ischaemia, severe distal 123*f*

K

Kaplan-Meier life-table analysis 80
Kidney disease 43, 226
    Disease Improving Global Outcomes 229
Kidney injury 225

L

Lead apron 256*f*
Leg pain 199
Ligament, inguinal 278*f*
Limb
    ischaemia, critical 4, 39, 76, 90, 96, 134, 246
    size of 269
Lipids 37
Lipoprotein
    high-density 2, 38
    low-density 2, 38
Liposuction 281
Low profile modular bifurcated stent grafts 54
Lower limb 278*f*
    compression ultrasonography, value of 213
    deep venous thrombosis, acute 180
    ischaemia 77*t*
    lipoedema of 271*f*
    normal lymphoscintigram of 272*f*
    subcutaneous tissue of 274*f*
Lower lymphedoematous limbs 270*f*, 297*f*
Lung scintigraphy, role of 212
Lymph node 278, 282
    capsule, inguinal 277
    inguinal 277
Lymphadenectomy, inguinal 270*f*
Lymphatic
    fluid, stasis of 269
    free transplants of 282
    vessels 277
Lymphatico-venous microsurgical shunts 277
Lymphoedema 268f, 270, 271f, 274
    limbs 268
    lower

arm 268f
limb 281f
Lymphoedematous limb
  computer tomography of 274f
  lymphoscintigram of 272f
Lymphonodo-vein 277
Lymphoscintigram 279f
Lymphovenous microsurgical shunts 277f

M

Marfan's syndrome 63
Mastectomy 280f
Matrix metalloproteinases 7
May-Thurner syndrome 193
Mechanical thrombectomy 186, 208f
  devices 187
  percutaneous 186
Menorrhagia 297f
Microvascular lymph node transfer 282
Middle cerebral artery 150, 151f
  occlusion 151f, 152f
Mini stroke 137
Minimise fluoroscopy time 258
Mononuclear cells 4
Muscles 274
  compartment 274f
Myocardial necrosis 213
Myomectomy 294t

N

Nadroparin 204
National Health Service 89
National Institute of Neurological Disorders and Stroke 140, 146
Nephrogenic systemic fibrosis 230
Nephropathy, contrast induced 225, 227
Nephrotoxic medication 226
Newer oral anticoagulants 15
Nicotine replacement 139
Nitric oxide 37
North American Symptomatic Carotid Endarterectomy Trial 172

O

Oedema fluid flow pathways 278
Open surgery, role of 211
Oral anticoagulation schedule 217
Ostial stenosis, atherosclerotic 43
Oxidized low-density lipid particles 37

P

Paclitaxel coated balloons 120
Paclitaxel drug-eluting balloons 119
Pain
  abdominal 63
  severe abdominal 295f
Parenchyma 277
Parody antiembolisation catheter 164, 165t
Peak systolic velocity ratio 79
Pedal plantar loop technique 123f
Pedunculated fibroid 289f
Penicillium citrinum 38
Penumbra indigo vacuum assisted thrombectomy system 206f
Percusurge guardwire device 162f
Perforation 110
Pharmaceutical aneurysm stabilization trial 8
Pigtail catheter, rotational movement of 206f
Plaque, atherosclerotic 37
Pleuritic chest pain 199
Popliteal artery 132f
  occlusion of 123f
Popliteal vein access 189f
Porphyromonas gingivalis 8
Post-angioplasty angiogram 132f
Postmastectomy 268f
Post-thrombotic syndrome 180
Prothrombin complex concentrates 29
Proximal
  anterior tibial artery 123f
  balloon inflation 165f
  flow occlusion devices 163t
  occlusion devices 157, 162
    advantages 164
    disadvantages 164t
Pulmonary embolism 22, 180, 198, 214, 215
  acute 203, 211
  management 198
  severity index 215t
  thrombolysis 202
  triaging of 199

R

Radiation safety
  caps 256f
  glasses 256f

Real-time thermometry 287f
Recurrent acute dermato-lymphangio-
    adenitis 283
Renal
    artery 43
        interventions 167
        stenosis 43
    atherosclerotic lesions 43
    dysfunction, progression of 43
    insufficiency, chronic 244
    revascularisation 167t
Retrograde pedal access 123f
Rheolytic thrombectomy 205
Ring dosimeter 251
Rivaroxaban 17, 18, 24

S

Safety lead glasses 255f
Saphenous vein 277, 278
    bypass graft 167
Scar, abdominal 296f
Sepsis 226
Shock 200f
Silverhawk plaque excision system 89
Skin
    and soft tissue infection 268
    and subcutaneous tissue 269f
    fragment of 270f
Society of Interventional Radiology 250
Society of Vascular Surgery 39
Standard percutaneous transluminal
    angioplasty 80
Stem cells
    adipose derived 6
    embryonic 4
Stenosis 132f, 133f, 168f
    level of 132f
Stent placement 43
Stroke 137
    ischaemic 137, 147
    prevention 42, 138
    primary prevention of 138
    secondary prevention of 139
    treatment 140, 141
Subepidermal lymphatic plexus 273f
Subintimal angioplasty 81, 96, 108
Suction thrombectomy 206
Superficial femoral artery 77f, 96
    endovascular treatment of 76
    lesions 75

nitinol stent trials 82
treatment of 75
Super-microsurgical lymphatico-venous
    shunts 278
Symptom severity score 294f, 295f
Syncope 199
Synthesis 141
Systemic thrombolysis 182, 203

T

Thermal therapy 286f
Thoracic
    aneurysm 63
    endovascular aortic repair 68
Thrombectomy
    devices 188
    percutaneous 186
    surgical 182
Thrombin 15
Thrombocytopenia, heparin-induced
    28
Thrombolysis 141
    flow-directed 182
Thrombosis 274f
Thrombus fragmentation 205
Thyroid disease 252
Tibial artery, anterior 98f
Tibial vessel
    CO_2 angiogram of 242f
    disease 117
    subintimal angioplasty of 106
Tinzaparin 204
Tissue plasminogen activator 204
Toe brachial pressure index 4
Total contralateral internal carotid artery
    160
Transatlantic Inter-Society Consensus
    Classification 76
Transcatheter aortic valve implantation
    168, 169t
Trans-collateral angioplasty 124f
Transfemoral suction thrombectomy 86f
Transluminal angioplasty, percutaneous
    82
Transoesophageal echocardiography 63
Transthoracic echocardiography 63
Trauma 268
Trellis device 190f
Trellis peripheral infusion system 189

U

Ultrasound accelerated catheter-directed thrombolysis 207
Uterine
  artery embolization 285, 294
  fibroid 288, 294

V

Vascular
  disease, peripheral 37, 244
  endothelial growth factor 4
  smooth muscle cells 37
Vein
  femoral 277
  graft 130, 132*f*
    occlusion 133
Venous cannula, peripheral 183*f*
Venous thromboembolism
  management of 22
  prevention of 18
Venous thrombosis, acute 188
Veterans Affairs Cooperative Study 172
Vienna nomogram 218*f*
Vitamin K antagonist 15, 20, 132

W

Wells' criteria 181*t*
Wells' scoring system 212*t*

EU GSPR Authorised Reprsentative
Logos Europe, 9 rue Nicolas Poussin
1700, La Rochelle, France
Phone: +33 (0) 6 67 93 73 78
E-mail: contact@logoseurope.eu